Clinical Exercise Testing

Clinical Exercise Testing

Fourth Edition

Norman L. Jones, MD
Ambrose Cardiorespiratory Unit
Department of Medicine
McMaster University
Hamilton, Ontario, Canada

W.B. Saunders Company
A Division of Harcourt Brace & Company
Philadelphia London Toronto Montreal Sydney Tokyo

W.B. SAUNDERS COMPANY
A Division of Harcourt Brace & Company

The Curtis Center
Independence Square West
Philadelphia, Pennsylvania 19106

Library of Congress Cataloging-in-Publication Data

Jones, Norman L.

Clinical exercise testing / Norman L. Jones.—4th ed.

p.   cm.

Includes bibliographical references and index.

ISBN 0–7216–6511–X

1. Exercise tests.   2. Heart function tests.   I. Title.
[DNLM: 1. Exertion.   2. Exercise Test.   WE 103J78c 1997]

RG683.5.E94J66 1997   616.07′54—dc20

DNLM/DLC   96–9821

CLINICAL EXERCISE TESTING, fourth edition   ISBN 0–7216–6511–X

Printed in the United States of America.

Last digit is the print number: 9   8   7   6   5   4   3   2   1

Notice

Pulmonary medicine is an ever-changing field. Standard safety precautions must be followed, but as new research and clinical experience broaden our knowledge, changes in treatment and drug therapy become necessary or appropriate. The editors of this work have carefully checked the generic and trade drug names and verified drug dosages to ensure that the dosage information in this work is accurate and in accord with the standards accepted at the time of publication. Readers are advised, however, to check the product information currently provided by the manufacturer of each drug to be administered to be certain that changes have not been made in the recommended dose or in the contraindications for administration. This is of particular importance in regard to new or infrequently used drugs. It is the responsibility of the treating physician relying on experience and knowledge of the patient, to determine dosages and the best treatment for the patient. The editors cannot be responsible for misuse or misapplication of the material in this work.

The Publisher

Preface

The fourth edition of *Clinical Exercise Testing* represents an evolutionary jump relative to the previous editions. The first edition, written 25 years ago and published in 1975, argued for exercise testing as a way of measuring the responses of physiological systems to the metabolic demands of exercise. It stressed the fact that integration and cooperation between systems was of prime importance in maintaining a normal exercise capacity. Thus, although blame for a limitation in capacity might be attributed to one system, other systems could maintain the capacity of the whole through adaptive changes, or add to the incapacity if their function also was suboptimal. The argument was made for the application of simple noninvasive measurements to assess the metabolic, cardiovascular, and respiratory responses to incremental exercise up to the maximum the subject could tolerate.

In the late 1960s and 1970s many advances in exercise physiology and pathophysiology were made, and the second edition (1982) reflected our increased knowledge; however, exercise was still not widely used, apart from its use in the diagnosis of coronary artery disease and in deciding whether the heart or lungs were causing disability. Basically, the approach in the second edition was similar to that in the first edition. Improvements in technology made exercise measurements more reliable and simpler to obtain, and they allowed faster and more elegant presentation of results. These aspects were included also in the third edition (1988).

However, automated exercise systems are now so widely available that the "horse and buggy" measurements included in the early editions have reluctantly been omitted from the present. During these intervening years our laboratories at McMaster University have amassed a large data base of results obtained during incremental exercise in health and a wide range of clinical conditions. This has allowed us to refine normal prediction equations and to identify more clearly the factors that may contribute to disability. Partly because of this have moved farther and farther away from the use of exercise testing to identify single factors, such as impaired function of the heart or lungs, as those limiting exercise capacity. What has become abundantly obvious is that it is symptoms—mainly muscular effort, shortness of breath, and pain—that limit the subject's willingness to continue to exercise.

Until recently the sensory aspects of exercise have been largely ignored, dismissed as too "subjective" and unable to be measured. However, the work of the Swedish psychologist Gunnar Borg, building on the seminal work of S. S. Stephens, the father of the discipline of psychophysics, has established validated methods for the measurement of sensory intensity during exercise. In our own group, Kieran Killian has used Borg's method to measure the intensity of effort and breathlessness, using the measurements as dependent variables to quantify the underlying mechanisms. Killian masterminded the incorporation of the Borg scale into routine incremental exercise tests. This proved to be the breakthrough that allowed us to move away from the previous method of identifying single factors limiting exercise using arbitrary criteria. Now we use the results to provide a description of factors contributing to limiting symptoms. Many of the changes in the present edition reflect this change in emphasis and provide a more detailed background and examples. These changes to some extent take the place of technical details, which are now less necessary because of the improvements in exercise testing equipment.

This edition is dedicated to present and past members of the Ambrose Cardiorespiratory Unit in the McMaster University Medical Centre, with whom it has been my privilege to work for the last 25 years. It is a particular pleasure to acknowledge the generous help I have had through the years from my colleagues Moran Campbell, Kieran Killian, and George Heigenhauser.

NORMAN L. JONES

Acknowledgments

This book was conceived in the mid-sixties at the Royal Postgraduate Medical School of London, when my colleagues and I began to use exercise in the clinical assessment of patients with cardiac and pulmonary disease. At that time many colleagues contributed to the book directly or indirectly. Richard Edwards and Denis Robertson worked with Moran Campbell to produce the first edition. Ross McHardy provided much of the early momentum to the development of rebreathing methods. Brenda Higgs, Marie Clode, Stan Freedman, Tim Clark, Simon Godfrey, Gabriel Laszlo, Neil Pride, and Arnold Naimark all made notable contributions to our early ideas and methods. Ted Davies and Ray Fautley solved many technical problems with inventive genius. The first edition was finally born at McMaster University with a great deal of help from colleagues in the Cardiorespiratory Unit, who have also aided in the production of subsequent editions. John Sutton, who sadly died in 1996, made many suggestions and helped with the electrocardiography section. Kieran Killian established a routine for recording symptom intensity and then used the large data base that we accumulated in the clinical exercise testing laboratory to derive normal predictive values and research the mechanisms contributing to disability in patients with cardiorespiratory disorders. Many technologists have contributed to our research and clinical endeavors. Jim Kane has been our Chief Technologist and Manager from our earliest days, and the laboratory staff has included our Nurse Specialist Suzanne McCollum, Edie Summers, Adrian Mellon, Catie Creighton, Vera Hyatt, Leslie Montgomery, Susan Radford, and Rick Watson. Colleen Conolly and Ellen Dixon have coordinated the cardiac exercise program, under Neil McCartney's direction. Our progression through larger and larger computer data bases has been guided by George Obminski. Many other colleagues have supported and encouraged us in many ways. Finally, Judith Fletcher, Senior Medical Editor at W.B. Saunders Company, and her staff made light the task of making many small and large changes to the text, in producing what we hope is a more comprehensive and clearer coverage of the topics that make up this fascinating subject.

Contents

1

An Introduction to Exercise Testing

A number of points need to be made at the outset, some of which are developed in more depth elsewhere but which should be borne in mind from the beginning.

WHY USE EXERCISE TESTING?

Disease of an organ or system reduces its reserve capacity—its ability to respond to increasing demands. Most organs have a large reserve, and clinical manifestations occur only when their capacity is greatly reduced. Thus, the relationship between a clinical symptom and the severity of the underlying function derangement is not simple. Furthermore, symptomatic limitation of exercise tolerance depends on the function of the whole organism, including the subjective response to stress. Let us examine these points in greater detail.

Clinical Assessment of Exercise Tolerance

Clinicians are frequently faced with contrasts between the clinical severity of a disorder and its expression in the extent of the patient's disability. Clinical severity is measured by impairment in function, whereas disability and handicap are the result of a complex interaction between impairment, the person, and the environment. Exercise testing has the potential to increase our understanding of such contrasts and to assess various factors that contribute to disability. Although most clinical investigators appear to agree that exercise testing and interpretation need to be based on an approach that explores the integration between systems, this concept is often ignored or given lip service only. There has been a reluctance to use such an approach routinely in cardiac exercise testing laboratories, where undue emphasis on the electrocardiographic changes means that a limited exercise capacity unrelated to myocardial ischemia may be ignored. This leads to the frustration experienced by referring physicians when they receive a report indicating limited capacity and "submaximal effort." Leaving aside the fact that such patients would probably not agree that their effort was submaximal, the opportunity to understand the factors underlying

disability has been lost for the sake of a few simple measurements and questions regarding limiting symptoms. Measurement of ventilation and gas exchange during exercise is now technically feasible on a routine basis and provides a more complete analysis of effort intolerance.

Exercise Tolerance Depends on Reserve Capacity

Many measurements made at rest inadequately reflect the reserve capacity of physiological systems that contribute to exercise tolerance. Exercise testing uses the increased metabolic demands of exercise to stress the systems and so establish their capacity to respond. The reserve capacity that is normally available in the circulatory and respiratory systems is so large that the demands of daily living do not become compromised until function has been greatly impaired; thus, exercise testing may reveal abnormality at an earlier stage of cardiopulmonary disorders. Once disability is apparent, an opposite effect may be demonstrated; a small increase in the clinical severity of a disorder may then be accompanied by a relatively marked increase in disability.

These concepts are expressed diagrammatically in Figure 1–1, in which the ordinate clearly depends

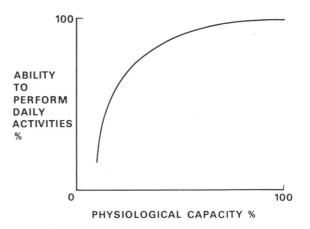

Figure 1–1. Curve showing physiological capacity versus ability to perform daily activities.

on the person, activities, and culture but might extend to walking quickly, to cycling or swimming, or even to competitive athletics. On the abscissa, physiological capacity may represent the maximum capacity to breathe, to transfer oxygen in the lungs, to increase cardiac output, and so on. Whatever the detailed variations in the axes, the general shape is certainly convex upward, with a flat upper part in which major changes in the functional capacity of organs cause few symptoms unless strenuous exercise is taken, and a lower steeper part in which major changes in symptoms may signify little change in the function of the affected organ.

Exercise Tolerance Depends on Many Systems

Limitation of exercise, in both health and disease, is never due to a single mechanism acting alone. The principle of integration rather than the identification of a limiting system, such as the heart or lungs acting alone or in a dominating role, becomes self-evident when a few facts are considered.

First, a limitation in one mechanism often leads to an adaptive response that tends to maintain exercise capacity. This phenomenon may occur within a system, such as the increase in cardiac stroke volume that tends to maintain exercise in the presence of an impaired heart rate response but that may be absent, for example, if myocardial contractility is also impaired. A patient with expiratory airflow limitation may adapt by changes in the pattern of breathing and in the operative lung volume, changes that may be absent if the respiratory muscles are also weak. Other adaptations may involve cooperation between systems; examples include changes in muscle blood flow and oxygen extraction in patients with an impaired cardiac output, and increases in cardiac output in patients who become hypoxic as a result of impaired pulmonary gas exchange.

Second, more than one system may be impaired; in pulmonary vascular obstruction due to multiple pulmonary emboli, for example, a limited cardiac output and ventilation-perfusion mismatch may combine to limit exercise to a far greater extent than if only one of these abnormalities were present, because of their separate contributions to severe breathlessness.

Third, many chronic conditions (those lasting more than a few weeks) are accompanied by a curtailed activity, leading to changes in systems other than the one mainly involved; patients recovering from a myocardial infarction are after a few weeks found to be limited by leg muscle fatigue secondary to reductions in enzyme activities and other changes in muscle.

An important practical corollary to the physiological truism stated above is that clinical improvement may depend on attention to other mechanisms in addition to that primarily affected by disease. There is no need to belabor the point that symptoms arising from the same limitation vary in different subjects and in the same subject at different times, depending on many factors. The need for objective assessment is obvious.

Exercise in Everyday Life Is an "Un–steady State" Affair

Examined broadly, a review of exercise performance might range from studies of single motor unit contractions, through maximal brief muscle contraction and isometric power of several muscle groups, to dynamic exercise of long duration. However, in this book, we are concerned with dynamic exercise involving large muscle groups for at least several minutes and requiring complex energy supply mechanisms. Many activities in everyday life are brief, particularly those involving a high power and in which many of these mechanisms do not fully adapt during the time of the exercise; in this sense, the mechanisms never reach the "steady state" beloved of exercise physiologists. The standard clinical questions "How far can you walk?" and "How many stairs can you climb?" seek information regarding maximal performance in what is usually "un–steady state" exercise. Consider stair climbing: the power output achieved in climbing is usually beyond the ability of the respiratory and circulatory systems to sustain in a steady state, although we know that one or two flights can be climbed without even taking a breath. The answer to the common clinical question "How many stairs can you climb without getting short of breath?" must lie somewhere between 30 and 120 stairs, or two and six domestic flights. Less than this can be accomplished without using the heart or lungs, and more is within the compass of an athlete only. Of course, this argument is a caricature. Although we may climb 30 stairs at a rate in excess of our ability to meet the energy demands, we do not have to meet the cost immediately; we "buy now and pay later." Patients often estimate the cost of exercise from their experience of the difficulty they have in paying the bill later, when the severity of dyspnea indicates how close they are to the limit of their ability to repay. Nevertheless, the evaluation of exercise tolerance by questioning alone leaves much to be desired; it becomes increasingly unrealistic as limitation becomes increasingly severe and even minor activity becomes limited by the patient's willingness to tolerate (Campbell, 1967).

Having made these points, we do not want to imply that testing patients during exercise necessarily is superior to testing based on their stated ability to perform certain activities; the two are complementary, the information of each being directed toward a different end. Exercise testing is directed toward measurement of individual components of the system; the symptoms experienced by a patient when he performs a certain activity depend on the way the whole person responds to the environment.

Exercise Tolerance Depends on the Whole Organism

By objectively assessing the contributions of physiological systems with exercise testing, we may close the gap between the patient's disability and the impairment in exercise capacity. We are then better able to explain the disability in physiological terms, more precisely than by clinical examination and by investigations made at rest. However, there are always situations in which a contrast remains, partly because disability in everyday life depends on the demands made on the person and partly because the appreciation of the effort or distress encountered in meeting them varies from one person to the next. Sometimes, there may be a suspicion that disability is being exaggerated for some reason, and this may not be helped by a feeling that the person lacks motivation or has not tried during the test. It is often possible to resolve these apparent discrepancies through careful observation of the subject during the test and by an estimate of the intensity of sensations, such as effort, dyspnea, and pain, while the test is proceeding. The measurement of sensation will take us briefly into the realm of the psychophysicists; sensations may be quantified at least as precisely as most of the other measurements made during exercise.

PRELIMINARY CONSIDERATIONS IN EXERCISE TESTING

How May Exercise Testing Be Most Effectively Used?

Exercise testing must examine all component systems and the integration and interaction between them. An exercise test should not only reveal the primary malfunction but also demonstrate whether other mechanisms are hiding, disguising, or aggravating the primary defect. This information provides the added benefit that the performance of the systems can be examined in relation to one another rather than in relation to established normal standards alone. Accomplishing this requires testing at several work rates. Exercise testing based on the use of a single standard level of exercise may add little to studies made at rest, for it may represent no stress for one patient but may be too high for another.

Exercise Testing Should Be "Cost Effective"

There has been much concern regarding the cost of patient investigation in relation to its value in diagnosis or treatment. Few investigations have been realistically assessed in this way, and, indeed, such an assessment often may be impossible. However, the responsibility should not be shirked, and as a first step, the desired information should be provided with the least cost. As with many other disciplines in medicine, technical innovation has led to the development of complex and expensive procedures, which are used in many cardiorespiratory laboratories. Although exercise testing may be added to these procedures, their complexity may make it difficult to obtain simpler information that is more applicable to the functional assessment of the patient. Hence the "cost" of this approach is compounded. On the other hand, innovation has brought practical benefits in terms of measurement, on-line calculation, report generation, and data storage. The results of exercise tests are thereby more reliable than they were 20 years ago, and it is now possible for the patient to undergo a test and walk out of the laboratory with the results and a report an hour later. Thus, although the capital outlay on a modern exercise testing system may appear high, the systems now function more reliably for longer, and such costs are soon recovered.

A major underlying motive has been to extend the benefit and lessen the cost of simple noninvasive tests so that the simplest and least invasive technique that gives the required information can be applied. The object is to describe the available choices for those wishing to use exercise testing as part of clinical investigations. It has been our experience that physicians may make extensive use of exercise test results, particularly if these are presented in a standardized and informative manner.

Exercise Testing Is a Clinical Procedure

As with any investigative technique, the information yielded by exercise testing needs to be usable by a referring physician in the clinical context; something must be learned about the patient that is readily applied to the management problem. A corollary to this maxim is that the information should be readily understood and relevant; with the present trend for computer-generated results, it is too easy to supply more information than is wanted. Confusion is apt to result, and exercise testing may be relegated to irrelevancy, the hobby of physiologists in their ivory laboratories.

"Routine" exercise tests are valuable, and it is certainly necessary to have a routine, but a test is more informative if it is addressed to a particular clinical problem and conducted in such a way as to yield a specific answer.

If exercise is used as part of the assessment of certain clinical problems, it soon becomes clear that it is of greater value in early than in advanced disease. In a patient who is so limited as to be capable of very little exercise, the results are largely predictable and may add little to the clinical examination, apart from an objective assessment of symptoms.

Finally, a change in a simple measurement repeated over a period of time is often more helpful than a more complicated measurement made once in the course of the patient's illness. If assessment is based on simple techniques, it is possible to study patients more frequently.

A common practice in pulmonary function testing is to supply the referring clinician with a battery of numbers (often expressed as "percentage of normal"), followed by an expert interpretation that is usually descriptive, and rarely as clinically useful as it ought to be. An objective of this book is to increase the clinically relevant functional information obtained from exercise tests.

The information we aim to provide does not depend on advanced theory. We seek to answer such simple questions as "How much air does this patient breathe?" "How much blood does his heart pump?" "Is he limited more by his ability to breathe, or by his ability to pump blood?" "Is the volume of air she is breathing or blood she is pumping more or less than it should be or used to be when stressed by exercise?" It is hoped that this book will provide clinicians with the information necessary to answer such questions from measurements made during exercise.

Exercise Testing: Steady or Unsteady?

Having made the point that exercise in everyday life is seldom steady state, I also propose an exercise testing protocol that uses regular increases in intensity up to the subject's tolerable maximum. A steady state is not maintained in this type of test, but the advantages of measurements made at many levels outweigh the possible disadvantages of the unsteady state. Furthermore, recent work has shown that few measurements require a steady state in order to be valid. I defend the approach in detail in considering the available choices; the protocol represents a compromise between the demands of the measurements for a relatively steady state and the need for the test to be completed within a reasonable time.

WHAT IS A "NORMAL" RESPONSE TO EXERCISE?

A problem discussed extensively in the literature during the past few years has been the definition and prediction of the normal responses to exercise, with which measurements made in patients can be compared. It might appear to be a question that would be settled easily by population studies carried out by those who conduct exercise tests and who then use the data to interpret their results. However, the problem is in fact more difficult, and, paradoxically, the solution is easier than this simple approach would indicate. Defining a "normal" population is a complex task. The exercise performance of most people in the Western world can be improved by regular exercise. One might, therefore, take for normal values the results of studies of those who take exercise regularly, but such standards might not be easy to apply to the results of a test performed in a patient who has not taken any exercise for years. Even if results from an appropriate population are available, the problem of defining limits remains with the attendant risks of including false positive and false negative results. Fortunately, the situation becomes less troublesome with increasing familiarity as the clinician uses the numerical values to complement other clinical investigations and finds that more information is obtained from the relationship between variables than from the value of each considered by itself.

Publications presenting prediction equations are few, and striking differences may exist between the equations from different groups, particularly when they are applied to subjects at the extremes of stature and age. Several reasons for the variation may exist. First, differences in the manner of selection of the reference population may lead to equations that are unrepresentative because of unequal numbers in cells containing subjects of different ages, stature, gender, and activity (or "fitness"). Second, equations have been applied that mathematically are not in accord with what we know of the physiological effects of these parameters; for example, many equations in current use employ linear functions to describe the influence of age, height, or weight, whereas we know intuitively and experimentally that these parameters cannot be expressed as linear functions.

This topic is dealt with extensively in Chapter 8, but, to summarize our approach briefly, we decided to base our standards on subjects referred for exercise testing (Jones et al., 1989), as well as on a recruited population (Jones et al., 1985). The referred subjects had no definite diagnosis, were receiving no drug treatment, and had normal spirometric and electrocardiographic results and a response to exercise that was consistent with that of the recruited subjects. This strategy allowed us to increase the reference population, especially in those combinations of age and stature that are hard to find in recruits. We were then able to calculate the mean response in each combination of age (5-

year increments) and height (5-cm intervals) and to calculate nonlinear equations in which the weighting of age and height were equal throughout the whole range of age and stature encountered in patients referred for exercise testing.

INDICATIONS FOR EXERCISE TESTING

A brief review of the clinical uses of exercise testing underlines some of the book's major objectives. We can gain an assessment of the impaired function in various systems, the extent of disability, and the reasons for handicap experienced in the patient's everyday life. Although clinicians often hope to obtain a diagnosis from the results of exercise testing, diagnosis almost always involves integration of the test results and other clinical information; the test rarely provides a pathognomonic response.

Impairment, Disability, and Handicap

These three terms have been used by the World Health Organization (1980) in a working manual on occupational disability assessment; they are helpful in clarifying effects that are often confused in physicians' minds, and for which exercise testing makes separate and important contributions.

Impairment is defined as "any loss or abnormality of psychological, physiological, or anatomical structure or function." In these terms, functional impairment may be assessed from the responses of a system to exercise. For example, the severity of impaired pulmonary gas exchange is reflected in decreases in arterial oxygen saturation relative to increasing oxygen intake, and in increases in ventilation relative to carbon dioxide output; impaired ventricular function is reflected in increases in cardiac rate relative to oxygen intake. An exercise test should provide quantitative information regarding the following systems and processes: ventilation and pulmonary gas exchange, central and peripheral circulation, blood gas transport, peripheral gas exchange and metabolism, and muscle function. This information often helps in the treatment of a patient with exercise intolerance or suspected heart or lung disease. Occasionally, it is possible to demonstrate the absence of malfunction when symptoms have made the patient fear, and the clinician suspect, serious disease, leading to reassurance and advice.

Disability is defined as "any restriction or lack (resulting from an impairment) of ability to perform an activity in the manner or within the range considered normal for a human being." A reduction in exercise capacity may be used to measure disability as long as the capacity expected for the individual may be defined with sufficient accuracy. This places considerable importance on predictive algorithms,

and especially on appropriate scaling, a topic that is dealt with in Chapter 8. Normal standards remain a worry for anyone carrying out tests in a population in which stature, age, and disability vary widely.

Handicap is defined as "a disadvantage for a given individual, resulting from an impairment or a disability, that limits or prevents the fulfilment of a role that is normal (depending on age, sex, and cultural factors) for that individual." This assessment involves the application of information regarding exercise-related symptoms to the energy demands experienced in daily living. This is a clinical exercise that requires a knowledge of the activities in the patient's normal occupation and leisure. The patient's weight may exert a large effect because an overweight individual may have a normal exercise capacity and thus may not be disabled, as defined above, while experiencing considerable handicap during activities in which weight bearing and walking uphill are inevitable. An important consideration in exercise testing is the measurement of symptom intensity experienced in the complete range of exercise from rest to maximum effort. This measurement is practically feasible if a quantitatively valid psychophysical scaling method is used; this topic is considered in Chapter 3.

The Diagnostic Uses of Exercise Testing

Having emphasized that the proper concern of physiological tests is with functional changes, I recognize that the problems that lead a clinician to ask for an investigation are couched more often in structural or causal than in functional terms: the question asked is more frequently "What is causing this patient's symptoms and how bad is it?" rather than "What is the matter, how is it affecting function, and how is the body responding to it?" Physiological findings may have structural implications that can be useful, either because the response is diagnostic or, more commonly, because the response indicates a functional abnormality that can be used diagnostically with other clinical information. This raises the topic of the specificity-sensitivity of exercise tests, which has been hotly debated with respect to coronary artery disease; this is discussed later in the book. For the moment, let us say that to be strictly diagnostic, an abnormality has to be as close as possible to 100 per cent specific for the given diagnosis.

Conditions in which an exercise test result may be specific include the following:

- Myocardial ischemia
- Peripheral vascular disease
- Exercise-induced asthma
- Unfitness

- Psychogenic dyspnea
- Muscle phosphorylase deficiency

I do not detail the abnormalities found in these conditions but make a few observations at this point. Unfitness is common in urban men and women and may make the quantitative assessment of other conditions difficult. Psychogenic dyspnea is common in organic disease and can compound the physician's and patient's assessment of severity. An exercise test often allows an assessment to be made of the relative importance of unfitness or psychogenic dyspnea in a mixed situation.

There has been a recent tendency to suggest that arteriographic changes should replace other diagnostic criteria of myocardial ischemia. However, the presence of narrowing or obstruction of major coronary arteries may not be a reliable indication of inadequate myocardial blood flow, which is more realistically assessed during exercise, when the myocardial oxygen needs are increased. The same arguments apply to peripheral vascular disease.

In muscle phosphorylase deficiency (McArdle's syndrome), impaired glycogen breakdown results in extreme fatigue without lactate accumulation. This rare combination is virtually pathognomonic, although recently, other muscle enzyme defects have been discovered.

Conditions That an Exercise Test Can Detect or Exclude

Conditions that an exercise test can detect or exclude are those that cause an abnormal exercise response but do not cause a diagnostic pattern of abnormality. Hence in this category, there should be no false-negative results, but a positive result may be nonspecific. The test result should be sensitive but need not be specific. Virtually all diseases affecting the airways, lungs, pulmonary circulation, heart, systemic circulation, and blood could come under this category, but for the sake of clinical practice, the following is a conservative list of conditions in which abnormalities in an exercise test are likely to be diagnostically helpful:

- Chronic bronchitis
- Pulmonary emphysema
- Pulmonary infiltration, alveolitis, and fibrosis
- Pulmonary thromboembolism and hypertension
- Congenital cardiac abnormalities
- Cardiac valvular obstruction or incompetence
- Primary myocardial disease
- Generalized neuromuscular disorders

I re-emphasize the concept that proper application of exercise tests is not so much in the narrower sense of diagnosis of these conditions, but in a wider sense of assessing them. When used in this manner, their diagnostic value may be increased indirectly in two ways. First, the response to exercise may be at variance with the clinical impression and may indicate the need for other investigations, for example, a patient thought to have asthma in whom exercise reveals a cardiac limitation resulting from thromboembolic pulmonary hypertension. Second, exercise may allow a diagnostic weighting in a patient with more than one disorder; for example, a patient with valvular heart disease and chronic bronchitis in whom the ventilatory impairment exceeds the cardiac, leading to a change in therapeutic emphasis.

The Use of Exercise Testing in Clinical Management

Many techniques used in clinical assessment become more valuable when repeated on several occasions in any one patient for the purpose of following the natural history of a condition or the effect of therapy. This is particularly true of exercise testing, in which a change in overall performance or in the performance of a single mechanism carries greater weight than an absolute value at a single point in time. One obvious application is in the use of regular exercise in rehabilitation programs. The initial exercise test allows accurate prescription of the activity, so as to be safe yet effective, and direct attention to mechanisms requiring particular care. Repeated testing provides objective evidence of improvement and identifies the mechanisms that underlie any change. It also provides a valuable tool for the physician to use in motivating the patient to continue the activity and in changing the activity to keep it at an optimal level. Many types of activity programs are in their infancy: assessment of their values must include objective evidence of improved function before they can be applied on a wider scale.

The results obtained from an exercise test may help in a number of other clinical situations as well, such as myocardial infarction, before hospital discharge; the assessment of disability for industrial compensation; and deciding if occupational demands may be safely met. They may also be used as a basis for reassurance when the possibility of serious disease is excluded by the results.

THE DESIGN OF A PRACTICAL EXERCISE PROTOCOL

Many exercise tests have been advocated in the 75 years or so that exercise has been applied to clinical problems. Although the background to the development of our approach is provided in Chapter 5, some concepts are worth identifying at the outset. First, the arguments for and against the use of cycles, steps, or treadmills are not really important if the protocol allows measurements to be easily obtained at a range of power outputs that spans energy levels from rest to maximum effort. Second, the decision regarding increments in power and the time for which each is maintained is almost impossible to resolve, and an arbitrary decision has to be made that is mainly based on practicality. In an ideal situation, probably the increments would be an equal proportion of the patient's maximum capacity, but we do not know this before the test and cannot guess it with any confidence from clinical information. Large increments and short durations risk early fatigue and mainly test muscle strength and anaerobic metabolic processes. Long durations and small increments, although allowing time for gas exchange processes to adapt fully, assess mainly aerobic metabolic processes and the size and availability of energy stores but risk boredom and require a total duration that is unacceptable both to the patient and to the laboratory schedule. A compromise is reached by choosing standardized increments in power, each maintained for 1 minute, such that the total duration in most individuals is 10 to 20 minutes. In very disabled individuals, this leaves the option of choosing a smaller increment and repeating the test if the first effort lasts for only a minute or two.

As to the measurements to be made at each load, there is agreement that these should include noninvasive recording of metabolic, cardiovascular, ventilatory, and pulmonary gas exchange variables; we would add to these the scaling of symptom severity. Although capillary or arterial blood sampling and cardiac output measurement are feasible during routine incremental exercise testing (McKelvie et al., 1987), they add a complexity and cost that is not justified in most studies. Our own practice has been to reserve such measurements for problems in which these measures are clinically justified and important and in which the noninvasive results have left questions to be answered. These considerations led to a staged approach to testing (stages 1–4), which has allowed us to be cost-effective in terms of time and resources; most referred patients undergo the simple noninvasive study (stage 1), leaving fewer than 5 per cent who go on to the more complex or invasive assessments (stages 3 and 4). The remaining procedure (stage 2) was designed at a time when blood gas and cardiac output measurements were more difficult than they are now; we seldom use it except as a model of physiological and mathematical integration between systems, in the classic lineage of Douglas, Barcroft, and Margaria (see Chapter 11). It remains a useful tool in teaching concepts of integration in physiology.

AN ASSESSMENT OF THE CLINICAL VALUE OF EXERCISE TESTING

Throughout the book, there is a largely undefended belief that exercise testing can contribute to the management of many clinical disorders. Although the clinical usefulness of exercise testing in the diagnosis of coronary artery disease has been widely studied and debated, the value of the wider uses of exercise in clinical medicine remains hard to measure and has not been formally attempted. To remedy this, at least for my own practice, the physicians who referred patients for 100 consecutive tests in our laboratory were surveyed. By use of questionnaires, information was obtained regarding the clinical reasons for the request before the test was performed and the clinical use subsequently made of the results. The initial questionnaire was completed for 84 patients and exercise studies were performed in 72, the second questionnaire being completed for all these patients. Ten patients did not appear for their tests, one refused after reading the consent form, and one showed a resting electrocardiogram of recent myocardial infarction. The physicians surveyed consisted of 14 family physicians, 14 internists, and three residents in specialty training programs. Although there were many reasons for exercise testing, chest pain and dyspnea were the most common symptoms under investigation (Table 1–1).

Table 1–1. REASONS FOR EXERCISE TESTS IN 72 PATIENTS	
Reason	No. of Patients
Chest pain on effort	31
Postbypass surgery	4
Postmyocardial infarct	4
Noncoronary cardiac disease	9
Arrhythmias	9
Hypertension	9
Dyspnea	23
Airway obstruction	7
Nonobstructive pulmonary disease	3
Obesity	5
Diabetes	1
Growth hormone deficiency	2
McArdle's syndrome	1
Anxiety	2
Claudication	2

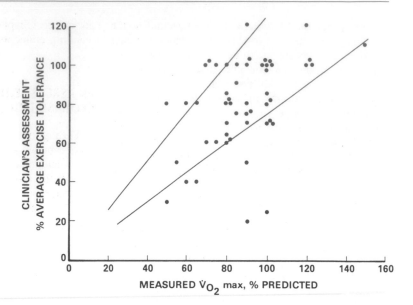

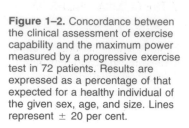

Figure 1–2. Concordance between the clinical assessment of exercise capability and the maximum power measured by a progressive exercise test in 72 patients. Results are expressed as a percentage of that expected for a healthy individual of the given sex, age, and size. Lines represent ± 20 per cent.

For each patient, the referring physician was asked to scale the patient's effort tolerance on clinical grounds; this estimate was later compared with the objectively measured exercise capacity. Although the concordance was perhaps surprisingly good, the clinical estimate tended to be lower than the measured value, sometimes to a marked degree (Fig. 1–2). On the other hand, clinicians seldom overestimated the patient's exercise capacity. Large discrepancies between the clinical assessment and the exercise test results were usually explained by a clinical diagnosis that did not allow a good exercise tolerance. In one patient, a clinical diagnosis of McArdle's syndrome had been made; the exercise test showed a normal exercise capacity, and the diagnosis was excluded. Two patients shown by coronary angiography to have severe three-vessel narrowing and who were thought to be severely impaired were also found to have normal exercise capacities. In two patients with severe chronic airway obstruction demonstrated by pulmonary function tests, exercise performance was less impaired than expected on clinical grounds. In several other instances, the test results demonstrated that a diagnosis was not necessarily associated with a significant exercise limitation—for example, in aortic stenosis and sarcoidosis.

Although in a narrow diagnostic sense the results of exercise tests were supportive of the clinical assessment, the emphasis placed on a given diagnosis in limiting exercise was changed sufficiently often to make this type of information of clinical value. Physicians reported a change in their management approaches after the exercise test results in 13 patients (Table 1–2). The results were used by physicians to give advice on activity and occupation, to explain the reason for symptoms, and to discuss the demands of exercise with greater confidence. A more positive attitude was often taken on the basis of test results—reassurance regarding the absence of any serious condition (eight patients); positive encouragement to enter an exercise program (eight patients); and advice regarding occupational capability (two patients). Three patients with

Table 1–2. CLINICAL USES OF TEST RESULTS IN 72 PATIENTS	
Clinical Use	**No. of Patients**
Confirmed clinical diagnosis	42
Revealed performance worse than suspected clinically	8
Revealed performance better than suspected clinically	25
Confirmed limiting factors to exercise	36
Changed clinical impression regarding limiting factors	6
Revealed unsuspected limiting factors	2
Changed clinical management	13
Used to advise on activity and/or occupation	41

symptomatic angina underwent further investigation on the basis of completely normal exercise test results, leading to final diagnoses of duodenal ulcer in one patient and hiatus hernia in two.

The test was judged unhelpful in only one instance because the report did not contain a comparison with results obtained in a previous test; otherwise, the physician classed the information as ''helpful'' or ''very helpful.''

The assessment of the clinical value of investigations presents notorious difficulties that were not avoided in this small study; nevertheless, the enthusiastic response from physicians with varying clinical practices tended to support the value of a simple test that might be applied to many situations. In particular, it supported our contention that the commonplace separation between ''cardiac stress tests'' and ''pulmonary exercise tests'' has outlived its usefulness.

REFERENCES

Campbell EJM. Exercise tolerance. Sci Basis Med Annu Rev 1967;8:129–144.

Jones NL, Makrides L, Hitchcock C, et al. Normal standards for an incremental progressive cycle ergometry test. Am Rev Respir Dis 1985;131:700–708.

Jones NL, Summers E, Killian KJ. Influence of age and stature on exercise capacity during incremental cycle ergometry in men and women. Am Rev Respir Dis 1989;140:1373–1380.

McKelvie RS, Heigenhauser GJF, Jones NL. Measurement of cardiac output by CO_2 rebreathing in unsteady state exercise. Chest 1987;92:777–782.

World Health Organization. International Classification of Impairments, Disabilities, and Handicaps. A Manual of Classification Relating to the Consequences of Disease. Geneva: Schuler AG; 1980.

2

Physiology of Exercise

This chapter sets the scene for the chapters that follow by briefly reviewing the physiology of muscular exercise in health and disease. Before this is done, some units of measurement require explanation, and the types of exercise considered later need to be described.

FORCE, WORK, AND POWER

The unit of force is that acting on a mass of 1 kg to produce an acceleration of 1 m·sec^{-2} and is called the newton (N). An object falling freely increases its speed by 9.80 m·sec^{-2}, and because the only force acting is gravity, the acceleration is constant. The gravitational force acting on a stationary mass of 1 kg is 9.80 N; this force is also called the kilopond (kp).

A unit of work is done when a force of 1 N acts through 1 m and is called 1 newton-meter, or 1 joule (J). If a mass of 1 kg is moved through a vertical distance of 1 m against the force of gravity, the work performed is 9.80 J; this is more widely called a kilopond-meter (kpm).

Throughout this book we will be concerned with dynamic exercise performed by large muscle groups. The external expression of this action is power, which is work performed per unit of time. The unit of work is the joule, and the unit of power is the joule per second, or watt (W). Many physiologists use the kilopond-meter as the unit of work, in which case the unit of power is the kilopond-meter per minute (kpm/min). This equals 9.80 ÷ 60 watts, or 0.1635 W (an easier conversion to remember is that 600 kpm/min is about 100 W).

The adoption of the SI system (International System of Units) of notation has been well argued (Piiper, 1973), but we have not used it in the text; a table given in Appendix C allows the reader to convert measurements if required.

The work performed and the energy liberated by chemical processes may both be measured in the same units (joules), but because the free-energy changes associated with metabolic processes were initially measured as heat liberated, a thermochemical equivalent is also widely used—the calorie (4.184 J). Because muscle contraction is accompanied by adenosine triphosphate (ATP) hydrolysis, an ATP equivalence is another way of quantifying energy liberation; the net free-energy release that accompanies the hydrolysis of 1 mole of ATP is 17.5 to 18.5 kilocalories (kcal) (73–78 kJ [kilojoule]). For many physiological studies, oxygen intake is used as a measure of power, but the conversion of power to oxygen intake is not a constant, varying with the type of exercise being performed.

The Oxygen Equivalence of Power

When a fuel is oxidized, oxygen is used and heat is liberated; the classic experiments with bomb calorimetry are the basis for the caloric equivalents of food that appear in popular diet books. Thus, it is almost common knowledge that the combustion of 1 g of protein yields 4.32 kcal of heat and uses 4.46 kcal/L of oxygen; the corresponding values for fat are 9.46 and 4.69 kcal, respectively, and for starch, 4.18 and 5.05 kcal. Thus, for these reactions about 20.1 kJ is equivalent to 1 L of oxygen. These values became the basis for indirect calorimetry, in which the oxygen used was converted into heat units; measurement of the respiratory quotient (RQ) was used to obtain the proportion of fats and sugars and urinary nitrogen excretion used to derive protein metabolism. There are several limitations to indirect calorimetry—the critical review by McGilvery (1979) is recommended—but the technique established values for the basal metabolic rate and led to studies of the "efficiency" of muscular exercise. *Efficiency* in this context is the ratio of the oxygen equivalence of the energy expended to the measured oxygen intake at that power. For exercise not requiring much skill and using large muscle groups (as in cycling or treadmill walking), values of around 20 per cent are obtained—that is, the measured oxygen intake is some five times larger than the oxygen used to generate an equivalent amount of energy by oxidizing mixed fuels. The efficiency calculated in this way may be affected by many factors; it is less with smaller muscle groups (e.g., arm work), with highly skilled exercise (e.g., swimming, wheelchair propulsion), and with excessive oxygen demands (e.g., owing to obesity, severe lung disease, and some metabolic disorders). However, with exercise using large muscle groups, as in treadmill walking and cycle ergometry, the increase in oxygen intake for a given increase in power may be predicted with reasonable accuracy ($\pm$ 10 per cent).

Another unit of power in common usage is the "met," defined as a multiple of the resting metabolic oxygen requirements (3.5 mL/min/kg). This unit has its main application in describing the energy cost of activities—for example, occupational demands and intensity of exercise training programs. The concept of the met is easy for patients to understand during an explanation of exercise test results and the prescription of activity. Also, the met may be directly and simply related to the maximal oxygen intake ($\dot{V}O_2$max); a $\dot{V}O_2$max of 35 mL/min/kg is 10 mets. The met is not recommended, however, as an independent measure of exercise demands to which other measurements can be related; measurements of the absolute oxygen intake or the carbon dioxide output are preferred because these are the "loads" presented to physiological mechanisms. Also, it will become apparent that the division of $\dot{V}O_2$ by body weight represents an erroneous scaling of this variable and thus should not be used.

MUSCLE CONTRACTION

Although this publication is not the place to attempt a description of the intricacies of muscle structure and the mechanisms of muscle contraction, some features of the structure-function relationships are relevant to the maximum exercise capacity in health, the design of exercise tests, and the impairment in exercise capacity seen in many disorders, not only those affecting muscle. The contractile unit of muscle is the myofibril, but in many ways, it is more logical to think in terms of the motor unit, which consists of a motor neuron together with the fibers innervated by it; this is because all the fibers in a motor unit are homogeneous and are activated synchronously. Under most conditions, muscles contract tetanically, and the force developed in a given muscle is dictated by the recruitment of fibers, which is directly related to the extent of activation of the motor neurons supplying it. There are large variations between different muscles in the capacity to generate power that are accounted for by variations in their structure and fiber type composition (Larsson et al., 1979). The structural differences between muscles are seen in differences in the arrangement of fibers (for example, the contrast between strap and pennate muscles) and in their length and cross-sectional area. Fibers may be classified as fast or slow contracting, related to their motoneuron characteristics, and

these contractile properties are accompanied by differences in metabolic properties. Power in the context of the single fiber may be considered in terms of the capacity to generate both force and velocity of contraction; the former is largely dependent on the fiber's cross-sectional area (Maughan et al., 1983), and the latter, on its twitch characteristics (slow or fast contracting). The power generated by a complete muscle is related to the recruitment of motor units, both number and type; within limits, recruitment follows the "size principle" of Henneman and colleagues (1965), with the smallest motoneurons being activated by the lowest excitatory stimuli. Thus, with increasing motoneuron stimulation frequency, there is an increase in the resulting force, but the slow-twitch fibers (small motoneurons) reach their peak tension at a much lower frequency than fast-twitch fibers. In a muscle with a mixed fiber population, the slow-twitch fibers may perform all the work at a low proportion of their capacity, and some fast-twitch fibers, supplied by the largest motoneurons, may fire only with extreme effort.

Speed of contraction is measured as the time taken to shorten or develop tension. All fibers possess a hyperbolic force-velocity characteristic, but at a given relative force, fast-twitch fibers generate a greater velocity of contraction than slow-twitch fibers and thus also generate a greater relative force at any given velocity of contraction. Although slow-twitch fibers are often long and fast-twitch fibers usually short, these differences do not account for the different characteristics of force and velocity. The fast-twitch fibers have a greater myosin ATPase activity, as well as a larger number of binding sites for calcium; the types are probably defined by isoforms of the myofibrillar proteins that are the products of different genes (Whalen, 1985). However, it is intriguing that the frequency of neural impulses appears to control gene expression; nerve transplantation can change the dominant fiber population in a given muscle, and certain types of repetitive exercise may lead to small changes also (Schantz et al., 1982). Associated with the differences in ATPase activity are a number of other differences between the fiber types related to their metabolic requirements; these differences influence the capacity of the fiber types for prolonged contraction (endurance). Such differences have allowed the identification of at least three main fiber types (Peter et al., 1972), slow oxidative (SO), fast oxidative–glycolytic (FOG), and fast glycolytic (FG), as described later in the chapter.

The sliding filament hypothesis of the Huxleys is now accepted as the mechanism of myofibril shortening, with filaments of myosin and actin sliding past each other (Huxley, 1985). The reaction between actin and the myosin heads containing activated MgATP is the final process in contraction, which also involves the other two proteins of the myofibril, troponin and tropomyosin. Depolarization of the motor end-plate leads to propagation of an action potential through the T-tubules of the sarcolemma that extend the extracellular space deep into the myofibrils to intracellular terminal cisternae where Ca^{2+} is released (Peachey, 1985). The increase in Ca^{2+} concentration (from 10^{-7} to 10^{-5}) leads to saturation of binding sites on troponin-C. The position of tropomyosin is such as to obstruct interaction between actin and myosin, but the binding of Ca^{2+}-activated troponin leads to a realignment that allows the reaction to proceed with hydrolysis of ATP and release of free energy. The compact head of the myosin molecule contains a binding site for ATP and one for actin, to enable the transmission of force; the proximity of the binding sites presumably enables conservation of part of the free energy for mechanical work. As the spacing between cross-bridges amounts to only 5 per cent of the contractile element, but muscles can shorten by as much as 30 per cent, a succession of attachments, releases, and reattachments occurs between the individual force generators to produce a smooth contraction that continues until Ca^{2+} is removed from troponin. Thus, relaxation is associated with resequestration of Ca^{2+} in the intracellular vesicles; as this movement is against an electrochemical gradient, the process requires ATP. Myosin is then left activated by the products of ATP hydrolysis and ready for the next contraction; in the absence of ATP, myosin would be left attached to actin, and the muscle would be in rigor.

The importance of Ca^{2+} in contraction is not limited to the binding by troponin, as it is the central regulator of many metabolic reactions, acting in this way as a coordinator between contraction and metabolic activity. It has been calculated that 20 to 30 per cent of the ATP flux in muscle is required for the maintenance of Ca^{2+} gradients (Kushmerick, 1977), and other ion pumps function to maintain other concentration gradients. Thus, at high energy demands there may be competition for ATP that becomes self-limiting; furthermore, in heavy exercise a low muscle pH may act to impair the ion pumps and thereby contribute to muscle fatigue.

With cross-bridge formation, the myofibril shortens, or develops tension, or resists externally imposed tension, at a rate determined by the turnover of ATP; any given muscle may be characterized by its capacity to generate force at varying velocities and lengths—the force-velocity and length-tension characteristics.

The relationships between force and velocity of contraction mean that for any muscle fiber, there is an optimal velocity of contraction for generation of power. Maximal velocity is achieved in the un-

loaded state, and maximal force is developed at zero velocity; as power incorporates both force and velocity components, a compromise is achieved at the submaximal velocity at which maximal power is generated (Edgerton et al., 1986). Although it is difficult to translate this concept into human exercise performance in any strict sense, it may be possible to identify an optimal velocity for different activities, such as cycling (McCartney et al., 1983), and to show that different muscles in a given subject, or even the same muscles in different subjects, achieve maximal power at their own unique contraction velocity.

In terms of the length-tension relationship, a muscle length may be identified at which peak force may be generated; the development of force depends on the extent of overlap between crossbridges, which is maximal at about twice the resting sarcomere length (Gordon et al., 1966). Again, one cannot translate the information obtained in a single muscle fiber to the intact muscle in vivo, but studies of tension development in the calf muscles, at varying angles of the ankle, do show that the principle holds (Fitch and McComas, 1985).

MUSCLE FATIGUE

This brief discussion has an important, albeit obvious, implication. When we are asked what limits exercise capacity, or what underlies the fatigue experienced in a given person, the answer is never simple and always leads us to consider various aspects of muscle structure and function in relation to the type of activity and its duration. At one end of the spectrum, we have high force generation for brief periods, and at the other, long-term endurance. In the former, muscle structure dominates; in the latter, the mechanisms responsible for ATP supply and ultimately the size of muscle glycogen stores and the ability to mobilize free fatty acids; between, the complex interaction of many factors may never allow us to be confident that this or that mechanism is "limiting." Thus, in designing an exercise protocol and in interpreting the results of exercise testing, the nature of the curve expressing the relationship between power and the time for which it can be maintained has to be kept in mind (Fig. 2–1) (Dawson, 1985). The curve has the form

$$W = E + S/t$$

Equation 1

where W is maximal power that can be sustained for time (t), E represents power that can be maintained indefinitely (endurance), and S represents peak instantaneous power (strength) (Wilkie, 1980). Thus, the left end is dominated by muscle crosssectional area, motor unit activation, and excitation-

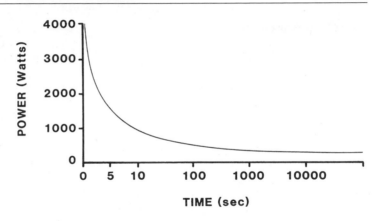

Figure 2–1. Schematic diagram showing the power (J/sec = watts) that can be maintained by athletes in maximal running or cycling.

contraction coupling, and the right end is dominated by muscle glycogen content, fat utilization, and maintenance of blood glucose level. Between these extremes is a complex interaction between high-energy phosphates, activation of regulatory enzymes that determine the relative use of glycogen and fat and the extent of lactate formation, and muscle blood flow providing oxygen and removing carbon dioxide and lactate. The importance of each of these mechanisms varies from subject to subject and determines the shape of the power or fatigue curve. The form of the curve varies in persons undertaking a given activity; for example, in running exercise, sprinters have a high value for S but E may be small, whereas marathoners may lack strength but show high values for E. In a given person, we may need to define performance at several points on the curve to understand his or her ability or lack of it. Wilkie (1960), who has long emphasized the importance of these relationships to human performance, interprets the steep left part of the curve as the total amount of metabolic work; at any point, power/time is a constant. The form of the curve defines the capacity of a given muscle or a given person. Muscle fatigue is defined as a failure to maintain a given or expected power output (Edwards, 1981). In various experimental models, fatigue may be shown to be due to failure at a number of points in the pathway between the cerebral cortex and external power—in synapses, at the neuromuscular junction, in T-tubule propagation, in the cellular ionic environment, and in the provision of ATP for contraction and ionic pumping. In many human situations, it may be impossible to separate contributory factors; indeed, there is good reason to believe that more than one is involved in most cases. For example, the development of a severe intramuscular acidosis impairs ATP production by inhibiting glycolysis, inhibits the Na^+/K^+ and Ca^{2+} ion pumps, and impairs T-tubule propagation. Many of the mechanisms proposed as important in determining muscle fatigue remain controversial; the

reader is referred to Fitts' excellent review of this topic (1994).

MUSCLE STRENGTH

Although this section may appear to have little clinical relevance, it should be remembered that muscle may be the most plastic of tissues. Any condition associated with limitation of exercise and thus of muscle activity after just a few weeks becomes associated with reductions in muscle strength and metabolic function, which in their own right contribute to disability. Reductions in muscle strength in patients with cardiac and respiratory impairments have been shown to contribute up to half of the reduction in exercise capacity and to the symptom of increased effort (Hamilton et al., 1995). Because muscle strength may be improved by specific measures in such patients, with corresponding increases in exercise capacity and reductions in symptom intensity (McCartney et al., 1991; Simpson et al., 1992), this factor is worth assessing as part of an exercise assessment.

For many years, it was felt that muscle strength played only a minor part in determining exercise capacity; this was because strength, represented by the extreme left side of the power curve (see Fig. 2–1), is so much greater than the power that can be achieved in an exercise test lasting several minutes. However, for an individual, the curve is continuous and to a large degree influenced throughout its extent by the strength of the muscles taking part in the task. This is not to say that the curve may be defined by one measurement; indeed, typically subjects capable of generating high short-term power fatigue rapidly and vice versa, typified by comparisons between sprinters and marathon runners (Thorstensson et al., 1977; McCartney et al., 1983). Rather, strength to one extent or another influences the capacity to exercise and needs to be assessed.

Strength Measurement

Having identified the need to assess muscle strength, we have to decide how to do it. The choice is wide and not easy to make (Sale, 1991), ranging from observations of weight lifting (virtually static) to a full examination of the dynamic force-velocity relationships for different joints. For some applications, such as the assessment of elite athletes, the methods are complex and costly and not easily reproducible in naive subjects. Testing that is relevant to exercise capacity needs to be dynamic and related to the muscles acting on large joints, such as the knees and elbows, but does not require great precision. Thus, for routine testing, we have chosen a relatively cheap method that provides a measurement of strength at different velocities of contraction in knee flexion and extension and in arm (shoulder and elbow) flexion and extension. For a helpful and comprehensive review of this topic, the reader is referred to Sale (1991); methods are briefly reviewed in Chapter 14.

MUSCLE METABOLISM

Although the relevance of muscle metabolic processes to an understanding of exercise capacity in most patients referred for exercise testing may appear somewhat strained, there are a number of reasons for keeping them in mind in this context. First, the metabolic demands of exercise impose stresses on the mechanisms responsible for oxygen delivery, carbon dioxide removal, and acid-base stability; because these three functions may vary widely, even at a given exercise intensity, and often vary independently of one another in relation to the varying fuels used, metabolic changes may contribute to fatigue and to exercise impairment. For example, dietary inhibition of fat utilization in patients with respiratory disorders increases carbon dioxide production and thereby imposes a stress on ventilation that may be limiting in terms of $\dot{V}O_2max$. Second, metabolic factors may underlie the severity of exercise acidosis, which in turn may contribute to fatigue or other secondary effects, such as cardiac arrhythmias. Finally, manipulation of fuel choice may be one way to reduce disability in patients with very limited exercise capacity, in whom a small change in capacity may have important effects on the ability to carry out the activities of daily living.

The following topics are addressed: metabolic fuel pathways, fuel stores, regulation of metabolic pathways, mobilization and delivery of fuel to muscle, factors influencing plasma metabolite concentrations, integration between different fuels, and the "anaerobic threshold" concept. The discussion should allow the reader to identify which fuels are used in different activities and the interaction and "communication" between metabolites that facilitate the choice between the different sources of energy. The topic is complex and is rapidly evolving through research that is only partly possible in humans and thus uses information obtained from studies of isolated muscles, in vitro or in vivo, and of animals.

High-Energy Phosphates

The central need of muscle during contraction is the replacement of ATP at an appropriate rate. The rate of myosin ATP splitting varies greatly, being about 0.1 nmol/g/sec at rest and up to about 10 μmol/g/sec during maximal contraction; this means that there is only enough ATP to support about eight maximal twitches (Dawson, 1985) because the total concentration is only 4 to 8 μmol/g wet weight and much less than this at the site of contraction. The consumption of ATP may be described by the equation

$$MgATP^{2-} \rightarrow MgADP^- + Pi^{2-} + nH^+$$
$$\text{Equation 2}$$

which identifies the change in ionic charge during the reaction, with an accumulation of negatively charged ions being necessarily accompanied by an equivalent increase in protons (nH^+) to an extent (n) that is dependent on the initial pH and on the difference between the pK_a of ATP (6.97) compared with ADP (adenosine diphosphate) (6.75) and Pi (inorganic phosphate) (6.78) (Jones, 1980). The energy for ATP resynthesis is obtained from a variety of sources of varying availability and size. In maximal exercise, reductions of 50 per cent in ATP concentration may occur (Jones et al., 1985b), but in other situations, the reactions are capable of responding at appropriate rates.

Phosphocreatine (PC) is available in muscle at a concentration that is about four times that of ATP; the reaction is described by the equation

$$MgADP^- + PC^{2-} + nH^+ \rightarrow MgATP^{2-} + Cr$$
$$\text{Equation 3}$$

Again, a change in ionic charge occurs that is much greater than, and in the opposite direction to, that accompanying ATP hydrolysis. This is due to greater difference between the pK_a of PC (4.5) and the other reactants; thus, the breakdown of PC is accompanied by an alkalinization of muscle, as suggested by the absorption of H^+ in the aforementioned reaction. Because most metabolic reactions tend to acidify muscle, this effect is thought to help increase glycolytic enzyme activity at the onset of exercise. The mass action dissociation constant of the reaction favors the formation of ATP by at least two orders of magnitude, and increases in [H$^+$] also push the reaction to the right. PC is an important source of energy for ATP formation (Karlsson, 1971), but there is evidence that it also provides an extremely important link (or "shuttle") between myosin and the mitochondria, in which aerobic metabolic processes occur. Creatine moves to the mitochondrial membrane, and PC is reformed by the reversal of the reaction, leaving ATP to be itself reformed within the mitochondria. The presence of the same reactions in different sites in the muscle fiber makes the study of the processes in intact muscle difficult and the relevance of changes in concentrations, for example, of ATP, arguable at best. However, there is general agreement that PC may provide ATP at a rate of 3 to 6 μmol/g/sec.

The enzyme involved in the reaction, creatine kinase (CK), exists in different isozymic forms, which are bound close to the ATPase on the myosin heads and the mitochondrial membrane, and in association with the enzyme adenylate kinase (AK), which catalyzes the reaction

$$2ADP^{3-} \rightarrow ATP^{4-} + AMP^{2-}$$

Equation 4

The closeness of the enzymes and the fact that adenosine monophosphate (AMP) concentration varies very little have led to the theory that AK acts to link the CK and ATPase reactions, to maintain direction and optimal concentration of PC for ATP reformation (Bessman and Carpenter, 1985). A dynamic equilibrium may set up an ideal situation for the simultaneous regeneration of ATP at precisely the rate of hydrolysis and thus in parallel with the intensity of contraction. A given intensity of contraction is associated with a fall in PC concentration that is maintained as long as exercise is continued, and even into recovery, if the muscle is deprived of oxygen (Hultman and Sjöholm, 1986). This again identifies a more important role for PC than merely acting as a fuel store because in all but the most intense exercise, the capacity exists for PC to be maintained at its resting concentration.

The AK reaction is used only when high rates of ATP utilization occur, and then the AMP may be removed through the purine nucleotide cycle, leading to accumulation of inosine monophosphate (IMP) and ammonia:

$$AMP^{2-} + nH^+ \rightarrow IMP^{2-} + NH_4^+$$

Equation 5

leaving NH$_4^+$ to be metabolized or excreted.

Anaerobic Glycolysis

Glycogen exists in high concentration in muscle fibers (50–150 mmol/kg wet weight); the metabolic pathway by which it is hydrolyzed to pyruvate (Py$^-$) generates ATP without the need for oxygen.

$$Gly + 2 MgADP^- + 2 Pi^{2-} \rightarrow 2 Py^- + 2 MgATP^{2-} + nH^+ + 2 H_2O \ (+ 0.15 \ MJ)$$

Equation 6

where Gly represents a glucosyl unit of glycogen and n is usually taken to conform to stoichiometry at 2, because the pK_a of Py$^-$ is only 2.8. MJ signifies megajoule, 10^6 J; 1 MJ = 240 kcal.

Pyruvate may then enter mitochondria for aerobic oxidation or, if the flux in that pathway cannot be increased appropriately, may be converted to lactate in the cytoplasm. The flux-generating step in glycolysis is the phosphorylase reaction; the conversion of phosphorylase "b" to phosphorylase "a" is controlled by a specific kinase, itself activated by Ca^{2+} ions and cyclic AMP (Fitts, 1994); thus maximum rates of glycolysis may be achieved promptly at the onset of muscle contraction to provide ATP at a rate of at least 1 μmol/g/sec. However, at a concentration of 100 μmol/g of glycogen, the low yield of ATP means that the total capacity is only 200 μmol/g. Muscle biopsy studies in humans have shown that the concentration of pathway metabolites may increase by 10- to 20-fold within 10 seconds of the start of maximal exercise (Jones et al., 1985b), indicating rapid activation of phosphorylase. The other major rate-limiting step in the pathway is the phosphofructokinase (PFK) reaction (Fig. 2–2); PFK activity in a given muscle matches phosphorylase activity, and the two enzymes share important properties—activation by falls in ATP: ADP ratio and inhibition by falls in pH. PFK has additional properties that fit it to play a key role in regulating glycolytic flux; its product, fructose-1,6-bisphosphate, decreases the inhibition of PFK by ATP; its substrate, fructose-6-phosphate, decreases the inhibitory effects of falls in pH; and its activity is inhibited by citrate and by glucose-1,6-biphosphate. The activity of PFK clearly cycles markedly to regulate glycolysis and in particular tends to reduce glycolysis at high lactate concentrations (fall in pH) and in the presence of fat oxidation (high [citrate]). Its inhibition by falls in tissue pH acts to make glycolysis in heavy exercise a self-limiting affair.

If pyruvate concentration increases in the cytoplasm, lactate is formed; the concurrent regeneration of nicotine adenine dinucleotide (NAD) in the lactate dehydrogenase (LDH) reaction allows glycolysis to continue:

$$Py^- + NADH + H^+ \rightarrow La^- + NAD^+$$

Equation 7

The equilibrium constant favors the formation of

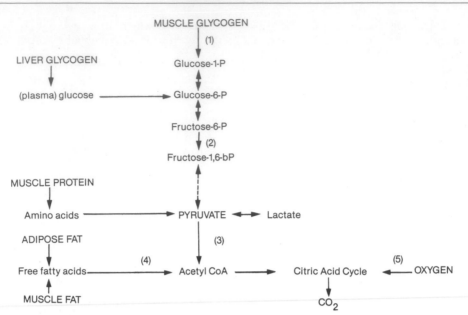

Figure 2–2. Metabolic pathways, showing main sites of regulation: 1, phosphorylase; 2, phosphofructokinase; 3, pyruvate dehydrogenase; 4, carnitine palmitoyl transferase; 5, cytochromes.

lactate (La^-), as does an increase in [H^+]. Thus, we may consider the reaction as consuming protons, rather than producing them.

In the twin concepts of the anaerobic threshold and oxygen debt, the limitation of oxygen supply does not allow sufficient NADH to be oxidized, its concentration rises in the mitochondrium and cytoplasm, and lactate production comes to the rescue. However, a cat has been set among these pigeons by recent estimates of mitochondrial [NADH]/[NAD^+] ratio (the "redox state"), which have not shown any shift to the reduced state in exercise that is associated with massive lactate production (Putman et al., 1995), calling into question the role of insufficient oxygen supply and suggesting an important role for a rate limitation in the flux through the pyruvate dehydrogenase complex (see below). Furthermore, studies in healthy subjects and patients with chronic heart failure have shown evidence of lactate production in the absence of a critical level of muscle Po_2 (Connett et al., 1986; Sullivan et al., 1990) and high activity of oxidative enzymes (Sullivan et al., 1991).

Usually the breakdown of glycogen is taken as resulting in lactic acid:

$$C_6H_{12}O_6 \rightarrow 2 \ (CH_3CHOHCOOH)$$

Equation 8

Although stoichiometrically neat, this equation should be viewed skeptically; an increase in [La^-] tends to increase [H^+], but the change depends on the existing pH as well as on the accompanying changes in weak acids (buffers). Because the LDH reaction is in equilibrium, an increase in [La^-] relative to [Py^-] drives the reaction to the left, allowing La^- to be oxidized to carbon dioxide. Thus, some fibers in a muscle may produce La^-, whereas others take up La^- and oxidize it, and the muscle as a whole appears to hydrolyze glycogen aerobically. Anaerobic glycolysis by some muscles acts to provide an aerobic substrate for others, indicating a wider role than just ATP regeneration.

The use of this metabolic pathway is recognized by changes in [La^-] in muscle or blood (Fig. 2–3). In heavy exercise, muscle [La^-] may rise to 40 mmol/kg before much rise in blood [La^-] has had time to occur. In progressive incremental exercise, [La^-] in muscle leads to increases in [La^-] in blood such that muscle [La^-] is about 1.5 times blood [La^-], and at maximum power outputs, blood [La^-] reaches 8 to 16 mmol/L. In steady state exercise, muscle [La^-] is always higher than arterial [La^-] because La^- produced by the active muscle is rapidly taken up by other muscles and by liver and other tissues; at low power outputs, a transient increase in blood [La^-] may be followed by a return to resting values, but at higher power, a constant [La^-] or a progressively increasing [La^-] to exhaustion may be seen (Åstrand et al., 1963). These changes in [La^-] have to be considered in terms of lactate production in muscle, its efflux into blood, and its uptake and aerobic metabolism by muscle and other tissues (Lindinger et al., 1995).

Finally, for one glycosyl unit metabolized to Py^- or La^-, only 2 mol of ATP are regenerated; no

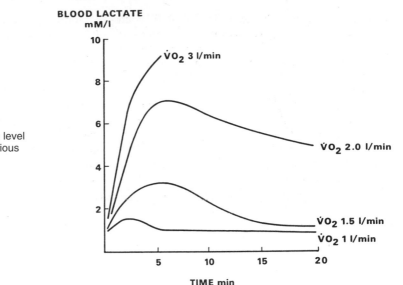

BLOOD LACTATE
mM/l

$\dot{V}O_2$ 3 l/min

$\dot{V}O_2$ 2.0 l/min

$\dot{V}O_2$ 1.5 l/min

$\dot{V}O_2$ 1 l/min

TIME min

Figure 2–3. Changes in blood lactate level found in one subject exercising at various power outputs.

oxygen is used, but if pH and P_{CO_2} are maintained constant, the associated acid-base interactions lead to the evolution of 2 mol of carbon dioxide.

Pyruvate Oxidation

The 2 mol of pyruvate formed from glycogen are transported into mitochondria and oxidized by means of the citric acid (Krebs') cycle to carbon dioxide and water, thereby providing energy for reformation of ATP through the electron carrier chain:

$$2\ CH_3COCOO^- + 36\ MgADP^- \\ + 36\ Pi^{2-} + nH^+ + 6\ O_2 \rightarrow 6\ CO_2 \\ + 36\ MgATP^{2-} + 36\ H_2O \\ (+ 2.82\ MJ)$$

Equation 9

or, starting at glycogen:

$$Gly + 38\ MgADP^- + 38\ Pi^{2-} \\ + nH^+ \rightarrow 6\ CO_2 \\ + 38\ MgATP^{2-} \\ + 38\ H_2O\ (+ 2.97\ MJ)$$

Equation 10

Thus, the aerobic oxidation of glycogen and glucose to carbon dioxide and water yields almost 20 times the ATP and energy per mol obtained from anaerobic glycolysis. Glucose effectively is not metabolized anaerobically; this is because its supply to muscle depends on the hepatic output and muscle blood flow and on the low activity of muscle hexokinase. Also, hexokinase is inhibited by increases in

glucose-6-phosphate concentration that invariably accompany heavy exercise. In heavy exercise maintained for longer than 10 minutes, plasma glucose level increases markedly as hepatic release exceeds muscle flux; in contrast, moderate exercise for several hours may be accompanied by hypoglycemia, owing to continued muscle uptake in the face of hepatic glycogen depletion.

The first step in Py^- oxidation, the formation of acetylcoenzyme A, is controlled by pyruvate dehydrogenase (PDH), a complex enzyme system bound to the inner mitochondrial membrane and existing in active and inactive forms. The activation of PDH at the onset of exercise is stimulated by Ca^{2+}, Mg^{2+}, and cyclic AMP and is strongly influenced by muscle activity and training (Ward et al., 1986). Thus, in heavy exercise, particularly in the unfit, Py^- may be presented to the PDH system at a rate that is higher than the maximal activity; an increase in $[La^-]$ is the result.

Although some rate-limiting steps may be present within the citric acid cycle (Newsholme and Start, 1977), flux is mainly governed by the supply of acetylcoenzyme A (CoA) and the availability of oxygen for the electron transport chain; an imbalance between the two, with insufficient oxygen supply, results in increasing concentrations of citrate and acetyl CoA and consequent inhibition of PDH and PFK; because the activity of PDH is so much less than that of PFK, an increase in $[La^-]$ first occurs, but inhibition of glycolysis soon follows. Thus, maximum aerobic oxidation of glycogen depends on full activation of PDH and an appropriate supply of oxygen; given these conditions, ATP may be formed in muscle at a rate of up to 0.5 μmol/g/ sec, and power output is maintained until muscle glycogen is depleted. Because 38 mol of ATP are regenerated for each glycosyl unit, the capacity of this reaction is large (3800 μmol/g), and sparing of muscle glycogen may be achieved by an additional supply of acetyl CoA from fats and of glucose from the liver.

We may summarize the aerobic metabolism of a glycosyl unit as generating 38 mol of ATP and 6 mol of carbon dioxide while requiring 6 mol of oxygen; thus, 6.3 mol of ATP are regenerated for each mol of oxygen and carbon dioxide.

In this brief discussion, it will have become apparent that the control within and between metabolic pathways is complex and is linked to associated changes in the intramuscular ionic state (Putman et al., 1995). Some changes that occur during muscle contraction activate all the flux-generating enzymes; the most important are increases in $[Ca^{2+}]$ and the ratio of $[ADP]$ to $[ATP]$. Other changes may inhibit some enzyme systems and may stimulate others. A fall in pH tends to reduce the activity of phosphorylase and PFK but increase the activity of PDH (Putman et al., 1995), thus providing feedback control that tends to limit the fall in intramuscular pH. Still other changes have more limited effects, such as inhibition of PFK by increases in citrate concentration. These mechanisms suggest a complex interaction that serves to optimize fuel utilization for continuing contraction of muscle while avoiding deleterious changes in its ionic state.

Fat Oxidation

Fatty acids may be fully oxidized to carbon dioxide and water, the final steps being through the citric acid cycle. For a representative fatty acid, the reactions may be summarized in the following equation:

$$Palmitate^- + 129\ MgADP^- + 129\ Pi^{2-}$$
$$+ nH^+ + 23\ O_2 \rightarrow 129\ MgATP^{2-} + 16\ CO_2$$
$$+ 146\ H_2O\ (+ 10.03\ MJ)$$
$$\text{Equation 11}$$

We may note from this equation that 5.6 mol of ATP are regenerated for each mol of oxygen used, and 8.1 mol for each mol of carbon dioxide produced; thus, the use of fat as a fuel may be considered costlier in terms of oxygen and less costly in terms of carbon dioxide than the oxidation of glycogen.

Fats are stored as triglycerides in muscle (2–10 μmol/g) and adipose tissue and thus represent the largest fuel store; whereas glycogen may supply enough energy to run for 2 to 3 hours at a marathon pace (60 to 80 per cent $\dot{V}o_2$max), fats could potentially support several days of continuous running.

Unfortunately, the maximum rate at which they can be mobilized and oxidized is equivalent to only about 40 per cent $\dot{V}o_2$max (or in terms of muscle ATP, a rate of 0.3 μmol/g/sec), and even this rate requires at least 20 minutes to reach its peak. The reasons for the slow rate of free fatty acid supply to muscle from adipose stores mainly reside in the control of lipolysis by catecholamines and insulin and of adipose capillary blood flow; once free fatty acids have been presented to muscle, they are rapidly taken up and oxidized. Mobilization of free fatty acids is markedly impaired by increases in circulating insulin, as well as by La^- and H^+, probably by increasing insulin binding or sensitivity in adipose tissue. Although there has been controversy regarding the availability of free fatty acids from muscle triglycerides, there is now no doubt that they are readily available (Spriet et al., 1986) and are probably used particularly when free fatty acids are not being supplied from the blood at the maximum oxidation rate. Once free fatty acids are available in muscle, the major limitation appears to be transport across the mitochondrial membrane, requiring activation of the enzyme acetyl carnitine transferase and the cofactor carnitine. In mitochondria, beta oxidation to fatty-acyl CoA (acetyl CoA) takes place, and entry into the citric acid cycle follows.

In terms of plasma concentration during mild exercise, there is an initial fall in free fatty acid, indicating a lag between uptake and mobilization, followed by a gradual increase; as glycerol is liberated during lipolysis, its concentration also rises.

Protein Metabolism in Exercise

Protein turnover is increased by exercise (Lemon and Nagle, 1981), which is accompanied by an increase in muscle amino acid production and a reduction in protein synthesis (Rennie et al., 1980) and in situations associated with low muscle glycogen (Lemon and Mullin, 1980) and acidosis. Muscle releases alanine and glutamine, derived from branched-chain amino acids, into the circulation, leading to increased plasma concentrations and to uptake by liver and other tissues. The fate of the amino acids is deamination, with subsequent oxidation in the citric acid cycle, or entry into the metabolic pool to end as glucose or ketoacids. Their oxidation accounts for 5 to 10 per cent of the total energy needs of prolonged exercise. Increased metabolism of proteins is accompanied by increased plasma levels and increased excretion of urea and ammonia-N. As for other substrates, the stoichiometry of the oxidation of mixed amino acids may be expressed approximately in the following equation:

$$Amino\ acid + 23\ MgADP^- + 23\ Pi^{2-}$$
$$+ nH^+ + 5.1\ O_2 \rightarrow 23\ MgATP^{2-}$$

$$+ 4.1\ CO_2 + 0.7\ urea + 28\ H_2O$$
$$(+ 1.99\ MJ)$$

Equation 12

The Balance Between Major Fuel Sources

The complexity of the control systems and the flexibility in the use of different sources of fuel for exercising muscle have made it difficult to assign a proportional usage of different fuels in a variety of exercise situations; even sophisticated radio-label techniques have provided an inadequate or controversial picture. In mild exercise (about 30 per cent $\dot{V}O_2$max), it seems likely that about 50 per cent of energy needs are obtained from carbohydrate, more or less equally shared by glycogen and glucose, and about 50 per cent from fat, again equally shared by adipose tissue and muscle (Havel et al., 1967; Ahlborg et al., 1974). At higher levels of power output and situations of hypoxia, acidosis, or impaired blood flow, relative contributions continue to be argued (Molé, 1983). The maximum utilization rates and the size of the fuel stores given earlier may be used to obtain theoretical balances between different fuels and to define strategies for the sharing of ATP regeneration and so enhance performance. For example, a need for ATP at a rate of 1 μmol/g/sec might be met for the first few seconds by 0.5 from PC and 0.5 from La$^-$ production, later by 0.5 from La$^-$ and 0.5 from aerobic glycogen, and later still by 0.1 from La$^-$, 0.5 from aerobic glycogen, and 0.4 from fat. The choice between these energy sources is largely determined by the extent to which different flux-generating and rate-limiting enzymes are activated (see below).

The many factors that influence the balance between different fuels make it impossible to apportion energy provision from the separate fuel sources in a person, although a reasonably clear picture has emerged to allow the effects of such factors as training, intensity and duration of exercise, and diet to be understood (Brooks and Mercier, 1994). The major mechanisms that influence choice between fuels are as follows:

1. Substrate availability—glycogen and lipid stores in muscle, glucose release from the liver and lipolysis in adipose tissue, and perhaps to a minor degree, glutamine and alanine production by muscle.
2. Oxygen availability for electron transport.
3. Activity of rate-limiting enzymes, including their concentration, the relative balance between inhibitors and activators, and the effects of feedback control. The main enzymes that regulate the flux in the pathways, and thus indirectly influence the relative use of different pathways, are phosphorylase (glycogen to glucose-1-phosphate), hexokinase (glucose to glucose-6-phosphate), phosphofructokinase (halfway down the glycolytic pathway at fructose-6-phosphate to fructose-1,6-bis-phosphate), pyruvate kinase (phosphoenol pyruvate to pyruvate), and pyruvate dehydrogenase (pyruvate to acetyl CoA). There is argument regarding the regulatory enzymes in the citric acid cycle. The regulatory enzymes of lipolysis are also debated, but there is little doubt that triglyceride lipase and carnitine palmitoyl transferase (which may control fatty acid transfer across the mitochondrial membrane) are important.
4. The plasma concentrations of several hormones change during exercise with predictable associated effects. However, as the concentrations represent the balance between the rates of secretion and clearance, interpretation of plasma changes in quantitative terms is difficult. Furthermore, there is evidence that exercise may change the binding characteristics of a hormone to a specific membrane receptor site, as demonstrated by LeBlanc and colleagues (1979) for insulin. Exercise is associated with increases in circulating norepinephrine (increased cardiac frequency and contractility) and epinephrine (increased glycogenolysis and lipolysis) (Galbo et al., 1977); with decreases in insulin (Pruett, 1970), tending to increase hepatic glucose release and increasing lipolysis; and with increases in glucagon (Bloom et al., 1976), stimulating hepatic glycogenolysis. Changes in other hormones—cortisol (Tharp, 1975), growth hormone (Sutton and Lazarus, 1976), and sex hormones (Jurkowski et al., 1978)—are of uncertain metabolic significance. The topic has been reviewed by Terjung (1979).
5. Changes in the H$^+$ concentration in blood and muscle may modulate the activity of rate-limiting enzymes (Trivedi and Danforth, 1966), may change the metabolic and physiological effects of hormones (Sutton et al., 1976), and may affect the exchange of ions across the muscle cell membrane (Aicken and Thomas, 1977). Furthermore, although these factors undoubtedly will be found to exert major influences on muscle

function in disease, the application of sophisticated biochemical techniques to diseased muscle is in its infancy (Edwards, 1979). For an authoritative review of the theories of metabolic control, the interested reader is referred to Newsholme and Start (1977).

The variety in these basic mechanisms underlies the variations in the metabolic pathways that exist between muscles of different fiber composition, during exercise of different intensities and durations, and after different dietary histories.

Variation in Metabolic Processes Among Types of Muscle Fiber

The source of energy for the resynthesis of ATP is not quantitatively the same in all muscles. In particular, the relative contribution of anaerobic and aerobic processes may vary considerably. The two extremes of this variation are seen in red muscle and white muscle (Gollnick et al., 1973). Red muscle fibers are slow contracting and are involved in continuous or sustained activity; they are found in the flight muscles of birds and the antigravity muscles of mammals. They have a high content of myoglobin and mitochondrial enzymes, a high fat content, and a high capillary density; their metabolic demands are met mainly through aerobic processes. White muscles, on the other hand, are subject to less continuous activity, are faster contracting, and have less myoglobin and more glycogen, and the activities of glycolytic enzymes (phosphorylase, phosphofructokinase) are higher than those of oxidative enzymes. Fiber types in human muscle are distinguished by histochemical techniques; their classification began by a division into the two types described above—red (or slow-twitch, or type I) and white (or fast-twitch, or type II). More recently, the histochemical techniques have shown some metabolic overlap between these two types, and at least three types are now recognized. These are termed slow oxidative–fatigue resistant (SO or type I), fast glycolytic (FG, or type IIB), and fast oxidative–glycolytic (FOG or type IIA). The reader is referred to the papers of Brooke and Kaiser (1970) and Petté (1985) for a discussion of fiber properties and their nomenclature. Most skeletal muscles in humans are composed of varying proportions of the fiber types, with a preponderance of type I fibers in muscles that are in almost constant use, such as the diaphragm, the postural muscles, and the soleus; the vastus, biceps, and triceps usually contain 50 to 60 per cent of type II fibers.

Variations Associated with Differing Intensity and Duration of Exercise

The discussion above provides some information to quantify the intuitively obvious concept that some fuels cannot be made available fast enough to provide all the energy required for intense exercise, and others are in amounts too small to sustain a given power output for a long time. It is intriguing that there is a roughly inverse relationship between the size of the store of fuel and its maximum utilization rate. The largest store, of triglycerides, takes time to be fully mobilized and even then can provide only a portion of the needs in heavy exercise; the smallest store, of high-energy phosphates, is immediately available at a high rate but is soon exhausted.

Because in most types of human exercise lasting for more than a few seconds most of the energy is provided by either anaerobic glycolysis or aerobic oxidation of glycogen and triglycerides, the distinction is often drawn between anaerobic and aerobic exercise, although both types of processes coexist in all forms of exercise.

Heavy Exercise, the Anaerobic Threshold, Oxygen Deficit and Debt

The concept of the anaerobic threshold implies that during exercise of increasing intensity, a point is reached at which aerobic processes give way to anaerobic processes. The point is defined in terms of power or $\dot{V}O_2$ and is usually termed the *anaerobic threshold*. Implicit in this concept is a dependency on oxygen supply; thus a point is reached in incremental exercise when oxygen intake is unable to meet all the energy demands and anaerobic glycolysis is recruited to provide all the energy for additional work. Because this leads to an increase in plasma lactate level and to associated increases in carbon dioxide output and ventilation, measurements of these variables are made to identify the threshold. The concept was first put forward 60 years ago and has been extensively applied in exercise research to investigate the mechanisms of tissue hypoxia, the effects of training, and the many clinical conditions in which oxygen transport is impaired (Wasserman et al., 1973). The identification of a threshold in this way has proved its value in these types of investigation, being reproducible and changing appropriately in most situations in which oxygen delivery mechanisms have been altered. Because of such studies, the anaerobic threshold is felt by many to be an important descriptor of exercise capability and even may be used as an alternative to $\dot{V}O_2$max. It must also be recognized that the concept, when applied literally (the "anaerobic," "threshold"), is fatally flawed from several points of view; the occurrence of a threshold may be due to many mechanisms that may be related or entirely unrelated to oxygen delivery. If an open mind is kept on the underlying mechanisms, then the need for the measurement may be assessed in its own right for any given application. The term itself has its own attraction; other terms, such as "OBLA" (for the onset of blood lactate accumulation) or "proportional limit" (for the change in ventilation), or even "Owles' point" (after the investigator who unwittingly started the controversy in 1930) (Owles, 1930), although freeing one from any mechanistic implications, seem unlikely to find general use.

A number of publications have critically reviewed the concept (Jones and Ehrsam, 1982; Molé, 1983); for this reason, the flaws, both conceptual and methodological, are listed only briefly here. At a trivial level, there is no "threshold" for muscle lactate production, and a lack of oxygen is not the only reason for it. Even resting muscle produces lactate, and although an oxygen supply is required for aerobic metabolism, even in its presence, lactate is formed if glycolysis produces pyruvate at a faster rate than that of the maximal activity of pyruvate dehydrogenase or other enzymes downstream to it (Ward et al., 1986). In recent studies in maximal exercise in healthy subjects (Putman et al., 1995) and in patients with cardiac failure (Sullivan et al., 1990), both situations associated with increased plasma lactate concentrations, independent evidence of tissue oxygen lack has not been found. The increase in lactate production by a muscle may be related more to the recruitment of fast-twitch fibers, having higher glycolytic than aerobic enzyme capacity, than to a limiting value for oxygen flow. In a given muscle, some fibers may be producing lactate, while others are taking it up and metabolizing it aerobically. A number of factors influence the rate at which lactate leaves muscle; $[La^-]$ and pH influence the activity of a specific transporter (Roth et al., 1990a, 1990b). Because blood lactate represents the balance between the rate at which lactate leaves muscle and the rate at which it is metabolized, lactate may be produced without any change in blood concentration; alternatively, an increase in concentration may be due as much to an inability to metabolize lactate as to an increase in its production. Thus, the rise in plasma $[La^-]$ at the anaerobic threshold is due in large part to a limit's being reached in La^- uptake and oxidation (Brooks, 1986).

The increase in ventilation that accompanies increases in blood $[La^-]$ has also been used to define an anaerobic threshold; the explanation that is usually invoked is an accompanying increase in carbon dioxide evolution according to the stoichiometry expressed in the following reactions:

$$La^- + H^+ + NaHCO_3 \rightarrow NaLa + H_2CO_3$$
$$H_2CO_3 \rightarrow H_2O + CO_2$$

Equation 13

Thus, a mol of carbon dioxide is evolved for every mol of La^- produced. Because increases in ventilation follow increases in carbon dioxide production very closely in exercise, the accumulation of La^- is followed by a relative increase in ventilation. The reactions stated above do not actually take place; as La^- diffuses out of muscle into extracellular fluid, it acts as a strong ion; if P_{CO_2} is maintained constant and other strong ions do not change much, a fall in $[HCO_3^-]$ occurs in order to maintain electrical neutrality. Carbon dioxide is excreted in an amount that is approximately equimolar to the increase in $[La^-]$ times its distribution volume in extracellular water, and ventilation increases in proportion to the relative increase in $\dot{V}_{CO_2}$. Thus, measurements of carbon dioxide output and ventilation give reliable indications of blood $[La^-]$ increases, as long as other acid-base changes are excluded but provide only crude estimates of muscle La^- production. Muscle $[La^-]$ may be 10 times higher than plasma $[La^-]$ in heavy exercise.

There are arguments regarding the best methods to detect the onset of blood La^- accumulation and its ventilatory equivalent. Although most studies that have used a measurement of the anaerobic threshold present a figure demonstrating a sharply defined increase in plasma La^-, others have shown the increase to be a smooth curve that makes it difficult to identify a clear "threshold." Indeed, an early study by Strandell (1964) emphasized the curvilinear increase and showed that blood $[La^-]$ increased as an exponential function of power or heart rate, a finding supported by Yeh and coworkers (1983). The more rapidly power is incremented, the sharper the inflection, due to a greater increase in the rate of La^- production than in that of lactate metabolism. Such problems lead to observer variation and account for the adoption of different criteria by different groups. Thus, in North America, the usual habit is to identify the $\dot{V}_{O_2}$ at which $[La^-]$ shows an upward inflection during an incremental exercise test in which the power output is increased quite rapidly, whereas in Europe, the $\dot{V}_{O_2}$ at which $[La^-]$ reaches an arbitrary value, usually of 4 mmol/L, is often preferred. For the ventilatory criteria, a method is usually used to identify the $\dot{V}_{O_2}$ at which pulmonary ventilation ($\dot{V}_E$) increases in relation to $\dot{V}_{O_2}$ without a change in the $\dot{V}_E/\dot{V}_{CO_2}$ relationship (Wasserman, 1984).*

---

*This topic has been made unnecessarily complex by some workers who recognize both aerobic and anaerobic thresholds; in their usage, the aerobic threshold is the same as the anaerobic threshold described above; the term *anaerobic threshold* is used for the $\dot{V}_{O_2}$ at which $\dot{V}_E/\dot{V}_{CO_2}$ increases.

The use of ventilation to identify La$^-$ accumulation has the advantage of being noninvasive; in sedentary subjects, it occurs at 57 per cent $\dot{V}O_2$max, but there is a large intersubject variability (Hansen et al., 1984; Jones et al., 1985a). However, here again, the identification of an inflection in a smooth curve is associated with considerable observer variation (Caiozzo et al., 1982; Gladden et al., 1985), leading some workers to doubt the utility of anaerobic threshold measurements and their application to clinical investigation (Yeh et al., 1983). We would not draw such a negative conclusion, but there is little doubt that changes in blood [La$^-$] and ventilation during exercise require careful interpretation in relation to $\dot{V}O_2$max and other variables.

Because the increase in carbon dioxide output that accompanies the fall in extracellular [HCO$_3^-$] is equimolar to the entry of La$^-$ in extracellular fluid, measurements of carbon dioxide output at several exercise levels can provide a quantitative measure of plasma [La$^-$] increases (see Chapter 10). This approach, described and validated by Clode and Campbell in 1969, has not been used by others but probably remains as valid as other approaches (see Chapter 11).

Linked to the anaerobic threshold, but subject to many criticisms at various times in the past 25 years (Harris, 1969), are the concepts of oxygen deficit and debt. Oxygen deficit implies that at the onset of exercise, the delay in oxygen delivery to muscle leads to breakdown of creatine phosphate and to anaerobic glycolysis with La$^-$ formation, which is maintained until oxygen delivery has increased sufficiently to meet the demand. Oxygen debt implies that the anaerobic metabolic processes called into play during exercise are reversed during recovery, leading to an elevated oxygen intake that is maintained until La$^-$ has been metabolized and PC has been resynthesized. Although studies in the past that established relationships between oxygen deficit and debt and changes in muscle metabolites tended to support both concepts, it now seems that other interpretations may be at least as valid. Thus, the initial rise in [La$^-$] and lag in oxygen consumption by muscle may be related to delays in enzyme activation, particularly PDH, and the postexercise increase in oxygen intake may be related to increases in metabolic rate related to increases in body temperature, catecholamine secretion, substrate cycling, and other factors.

Long-Duration or Steady-State Exercise and Aerobic Metabolism

Aerobic metabolic pathways take a variable amount of time to reach their maximum rate of flux, even if the demand for ATP is low enough to be fully met by them.

In heavy exercise, muscle glycogen concentration falls sharply, owing to anaerobic glycolysis; at lower work rates, the fall is more gradual (Bergström et al., 1967). This is due partly to the higher efficiency of aerobic glycolysis in regenerating ATP and partly to the greater use of free fatty acids. The turnover rate of glucose is increased during exercise. Glucose release by the liver increases during exercise and is matched by uptake by the muscles, with little change occurring in blood glucose level; however, in heavy exercise, a progressive rise in plasma glucose concentration to over 8 mmol/L may occur (Jones et al., 1980). It appears likely that this phenomenon occurs because a maximum rate of glucose uptake by muscle has been reached. About 20 per cent of the metabolic needs are supplied by glucose, with higher proportions after a high-carbohydrate meal. After exercise, muscle glycogen is replenished, and if glycogen stores have been severely depleted, muscle glycogen level increases during the next 3 days to above the pre-exercise level (Hultman et al., 1967).

Two sources of fatty acids are used in exercise—adipose tissue triglycerides and muscle triglycerides. In adipose tissue, free fatty acids are liberated by the hydrolysis of triglycerides and are transported loosely bound to plasma albumin. Uptake by muscle depends on the muscle blood flow and the blood level of free fatty acids. The mobilization of free fatty acids takes time; blood levels of free fatty acids fall during the first 5 to 10 minutes of exercise, owing to the rapid uptake by muscle, and then steadily increase because of mobilization (Havel et al., 1963). When exercise ceases, blood levels increase sharply as a result of the reduction in muscle uptake, and probably also as a result of an increase in fatty acids diffusing from muscle. Mobilization of free fatty acids is under complex hormonal control; catecholamines increase lipase activity in adipose tissue, and insulin exerts a powerful inhibitory effect on free fatty acid mobilization that almost ceases after a meal or a glucose infusion (Havel, 1965).

Hydrolysis of triglycerides in adipose tissue yields free glycerol, which cannot be rapidly reused, and leads to an increase in blood glycerol level; metabolism of glycerol occurs mainly in the liver. The part played by fatty acids obtained from triglycerides stored in the muscle cell is uncertain. Although this source has been thought to contribute little to muscle metabolism, studies using a biopsy technique suggest that it may be used when the supply of free fatty acids from blood is reduced (Carlson et al., 1971).

Although amino acids and ketoacids can be used by exercising muscle, their contribution is quantitatively small (Felig and Wahren, 1971). The role of the amino acid–glucose cycle is probably also of minor importance; alanine and glutamine are released by muscle in exercise and may then be used by the liver as substrates for gluconeogenesis (Felig and Wahren, 1971). Release of alanine and glutamine is one way that the muscles may get rid of protons.

From this brief review, it can be appreciated that the factors influencing the choice of fuels are complex and difficult to define precisely in all situations. Power output, duration of exercise, and diet are the most important factors. However, the ability of a muscle to use several fuels gives it a flexibility in maintaining ATP supply in a wide variety of situations. In heavy exercise, muscle glycogen is mainly used, anaerobic glycolysis being particularly important at the onset; thereafter, aerobic glycolysis is dominant. In moderate exercise of longer duration, half the needs are met by oxidation of carbohydrates (about 40 per cent from glycogen and 10 per cent from glucose) and half by free fatty acids (about 40 per cent from adipose tissue stores and 10 per cent from muscle fat) (Havel et al., 1967; Carlson et al., 1971). In exercise of several hours' duration, free fatty acids are used to an increasing extent (Young et al., 1967).

Ill health may influence the metabolic adaptations to exercise in a number of ways. Inactivity may lead to reduced levels of mitochondrial enzymes and energy stores, and interference with oxygen delivery leads to a greater use of anaerobic mechanisms. In addition, a few rare conditions are recognized in which absence of specific intramuscular enzymes affects the ability to perform exercise. The best studied example is that of McArdle's syndrome, in which muscle phosphorylase is absent. Because this enzyme catalyzes the breakdown of glycogen to glucose-1-phosphate, glycogen cannot be used for energy metabolism. For this reason, these patients are dependent on the supply of free fatty acids and glucose to muscle. The characteristic features are an inability to do heavy work, the absence of La^- in blood from working muscle, and the presence of a "second wind" phenomenon in which a gradual "warm-up" allows a work rate to be performed that is higher than that without warming up. This warm-up presumably leads to an increase in blood flow and delivery of free fatty acids and glucose (Pernow et al., 1967). The severe limitation in exercise tolerance that such patients experience emphasizes the importance of normal glycogen metabolism in exercise.

The Link Between Metabolism and Gas Exchange

From the stoichiometric relationships expressed in the equations above, the usage of different fuel substrates can be seen to influence the need for oxygen supply and carbon dioxide removal for a given energy yield. Also, the implications are different for the two gases, as expressed in the RQs for the different oxidations—1.0 for the aerobic oxidation of glycogen, 0.7 for fatty acids, and 0.8 for amino acids. Although the anaerobic breakdown of glycogen to La^- theoretically does not require oxygen or produce carbon dioxide, because La^- is a strong anion, acid-base homeostasis inevitably leads to carbon dioxide excretion, and the RQ is infinite.

We may quantify the implications of the differences between fats and carbohydrates in terms of the cost of the energy demands on the gas exchange systems. For each mol of oxygen used and each mol of carbon dioxide formed, 6.3 mol of ATP are reformed during carbohydrate oxidation; the corresponding figures for fat are 5.6 (129/23) mol ATP per mol of O_2 and 8.1 (129/16) mol per mol of CO_2. Although the oxidation of fat may be a little costlier to oxygen transport mechanisms, it more than makes up for this by sparing mechanisms that are more responsible for carbon dioxide, and ventilation may be markedly lower. Where fat utilization is inhibited, as after a recent meal, ventilation is higher (Jones and Haddon, 1973), and subjects who are limited by a reduced ventilatory capacity are unable to achieve their usual $\dot{V}o_2max$ (Brown et al., 1985). La^- production imposes a marked strain on carbon dioxide transport, even though it does not require oxygen; for each mol of carbon dioxide evolved, as little as 1 mol of ATP is reformed. It thus comes as no surprise that in exercise intense enough to require anaerobic glycolysis, the ventilatory demands are very high in relation to energy production (Fig. 2–4).

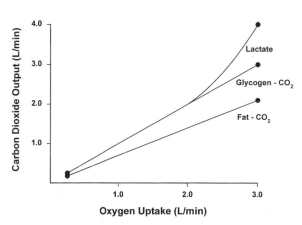

Figure 2–4. Schematic graph showing theoretical effects of different metabolic fuels on the relationship of CO_2 output to O_2 uptake. CO_2 output is lowest when only fat is used and increases with increasing use of carbohydrate and with the production of lactate.

PULMONARY ADAPTATIONS TO EXERCISE

Ventilation, pulmonary gas transfer, cardiac output, and peripheral blood flow all increase in response to the metabolic demands of working muscles. In disease, structural changes may interfere with these adaptations, causing reduced exercise tolerance, but various mechanisms help to compensate, tending to maintain oxygen supply and carbon dioxide excretion. Often, a patient's symptoms are related more to the compensatory mechanisms than to the initiating abnormality.

The transfer of oxygen from air to muscle cell and of carbon dioxide in the reverse direction can be considered as a series of cascades in which various mechanisms influence the differences in carbon dioxide and oxygen pressures in various sites.

The movement of oxygen and carbon dioxide may be considered in terms of pressure differences that drive the gases through a series of resistances and may thus be described in mathematical terms by equations analogous to Ohm's law; as well as describing the processes, the equations are those used to calculate the results of exercise tests.

Pulmonary Ventilation, Blood Flow, and Gas Exchange

Pulmonary ventilation ($\dot{V}E$) and its subdivisions—alveolar ventilation ($\dot{V}A$) and "dead space" ventilation ($\dot{V}D$)—are conventionally expressed in terms of carbon dioxide. The relationship between ventilation and carbon dioxide output is expressed in terms of the mixed expired carbon dioxide concentration ($FECO_2$):

$$FECO_2 = \frac{\dot{V}CO_2}{\dot{V}E}$$

Equation 14

Or, where expired carbon dioxide is expressed as a partial pressure:

$$PECO_2 = \frac{\dot{V}CO_2 \times K}{\dot{V}E}$$

Equation 15

In this equation, K converts fractional concentration to partial pressure and corrects $\dot{V}E$ to conditions at body temperature (BTPS): K is 0.863 when $\dot{V}CO_2$ is expressed in milliliters per minute STPD (standard temperature [0°C] and pressure [760 mm Hg] for dry gas) and $\dot{V}E$ in liters per minute BTPS (barometric pressure of 760 mm Hg and temperature of 37°C).

Similarly, alveolar ventilation for a given carbon dioxide output is defined by the alveolar PCO_2,

$$FACO_2 = \frac{\dot{V}CO_2}{\dot{V}A}$$

Equation 16

or

$$PACO_2 = \frac{\dot{V}CO_2 \times 0.863}{\dot{V}A}$$

Equation 17

Following the mathematical analysis of alveolar gas composition by Riley and Cournand (1949), arterial PCO_2 has been used as the closest "effective" estimate of the "ideal" alveolar PCO_2, representative of lung regions taking part in gas exchange.

$$PaCO_2 = \frac{\dot{V}CO_2 \times 0.863}{\dot{V}A}$$

Equation 18

Although this concept may be challenged on theoretical grounds because abnormalities in the distribution of ventilation-perfusion ratios lead to a difference between the PCO_2 of mixed alveolar gas and that of arterial blood, the effect is small and does not lead to important errors in clinical exercise testing (Farhi, 1966). If necessary, a correction may be applied using a second approximation procedure (Riley and Cournand, 1951) as outlined in Chapter 12.

The remainder of the ventilation is considered to be wasted, as if it were distributed to areas receiving inspired air but no blood. The total or "physiological" dead space has two components—the airway dead space and the alveolar dead space, owing to parts of the lungs with high ventilation-perfusion ratios ($\dot{V}A/\dot{Q}C$). Physiological dead space is expressed as the dead space–tidal volume (VD/VT) ratio, calculated by an equation first used by Christian Bohr (1889):

$$\frac{VD}{VT} = \frac{PaCO_2 - PECO_2}{PaCO_2 - PICO_2}$$

Equation 19

In this equation, the inspired carbon dioxide ($PICO_2$) is assumed to be so small (0.4 mm Hg) that it can be ignored.

The total blood flow ($\dot{Q}tot$) is defined by Fick's principle:

$$\dot{Q}tot = \frac{\dot{V}O_2}{CaO_2 - C\bar{v}O_2}$$

Equation 20

where CaO_2 and $C\bar{v}O_2$ are the concentration of oxygen in arterial and mixed venous blood, respectively. In the same way that ventilation was subdivided into alveolar and dead space portions, the total blood flow may be subdivided into the pulmonary capillary blood flow, which takes part in gas exchange, and a portion that is "wasted" with regard to gas exchange, either because it passes from the right to the left heart through an anatomical pathway or because it flows through areas in which the ventilation-perfusion ratio is low or the alveolar-capillary oxygen transfer is impaired. This portion is expressed as the venous admixture:

$$\frac{\dot{Q}_{VA}}{\dot{Q}_{tot}} = \frac{Cc'_{O_2} - Ca_{O_2}}{Cc'_{O_2} - C\bar{v}_{O_2}}$$

Equation 21

The similarity to V_D/V_T (Eq. 19) should be noted: Equation 21 calculates the extent to which the pulmonary end-capillary oxygen (Cc'_{O_2}) is altered by admixture of venous blood ($C\bar{v}_{O_2}$) to give the oxygen content in mixed arterial blood (Ca_{O_2}).

The ideal alveolar P_{O_2} determines the ideal end-capillary oxygen content, and the arterial oxygen content determines the arterial P_{O_2}. For this reason, the alveolar-arterial (A-a) P_{O_2} difference is used as a measure of venous admixture; arterial P_{O_2} is measured and alveolar P_{O_2} is calculated by use of the alveolar air equation, a simplified form of which is as follows:

$$P_{AO_2} = P_{IO_2} - \frac{Pa_{CO_2}}{R}$$

Equation 22

However, an increase in the A-a P_{O_2} difference needs to be interpreted with caution in exercise. Changes in alveolar ventilation influence P_{AO_2} (Eq. 22) and thus Cc'_{O_2} (Eq. 21); changes in cardiac output influence $C\bar{v}_{O_2}$ (Eq. 20) and thus alter Ca_{O_2} for a given value of $\dot{Q}_{VA}/\dot{Q}_{tot}$ (Eq. 21). A wide A-a P_{O_2} difference may be the result of alveolar hyperventilation and a low cardiac output rather than of a high $\dot{Q}_{VA}/\dot{Q}_{tot}$ ratio and therefore does not necessarily imply an abnormal dispersion of ventilation-perfusion ratios or impairment of alveolar-capillary oxygen transfer. Examples given later amplify the relation between the A-a P_{O_2} difference and $\dot{Q}_{VA}/\dot{Q}_{tot}$.

The two ratios, V_D/V_T and $\dot{Q}_{VA}/\dot{Q}_{tot}$, are used as indices of pulmonary gas exchange efficiency rather than as quantitative measurements of the dead space volume or the amount of right-to-left shunting of blood in the lungs. This use of the two ratios handles the complex relationships involved in pulmonary gas exchange in a simplistic way, in which the lung behaves as a three-compartment model. Although the approach may be criticized for

this reason, and more complex models may be developed in the future, this method allows the gas exchange abnormality in patients to be usefully quantified and has stood the test of utility for many years (Farhi, 1966).

The preceding equations recur in graphic form later in the text, in the discussion of the changes that occur in exercise.

Ventilation, Tidal Volume, and the Frequency of Breathing

Ventilation increases in a linear relationship to oxygen intake and carbon dioxide output up to power outputs of 50 to 60 per cent of the maximal $\dot{V}_{O_2}$. Above this point, sometimes termed the "anaerobic threshold," ventilation is more closely related to carbon dioxide output, which increases to a greater extent than oxygen intake. The P_{CO_2} of mixed expired gas (P_{ECO_2}) increases to a maximum at about 75 per cent of the maximal power output, above which P_{ECO_2} falls (Fig. 2–5). The linear portion of the ventilatory response is expressed by the following equation, obtained from studies in healthy subjects (Jones et al., 1985a):

$$\dot{V}_E = 23.9 \, \dot{V}_{CO_2} + 5.4$$

Equation 23

where $\dot{V}_E$ is expressed in liters per minute BTPS, and $\dot{V}_{CO_2}$ in milliliters per minute STPD. Within this relationship, there is variation among subjects, which is at least in part related to differences in the ventilatory response to a carbon dioxide stimulus (Rebuck et al., 1973). As expressed in Equations 15 through 18, P_{ECO_2} and Pa_{CO_2} express the response of $\dot{V}_E$ and $\dot{V}_A$ to metabolic carbon dioxide production. At submaximal power outputs, Pa_{CO_2} remains relatively constant, indicating that $\dot{V}_A$ increases in proportion to $\dot{V}_{CO_2}$. However, P_{ECO_2} rises toward Pa_{CO_2}, indicating that $\dot{V}_E$ approaches $\dot{V}_A$, owing to a fall in dead space ventilation. P_{ECO_2} falls in heavy exercise, owing to an increase in $\dot{V}_A$, as shown by the parallel fall in Pa_{CO_2}. This relative increase in $\dot{V}_A$ in heavy exercise is usually ascribed to the effects of the associated metabolic acidosis.

Equations 17 through 19 may be combined to yield

$$\dot{V}_E = \frac{(0.86 \, \dot{V}_{CO_2}/Pa_{CO_2})}{(1 - V_D/V_T)}$$

Equation 24

indicating that changes in several variables may increase ventilation during exercise—carbon dioxide production, alveolar ventilation, and dead space ventilation. A ventilation that is high for a given $\dot{V}_{CO_2}$ is an indication of an increase in either or

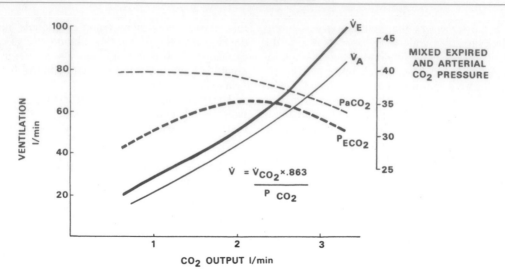

Figure 2–5. The ventilatory response to exercise. The thick solid line shows mean total ventilation ($\dot{V}E$) and thin line alveolar ventilation ($\dot{V}A$). Dotted lines show mean values for $PaCO_2$ (thick) and $PECO_2$ (thin).

both $\dot{V}A$ and VD/VT. On the other hand, a reduced total ventilation implies alveolar hypoventilation because there is a limit to the extent that VD/VT may be reduced. It is also apparent that a normal ventilation may be accounted for by a low alveolar ventilation and an increased VD/VT ratio in combination.

The Pattern of Breathing

At the simplest level, the pattern of breathing may be described in terms of tidal volume (VT) and frequency (f_b):

$$\dot{V}E = VT \times f_b$$

Equation 25

In these terms, in normal subjects, increases in $\dot{V}E$ are accomplished mainly by increases in VT at low and moderate exercise intensities; and at higher workloads, as VT approaches 50 to 60 per cent of vital capacity, f_b comes more into play (Jones and Rebuck, 1979). The shape of this curve appears to be determined by the hyperbolic relationship between volume and transpulmonary pressure and seems to optimize the mean force developed by respiratory muscles at any given level of ventilation. In healthy children, lung volumes are smaller than in adults, and the increase in ventilation is brought about more by an increase in the breathing frequency; values of up to 60 breaths per minute are commonly seen.

In patients with a reduced lung volume, the increase in ventilation during exercise is associated with high breathing frequencies and low tidal volumes, a finding that may be diagnostically useful.

Patients with chronic airway obstruction, on the other hand, breathe with tidal volumes that may be surprisingly high when considered in relation to measurements of airway obstruction, such as the one-second forced expired volume (FEV_1). These breathing patterns are those expected to minimize the sense of effort arising in respiratory muscles.

In interpreting ventilation during exercise, it is helpful to relate values to the maximal ventilation that can be sustained voluntarily. For many years, the index used for this value was the maximum breathing capacity as measured over 15 seconds. This "sprint" value is larger than the ventilation that can be maintained voluntarily for 1 to 4 minutes, a period more applicable to exercise. The maximal ventilation sustained voluntarily for 4 minutes (4 min MVV) has been extensively studied by Freedman (1970), who showed that it could be predicted in healthy subjects from the FEV_1 by use of the following equation:

$$MVV = 129 + 25\,(FEV_1 - 4.01)\ L/min$$

Equation 26

This relationship is approximated by $35 \times FEV_1$. In most healthy subjects, the ventilation in maximal exercise reaches values of around 70 per cent of the MVV. However, in patients with airway obstruction, ventilation during maximal exercise may equal the MVV, indicating that a ventilatory limit has been reached (Clark et al., 1969). Patients with severe airway obstruction ($FEV_1 < 1$ L) commonly achieve a maximal exercise ventilation that exceeds the $FEV_1 \times 35$ (Jones et al., 1971). The reason for this discrepancy is partly that the FEV_1 is a forced expiratory maneuver; ventilation during exercise is not associated with a maximally forced expiration and has both inspiratory and expiratory phases; many patients with chronic air flow limitation are capable of large increases in inspiratory flow in spite of severe expiratory slowing (Grimby and Stiksa, 1970; Stubbing et al., 1980b). Thus, a more complete description of the pattern of breathing may be obtained in terms of inspiratory and expiratory flow, tidal volume (VT), breathing frequency (f_b), and breathing "duty cycle" (TI/Ttot, the proportion of the breathing cycle during which the inspiratory muscles are active). Mean inspiratory flow ($\dot{V}I$) equals VT divided by inspiratory time (TI), and expiratory flow is VT divided by expiratory time (TE = Ttot − TI). As $\dot{V}E = VT \times f_b$, and $VT = \dot{V}I \times TI$, then

$$\dot{V}E = \dot{V}I \times TI/Ttot \times 60/f_b$$

Equation 27

Although this is a complex way to describe ventilation in exercise, the equation places emphasis on the importance of inspiratory flow, the duty cycle, and the frequency of breathing in the achievement of ventilation, and it is helpful in the understanding of dyspnea in both normal subjects and those with respiratory impairment. This is because inspiratory flow depends on the velocity of respiratory muscle contraction, the duty cycle represents the proportion of time that muscles are contracting, the frequency of breathing is equal to the frequency of their contraction, and the tidal volume is related to the extent of contraction.

Mechanics of Breathing During Exercise

Because elastance is expressed by pressure-volume and resistance by pressure-flow, we may consider the impedances and driving pressures required in meeting the demands of exercise in terms of the flow-volume and pressure-volume characteristics.

FLOW. The resting maximal flow-volume curve in healthy subjects is unchanged by exercise (Grimby et al., 1971; Stubbing et al., 1980a) and defines the limits of the tidal volumes and flows that may be recruited to meet ventilatory demands. Because of the linkage between tidal volume and flow, the curve also defines the maximal ventilatory capacity, the frequency of breathing, TI, and TE. In normal subjects with increasing intensity of exercise, expiratory flow increases progressively and approaches maximal levels, particularly at low lung volumes (Grimby et al., 1971) (Fig. 2–6). Inspiratory flow increases in a similar manner, but the maximum flow (measured at rest) is not reached; maximum exercise inspiratory flow seldom exceeds 75 per cent of the flow capacity measured at rest.

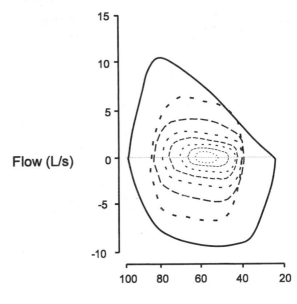

Figure 2–6. Changes in flow and volume during exercise in healthy subjects. Flow (in L/sec) is graphed as a function of total lung capacity (TLC) normalized between individuals as %TLC. The maximum flow-volume loop at rest is shown as a thick continuous line; loops adopted during spontaneous breathing at rest (dotted line) and six exercise levels of increasing severity (dashed lines) show that increases in tidal volume are achieved by both reductions in end-expiratory and increases in end-inspiratory lung volume, and that inspiratory and expiratory flows are increased equally within the maximum loop. (From Inman MD. The Role of Expiratory Muscle Activity in Ventilation During Exercise. Hamilton, Ontario: McMaster University; 1992, Ph.D. Thesis.)

To estimate the proportion of flow capacity used during exercise in patients with pulmonary impairment, mean inspiratory (VT/TI) and expiratory flow (VT/TE) may be related to the flow at 50 per cent vital capacity (VC) in the maximum flow-volume loop measured at rest. In patients with both obstructive and restrictive disorders, this flow capacity may be reached at maximum exercise.

VOLUME. In healthy subjects, increases in tidal volume are achieved by gradual increases in end-inspiratory lung volume to about 80 per cent of total lung capacity and reductions in end-expiratory volume to about 40 per cent of total lung capacity (see Fig. 2–6). The maximal observed exercise tidal volume (VTmax) in healthy subjects usually amounts to 55 to 60 per cent of the VC, but it is proportionally smaller in subjects with a smaller VC:

$$VTmax = 0.67\ VC - 0.64\ L$$

Equation 28

In patients with pulmonary fibrosis, in whom the capacity to generate increases in volume may be severely impaired, a greater proportion of VC may be recruited, but a limited V_T and high f_b is the characteristic breathing pattern.

INTRAPLEURAL PRESSURES. Increasingly negative esophageal pressures are generated during increasing exercise. The increases are related to increases in V_T and inspiratory flow, which are opposed by the impedance imposed by elastic and resistive forces. During expiration, pressures become more positive as high expiratory flows are generated and end-expiratory lung volume is reduced to below resting functional residual capacity. Measurements of esophageal pressure (Fitting et al., 1987) indicate that the high flow rates achieved in heavy exercise by healthy subjects (in whom V_T may exceed 4 L, and V_T/T_I may be 6 L/sec) are accompanied by intrapleural pressure swings between approximately -20 and $+20$ cm H_2O. The pressures developed, however, seldom exceed the maximum effective pressures that are required for the achievement of maximum flow.

Respiratory Muscle Capacity

The static (isometric) strength of the respiratory muscles is assessed by measurement of maximum airway pressures generated against a closed airway and standardized for lung volume. The static negative intrapleural pressures (-60 to -120 cm H_2O) that can be generated voluntarily at functional residual capacity by inspiratory muscles (Black and Hyatt, 1969) are more negative than those observed during exercise. However, with increasing lung volume, the capacity to generate maximum static inspiratory pressures is reduced because of the associated shortening of inspiratory muscles. Thus, the normal reduction in end-expired volume during exercise, to below resting functional residual capacity, can be viewed as unloading (shortening) the inspiratory muscles with a lowering of end-inspiratory volume; this option for reducing the sense of inspiratory effort is usually unavailable to patients with chronic airflow obstruction. Also, during exercise, increasing flow implies increasing velocity of respiratory muscle contraction, and, as with any muscle, the force generated falls with increasing contraction velocity, with a consequent reduction in the available inspiratory pressure. Similar considerations apply when expiratory pressures during exercise are related to those recorded during forced expiratory maneuvers at rest. Thus, when allowance is made for the effects of volume and flow, the pressures recorded during exercise are seen to be much closer to the pressure-generating capacity than might be expected from the static relationships. The relationship between the pressure generated and the capacity available is a dominant factor in the sensation of respiratory effort (dyspnea, breathlessness) during exercise. Recently, investigators have recognized that respiratory muscle weakness contributes to the limitation of maximum ventilation and exercise capacity and to dyspnea not only in patients with respiratory disorders (Killian and Jones, 1994) but also in those with cardiac failure (McParland et al., 1992).

Oxygen Cost of Breathing

The work of the respiratory muscles to achieve the high ventilations experienced by healthy subjects and against increases in pulmonary impedances in respiratory patients during exercise inevitably carries an increasing metabolic cost. For many years, there has been suspicion that the metabolic cost might eventually exceed the oxygen intake associated with the increase in ventilation, leaving none for any increase in muscle oxygen demands (Shephard, 1966). Although the oxygen cost of breathing is surprisingly difficult to study, it now seems unlikely that the oxygen cost can exceed 300 to 400 mL/min, even at very high ventilation and under conditions of severe respiratory loading (Jones GL et al., 1985).

Alveolar Ventilation

In health, arterial P_{CO_2} during exercise varies little from its resting values and seldom rises more than 1 to 2 mm Hg. Thus, by implication, at low and moderate levels of work, alveolar ventilation increases linearly with carbon dioxide output (Eq. 17) (see Fig. 2–5). The range of arterial P_{CO_2} during exercise is 35 to 45 mm Hg in healthy subjects. Many factors are thought to play a part in the control of breathing during exercise; in addition to neurogenic factors, changes in arterial carbon dioxide, oxygen, and pH also stimulate breathing, and complex mathematical expressions have been derived to describe their effects quantitatively (Cunningham, 1963). Above 75 per cent of the maximum $\dot{V}_{O_2}$, arterial P_{CO_2} shows a progressive fall, indicating that alveolar ventilation is increasing out of proportion to carbon dioxide output. Because the work rate at which this occurs is that at which blood lactate level rises, it is generally considered that the alveolar hyperventilation at high workloads is primarily due to the effect of the metabolic acidosis.

A low arterial P_{CO_2} is a common finding in patients with diffuse pulmonary infiltrative and fibrotic conditions, unless the ventilatory capacity is grossly impaired. The stimulus for alveolar hyperventilation is, at least in part, a fall in arterial P_{O_2}.

An impaired cardiovascular response to exercise may also be associated with hyperventilation; this is partly due to lactic acidemia. Severe hyperventilation associated with arterial P_{CO_2} of 20 to 25 mm Hg characteristically occurs during exercise in patients with obstructive pulmonary vascular disease (Jones and Goodwin, 1965). The observation of a reduction in ventilation and frequency after vagal blockade in such patients suggests that vagally mediated reflexes in the lungs or pulmonary circulation may be important (Guz et al., 1970).

Patients with severe chronic airway obstruction often exhibit a rise in Pa_{CO_2} during exercise that may amount to 20 mm Hg or more (Jones, 1966). This is probably due to a combination of an increase in the work of breathing and a reduced central responsiveness to carbon dioxide. The rise in P_{CO_2} is generally higher in patients with chronic obstructive bronchitis than in those with panlobular emphysema (Jones, 1964, 1966).

The VD/VT Ratio

The VD/VT ratio, which is normally 25 to 35 per cent at rest, falls to values between 5 and 20 per cent during exercise (Jones et al., 1966), leading to a narrowing of the difference between Pa_{CO_2} and PE_{CO_2} (see Fig. 2–5). The fall in VD/VT is due to the increase in tidal volume in exercise. Increases in end-inspiratory volume and transpulmonary pressure tend to increase the anatomical dead space, but this effect is small (Fig. 2–7). Although in healthy subjects at rest in the upright position there is a small contribution to the VD/VT ratio from alveolar dead space in apical regions of the lung, this disappears during exercise, when lung perfusion becomes more even (West, 1963). Harris and associates (1976) made a careful study of VD/VT in exercise, pointing out the important effect of changes in body temperature on the calculation of the Bohr equation.

The VD/VT ratio may be increased in disease for several reasons. First, a small tidal volume increases the VD/VT ratio. Second, the presence of high ventilation-perfusion ratios in the lungs leads to "alveolar" dead space. The highest values for the VD/VT ratio (> 50 per cent) are seen in patients with diffuse pulmonary fibrotic conditions, in whom the tidal volume is very small and ventilation-perfusion relationships are grossly abnormal. Widespread disease of the pulmonary vessels may lead to poor perfusion of large areas of lung, causing a marked increase in the VD/VT ratio. High VD/VT ratios are also observed in patients with severe chronic airway obstruction. In these patients, a normal value for the total ventilation should not be taken to indicate a normal pulmonary response to exercise without ensuring (through measurement of arterial or mixed venous P_{CO_2}) that it is not due to a combination of increased VD/VT and reduced $\dot{V}_A$.

Venous Admixture

The A-a P_{O_2} difference, normally about 10 mm Hg at rest, does not change at low exercise levels, but at heavy workloads, there is an increase to about 30 mm Hg (Fig. 2–8) (Hesser and Matell, 1965; Jones et al., 1966). Because the mixed venous oxygen content falls during exercise, the finding of an unchanged A-a P_{O_2} difference during moderate work indicates an improvement in oxygen transfer in the lung (fall in $\dot{Q}_{VA}/\dot{Q}_{tot}$ ratio) (see Fig. 2–8). This improvement is due to a more even distribution of ventilation-perfusion ratios in the lung (West, 1963; Hesser and Matell, 1965). The increase in A-a P_{O_2} during heavy work is a result of a rise in $P_{A_{O_2}}$ owing to alveolar overventilation, and of a low venous oxygen content; a variable but small contribution resulting from incomplete alveolar-capillary oxygen equilibration may also be present in healthy subjects at altitude and in patients with diffuse alveolar disease (McHardy, 1972; Torre-Bueno et al., 1985).

Impaired pulmonary oxygen transfer leads to an increase in the A-a P_{O_2} difference during exercise,

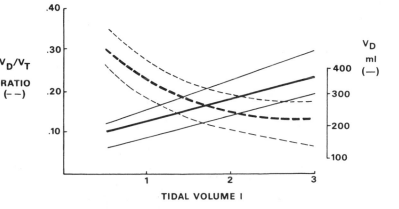

Figure 2–7. Physiological dead space (VD) and the VD/VT ratio (dashes), mean values for males (thick lines) and range (thin lines).

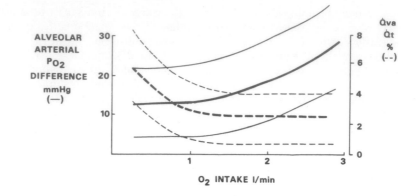

Figure 2-8. The alveolar-arterial Po_2 difference and venous admixture ($\dot{Q}va/\dot{Q}tot$). Mean values for males (thick lines) with range (thin lines).

ALVEOLAR ARTERIAL Po_2 DIFFERENCE mmHg (—)

$\dot{Q}va$ $\dot{Q}t$ % (- -)

O_2 INTAKE l/min

which may be an early indication of abnormal pulmonary function. Such an increase has been found in asymptomatic cigarette smokers, presumably owing to disease of small airways (Levine et al., 1970), and in patients in the early stages of diffuse alveolitis. Reduced ventilation of well-perfused areas in the lung is the main cause of an increased A-a Po_2 difference at rest. During exercise, the ventilation of these areas often increases owing to an increase in tidal volume, resulting in a fall in both the A-a Po_2 difference and the $\dot{Q}va/\dot{Q}tot$ ratio, as occurs in patients with chronic bronchitis (Jones, 1966). Thus, a wide A-a Po_2 difference at rest, although indicative of abnormal function, cannot be taken to signify an irreversible structural limitation of pulmonary oxygen uptake. However, in emphysema and pulmonary fibrosis, gas exchange does not improve with exercise; very wide A-a Po_2 differences are usually found at rest and during exercise.

Patients with a low cardiac output may show an increase in the A-a Po_2 difference during exercise partly because of the low mixed venous oxygen content and partly because of ventilation-perfusion mismatch (Mancini, 1995).

OXYGEN TRANSPORT IN BLOOD

Maximum oxygen transport in arterial blood is the product of $\dot{Q}tot \times Hb \times Sao_2$. The amount of oxygen carried by blood depends on the hemoglobin (Hb) concentration, the arterial Po_2, and the affinity of hemoglobin for oxygen. During exercise, an increase in temperature, a fall in arterial pH, and a rise in arterial Po_2 may all shift the oxyhemoglobin dissociation curve. The concentration of erythrocyte 2,3-diphosphoglycerate (2,3-DPG) has received attention in recent years but seems unlikely to be of importance during exercise. The level of 2,3-DPG formed in the red cells by glycolysis has a unique role in the regulation of oxygen transport: it shifts the oxyhemoglobin dissociation curve to the right and thus allows greater unloading of oxygen in the tissues. Although increased values of 2,3-DPG

have been found in conditions associated with hypoxemia, cardiac disease, and anemia (Lenfant et al., 1969; Shapell et al., 1970), the quantitative importance of this mechanism in the maintenance of oxygen delivery during exercise has yet to be established.

In patients with anemia (see Chapter 4), an increase in cardiac output maintains oxygen delivery, and only when anemia is severe (hemoglobin < 8 g/100 mL) or a cardiac impairment coexists is exercise much impaired. Studies of blood removal and reinfusion in athletes appear to show that maximal oxygen uptake can be directly related to the total available hemoglobin (Ekblom et al., 1972; Buick et al., 1980). Further evidence for the importance of the functionally available mass of hemoglobin has been provided by studies in which the oxygen capacity of hemoglobin was reduced by carbon monoxide administration (Ekblom and Huot, 1972).

CARDIOVASCULAR ADAPTATIONS TO EXERCISE

Cardiac Output

In health, cardiac output during exercise is linearly related to oxygen uptake (Eq. 20) (Fig. 2-9). At rest, cardiac output is related to body size, but during exercise, the change in cardiac output for a given change in oxygen uptake is little affected by such factors as sex, age, and size. Pooled results from a large number of studies (Wade and Bishop, 1962; Faulkner et al., 1977) in a variety of subjects exercising in the erect posture have shown that the relationship may be expressed by the equation

$$\dot{Q}tot = 4 + 0.006 \; \dot{V}o_2 \; (\pm SD \; 2) \; L/min$$
Equation 29

where $\dot{V}o_2$ is expressed in milliliters per minute. Values 2 L/min above this are found in patients in the supine position (Bevegård et al., 1960, 1963).

This relationship is supported by the findings of Faulkner and colleagues (1977), who made a careful

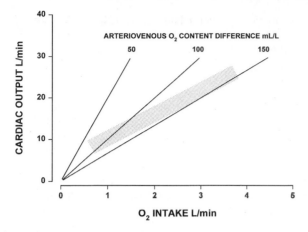

Figure 2–9. Cardiac output during exercise in healthy individuals, showing 95% confidence limits. Isopleths are the arteriovenous O_2 content difference, showing that increases in tissue O_2 delivery are accomplished by increases in both cardiac output and O_2 extraction.

study of the $\dot{Q}tot/\dot{V}O_2$ relationship in healthy subjects, examining the effects of age, sex, and fitness. They did not find significant effects of age, sex, and fitness; weight influenced the intercept of the relationship. They concluded that the slope of the relationship was between 5 and 6 L/min for 1-L increases in $\dot{V}O_2$ and that the intercept was about 65 mL/kg/min (i.e., 4.5 L/min for a 70-kg man).

Controversy has existed for many years regarding whether cardiac output reaches a maximum value in heavy cycling and treadmill exercise, which would imply that the cardiac pump is unable to increase further and is thus the main limiting factor to $\dot{V}O_2$max in healthy subjects. Rowell (1993) provided a review and concluded that the capacity of the peripheral circulation to reduce resistance to flow while maintaining an adequate driving pressure

is probably more important than the cardiac pump capacity. The addition of arm exercise to maximum cycling with the legs is accompanied by an increase in cardiac output (Andersen and Saltin, 1985). Similarly, recent work in patients with heart failure has questioned whether the lactate production seen at low workloads is a result of a reduced oxygen delivery due to a low maximum cardiac output; spectrophotometric measurements on active muscle have not shown a critically low tissue oxygen content (Gayeski et al., 1987), and reduced muscle oxidative enzyme activity is held to be more important (Sullivan et al., 1991). It has become increasingly clear in the past decade that increases in plasma lactate concentration cannot be taken to indicate a limitation in tissue oxygen delivery without other evidence of severe hypoxemia or impaired muscle blood flow.

The increase in cardiac output is associated with an increase in cardiac frequency but is not dependent on it (Segel et al., 1964). Maximal frequency is mainly influenced by age. This is the principal reason for the decline in maximal oxygen uptake that occurs with advancing age; at an age of 20 years, maximum frequency is 170 to 210, but it declines to 150 to 180 at age 60. The maximum cardiac frequency (obtained from many published studies reviewed by Lange-Anderson et al., 1971) is expressed by the following equation (Fig. 2–10).

$$\text{Max } f_c = 210 - 0.65 \times \text{age (y)}$$

Equation 30

Stroke Volume

Cardiac stroke volume increases to above resting values at low levels of work, but there is little or no further increase once cardiac frequency has risen

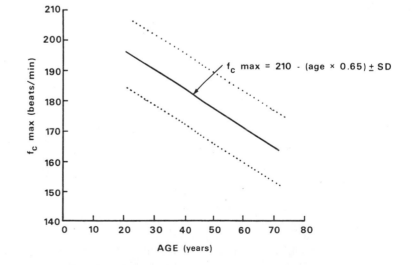

Figure 2–10. Maximum cardiac frequency in normal adults.

f_c max = 210 - (age × 0.65) ± SD

to 120 beats per minute. The increase in stroke volume is brought about partly by an increased ventricular filling owing to increased venous return and partly by enhanced contractility of the myocardium. Greater ventricular emptying leads to a fall in the end-diastolic volume.

Stroke volume in health mainly depends on heart size, which is therefore an important factor influencing maximal cardiac output. This explains the accuracy with which heart size, determined radiographically, can be used to predict maximum oxygen uptake and probably also accounts for the dependence of the heart rate-oxygen uptake relationship on body size. Stroke volumes are larger in men than in women and in athletes than in untrained subjects (Bevegård et al., 1963), both findings being explained to a great extent, but not entirely, by differences in heart size.

Patients with mild degrees of valvular heart disease may maintain a normal stroke volume but usually at the expense of an increase in ventricular volume and end-diastolic pressure. These changes may contribute to the maintenance of a normal relationship between cardiac output and oxygen intake, but in severer degrees of valvular dysfunction, stroke volume falls. At this stage, an increased heart rate response to a given oxygen intake is found; the increase in cardiac frequency often maintains a normal cardiac output in this situation, but the maximum cardiac output is low (Werkö, 1964). If the cardiac output response to increasing oxygen intake is low, tissue oxygen uptake may be maintained by an increase in extraction of oxygen from blood, resulting in a low oxygen content in venous blood. A further problem facing such patients is the competition between working muscles and essential organs such as the kidney or, particularly if there is a thermal stress, the skin; these organs normally operate at a high flow rate in relation to their metabolic rate. Patients with heart disease also may show a slow rate of adaptation of cardiac output to exercise, leading to an increase in plasma lactate concentration at the onset of exercise.

In patients with ischemic heart disease, stroke volume is often maintained, but left ventricular end-diastolic pressure usually increases (Parker, 1967). The onset of angina pectoris during exercise appears to be related to the myocardial oxygen requirements ($M\dot{V}O_2$). These are determined by the length-tension relationships of ventricular muscle and the heart rate (Sonnenblick et al., 1965) and are reflected clinically by measurements of the double product (systolic blood pressure × heart rate) or triple product (systolic blood pressure × heart rate × systolic ejection time). Although there is wide variation among patients in the relationship between these products and ST segment depression, they are helpful in assessing $M\dot{V}O_2$ in a given patient. For example, Redwood and associates (1972) showed that training may lead to an increase in the power output at which angina occurs, through reduction in blood pressure and cardiac frequency, without any change in the triple product at which angina occurs. The same authors were also able to show that the triple product was increased by treatment with coronary vasodilators and coronary bypass surgery. It is not uncommon in patients with ischemic heart disease to find that heart rate is low for a given power output or oxygen intake; the heart rate at maximal work is also low but is accompanied by a high blood lactate level, suggesting that the cardiac output has reached limiting values. This response suggests that ischemia has led to a reduction in the ability of the sinus node to increase its rate; usually, severe coronary atherosclerosis affecting the right and circumflex coronary arteries is present. It has been suggested that graded exercise tests be conducted up to a target heart rate based on the maximal rate found in healthy subjects, but this rate may be unrealistically high for many patients with ischemic heart disease. The electrocardiographic changes found in such patients is discussed in a later chapter.

Poor exercise performance in patients with heart disease may be difficult to distinguish from the effects of inactivity. Healthy subjects spending 3 weeks in bed have a reduced stroke volume, leading to a severe reduction in exercise performance, which takes several weeks to recover (Saltin et al., 1968). Furthermore, recent measurements on the muscles of patients with heart failure show an enzyme profile that is consistent with the effects of enforced inactivity (Sullivan et al., 1991).

Arteriovenous Oxygen Difference

The arteriovenous oxygen difference depends on the completeness of oxygen extraction from blood by muscle. This in turn is influenced by the metabolic rate, regional distribution of peripheral flow, local muscle capillary density and perfusion, changes in the position of the oxyhemoglobin dissociation curve, and probably the activity of muscle respiratory enzymes. Because maximal cardiac output depends on relatively fixed mechanisms governing stroke volume and heart rate, such factors assume important roles in determining maximum oxygen uptake in both health and disease. When these factors are poorly developed, work performance may be impaired.

In health, the arteriovenous oxygen content difference widens with increasing oxygen uptake from a resting level of around 50 mL/L to about 130 to 150 mL/L; the oxygen saturation of venous blood approaches 25 to 35 per cent in maximal work (see Fig. 2–9). In trained athletes, venous oxygen saturation may fall to 10 to 20 per cent (Pernow et al., 1965). These figures indicate a high utilization of transported oxygen in muscle, which is brought about by redistribution of blood to working tissue; up to 80 per cent of the increase in cardiac output during exercise is directed to muscle. Blood flow to brain and kidneys changes little during exercise, but flow to the liver and splanchnic region falls (Fig. 2–11) (Wade and Bishop, 1962; Rowell, 1993). Skin perfusion is also reduced unless work is performedin high environmental temperature, when it may amount to up to a quarter of the total cardiac output.

In patients with a cardiac limitation to exercise, more complete extraction of oxygen from blood perfusing muscle assumes an important role in the maintenance of oxygen delivery. Although the arteriovenous oxygen difference at a given oxygen intake is often increased, it seldom reaches the highest levels seen in athletes at maximum effort, probably because of the competition from essential organs with a high blood flow relative to their metabolic rate. Although their absolute blood flow may be small, it makes up a greater proportion of the total cardiac output. However, the arteriovenous oxygen difference and the venous oxygen content are influenced not only by the ratio of cardiac output to metabolic rate—distribution of blood flow between organs and tissues and the balance between mean blood pressure and peripheral vascular resistance are factors whose importance is difficult to quantify (Rowell, 1974). An increase in erythrocyte 2,3-DPG concentration may be important in some patients with a limited cardiac output, but this is not found invariably.

Intravascular Pressures

Systemic arterial blood pressure rises during exercise to levels around 200 mm Hg in maximal exercise. The rise is linearly related to exercise intensity but increases with increasing age (Jones et al., 1985a). The rise in diastolic pressure is much less (to around 90 mm Hg), and mean arterial pressure increases from 90 mm Hg at rest to 140 mm Hg in maximal exercise (Holmgren, 1956). This modest increase contrasts with the fivefold or more increase in cardiac output, implying a considerable fall in systemic peripheral vascular resistance that is presumably due to marked vasodilation in working muscle. Similarly, a considerable fall in pulmonary vascular resistance occurs during exercise; the rise in mean pulmonary artery pressure is 15 mm Hg or less in young subjects (Holmgren, 1956) but increases with increasing age (Fig. 2–12) (Tartulier et al., 1972; Ehrsam et al., 1983).

Although a limited stroke volume owing to cardiac disease may lead to a low systemic arterial pressure, this effect is seldom observed because of the compensatory vasoconstriction (Edhag and Zetterquist, 1968). Occasionally, a fall in arterial blood pressure may occur in patients with ischemic heart disease at the time that angina occurs. In systemic hypertension, the rise in systemic pressure usually parallels the normal rise (Sannerstedt et al., 1966). During treatment with hypotensive agents, blood pressure may fall in exercise. The measurement of blood pressure is an important part of the exercise evaluation of any patient with suspected cardiac disease or hypertension.

Patients with pulmonary vascular disease re-

Figure 2–11. Regional distribution of blood flow during exercise. (Data from Wade OL, Bishop JM. Cardiac Output and Regional Blood Flow. Oxford: Blackwell Scientific; 1962.)

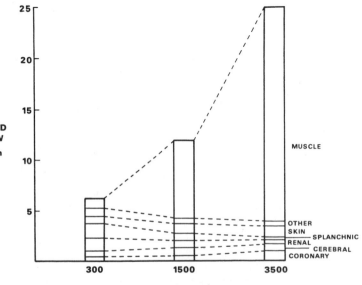

BLOOD FLOW L/min

MUSCLE

OTHER
SKIN
SPLANCHNIC
RENAL
CEREBRAL
CORONARY

300   1500   3500

O₂ UPTAKE ml/min

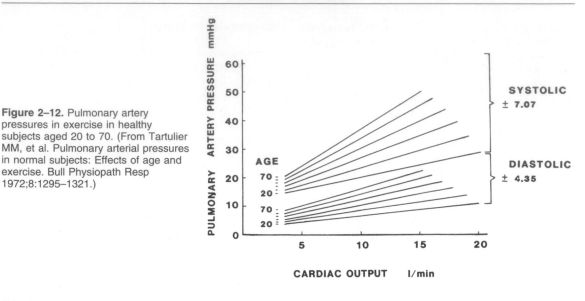

Figure 2–12. Pulmonary artery pressures in exercise in healthy subjects aged 20 to 70. (From Tartulier MM, et al. Pulmonary arterial pressures in normal subjects: Effects of age and exercise. Bull Physiopath Resp 1972;8:1295–1321.)

sulting from mitral stenosis, congenital septal defects, or pulmonary thromboembolism characteristically show marked increases in pulmonary artery pressure, sometimes to systemic levels, during exercise (Wilhelmsen et al., 1963).

Peripheral Vascular Changes

The capillary supply to muscles is dense but variable between muscles of differing fiber type distributions; a larger concentration of capillaries is related to oxidative SO and FOG fibers than is related to FG fibers. The capillaries run longitudinally alongside individual fibers, but many run transversely to form a tight mesh. During contraction, muscle shortening tends to lessen the distance between capillaries and increase their diameter (Groom et al., 1984). These changes tend to increase capillary volume despite increases in muscle pressure. Although cardiac output is the major determinant of muscle blood flow, capillary volume is also important. Furthermore, capillary volume is a critical factor in the maintenance of an adequate capillary transit time to enable diffusion of oxygen and carbon dioxide, uptake of blood-borne fuels, and removal of La^-. This is one aspect of the difference between untrained and well-trained persons; although cardiac output at a given oxygen uptake may be similar, femoral venous Po_2 is lower in the well-trained person, indicating a more complete oxygen extraction, owing to higher muscle flow and longer mean transit time. This concept has been elegantly strengthened by comparisons of trained and untrained legs in subjects who trained only one leg (Saltin, 1985).

An increase in muscle perfusion occurs extremely rapidly after the onset of muscle contraction (Honig et al., 1980). The mechanism is uncertain, but hypoxia and local changes in the concentration of lactic acid, ATP, and potassium have been implicated (Barcroft, 1963; Rowell, 1974). Where blood flow to muscle is limited locally, as in peripheral atherosclerosis, exercise is often limited by pain. Affected muscles exhibit a high oxygen extraction and increased lactic acid production.

In assessing the severity of the changes and in following the results of treatment, the clinician should choose a technique that ensures that the affected muscles are being exercised. Thus, although cycle ergometry is a good way of studying the effects of major leg vessel obstruction, walking or calf-muscle exercise may be better for distal peripheral vascular disease.

Electrocardiographic Changes

Careful recording of the electrocardiogram is a significant part of exercise testing. Changes in the ST segment are used as an important indicator of myocardial tissue hypoxia, which occurs when myocardial oxygen demands exceed oxygen delivery; the criteria are reviewed later (see Chapter 7). Tissue biopsy studies in experimental coronary occlusion showed that the earliest biochemical indices of impaired myocardial oxygen delivery—reduced lactate extraction and potassium release—correlate well with local ST segment changes recorded from the affected epicardium (Opie et al., 1973). The variation among different areas in the heart and the inconstant relationship between partial coronary arterial occlusion and an imbalance of oxygen supply and demand make it unlikely that any of the usual indicators—electrocardiographic, angiographic, or biochemical—will invariably identify myocardial ischemia. However, if care is taken with lead selection and recording (see Chapter 7), electrocardiographic changes during exercise correlate well with other indices.

BODY GAS STORES

Gas stores in the body act as important buffers in meeting metabolic demands that may be imposed more rapidly than the heart and lungs are able to increase oxygen and carbon dioxide transport. If the oxygen demands at the onset of exercise are not met promptly by increases in cardiac output and ventilation, oxygen "stores" in muscle and in arterial blood are drawn on to meet the oxygen deficit. Similarly, if carbon dioxide is not removed immediately, body carbon dioxide stores fill up so that the effects on venous PCO_2 and pH are minimized. The increase in carbon dioxide stores that normally occurs in exercise may be viewed as an important adaptive measure that reduces the load on ventilation. If no carbon dioxide was stored and tissue and venous PCO_2 were controlled at resting values, ventilation during exercise would need to be three to four times higher.

Oxygen stores in humans are small, amounting to about 25 mL/kg body weight. In muscle, oxygen is held in association with myoglobin; although the size of this store is difficult to estimate because of uncertainties regarding myoglobin concentration, the capacity to meet an oxygen deficit is limited. Carbon dioxide stores, on the other hand, are large. The carbon dioxide is in a variety of forms, but from the standpoint of exercise, the important component is the HCO_3^- in metabolically active tissues. At rest, the storage capacity is about 0.5 mL/kg/ mm Hg, but it increases to 2 to 3 mL/kg/mm Hg in moderate exercise, probably because the carbon dioxide originates in muscle in the first place, because muscle becomes much better perfused, and because reductions in muscle PC concentration reduce acidic (anionic) charge. Because it is impossible to measure carbon dioxide in all possible sites contributing to storage, the storage capacity has been examined in models of tissue gas exchange (Farhi and Rahn, 1960; Fowle et al., 1964; Cherniack and Longobardo, 1970). These studies, together with recent experimental work in humans, suggest that the relationship between changes in mixed venous PCO_2 and volume of carbon dioxide stored during exercise is similar to that expressed by the blood carbon dioxide dissociation curve, which becomes less steep as PCO_2 increases and muscle and venous pH falls (Jones and Jurkowski, 1979). Storage of carbon dioxide is important conceptually because it lessens the ventilatory demands, particularly at the onset of heavy exercise and in any

situation in which the circulation adapts slowly to the increase in metabolism. The practical importance of storage is related to the respiratory exchange ratio, which does not reflect the exchange at the tissue level if carbon dioxide storage is taking place. We meet this practical consideration again in the construction of a carbon dioxide balance equation to estimate La^- production (see Chapter 11).

ACID-BASE CHANGES DURING EXERCISE

Acid-base changes during exercise are another complex and interesting topic that has engaged the researcher's interest over many years and has stimulated much discussion regarding the mechanisms responsible for both the perturbation (acidosis) and the responses to it (Jones et al., 1977). Investigation has been hampered by difficulties in analysis, but the technique of magnetic resonance imaging has complemented data obtained by needle biopsy of muscle (Dawson, 1985), and there is a large degree of agreement as to the changes that occur in acid-base variables. In view of this, and also understanding of the basic physicochemical processes that determine hydrogen ion concentration, the ways in which they exert their effects in exercise are still surprisingly controversial. Superficially, the controversies appear to have a semantic basis and thus seem hardly worthy of further consideration; a deeper probing, however, reveals that there are major conceptual differences in the way that the topic is appreciated. Central to the discussion, and to paraphrase the controversy, is the distinction between the variables that are capable of acting independently and those that are dependent on the interaction of several systems, and thus cannot be viewed as independent, unless one makes the unreasonable condition of keeping other variables constant. The main variables in question are those appearing in Henderson's equation:

$$[H^+] = K (PCO_2/[HCO_3^-])$$
Equation 31

which is often used as a control equation—"$[H^+]$ is controlled by the balance between PCO_2 and bicarbonate concentration." In this concept, both PCO_2 and $[HCO_3^-]$ are viewed as acting independently; arterial PCO_2, at a given carbon dioxide production, is controlled by alveolar ventilation, and $[HCO_3^-]$ may be consumed (e.g., by titration with lactic acid) or conserved (e.g., by renal reabsorption). Hydrogen ions may also be treated as acting independently, when considered to be produced as an end product of metabolism ("the proton load"). Stewart (1981) made a plea for a more disciplined view, based on well-established physicochemical grounds, by pointing out that neither $[H^+]$ nor $[HCO_3^-]$ can act independently; both are the result of the interactions among several systems. Thus, Henderson's equation cannot be viewed as describing a control system; it needs to be solved simultaneously with other equations for a picture of all the variables involved to be obtained. In addition to Henderson's equation (which contains the independent variable P_{CO_2}), we must consider the balance between strong ions—those ions existing in a completely dissociated state—and the total concentration of buffers (weak acids and bases), in the context of water dissociation and the need for electrical neutrality (the total activity of positively and negatively charged ions must be equal).

The interacting systems are capable of rigorous quantitative description (Stewart, 1981; Jones, 1997), and although the measurements are not simple, the method may be applied to the changes occurring in several body fluid compartments—arterial and venous plasma, red cells, and active and inactive muscle. The changes occurring at all these sites have important implications for homeostasis, and the factors influencing $[H^+]$ in each are quite different. This makes a full description of the changes a daunting task, and only the concepts and more important factors are reviewed here because more detailed reviews have been published elsewhere (McKelvie et al., 1992; Lindinger, 1995; Lindinger et al., 1995).

In any given physiological fluid, several systems contribute to $[H^+]$, and their effects may be quantified in a series of equations.

1. Strong (fully dissociated) ions—positively charged cations (mainly K^+, Na^+, Ca^{2+}) always exceed the negatively charged anions (mainly Cl^- and La^-, plus, in muscle, PC^{2-}). The net effect of the charges may be expressed as the differences between their summed charges, known as the strong ion difference (SID), which thus by itself has an alkalinizing effect. However, a reduction in [SID], due to a reduction in $[K^+]$ or an increase in $[La^-]$, exerts a strong acidifying effect. As in any physiological fluid, electrical neutrality is maintained and the effect of changes in SID is measured in relation to all dissociated ions (see item 5 below).

2. Weak acids (HA) or buffers exist in partially dissociated form; their effect is quantified through their total concentration ([Atot]) and dissociation constant (K_a), which controls the extent of dissociation into H^+ and A^- at any given $[H^+]$, as described in

$$[H^+] \times [A^-] = K_a \times [HA]$$
$$[HA] + [A^-] = [Atot]$$

Equation 32

3. Carbon dioxide exists as dissolved CO_2, determined by its pressure and the solubility constant (s = 0.307 mmol/L/mm Hg), and as HCO_3^-; its effect on $[H^+]$ is expressed in Henderson's equation, with the apparent dissociation constant (K_c) determining how much of the total CO_2 content ([CO_2tot]) is dissolved and how much is present as HCO_3^-:

$$[H^+] \times [HCO_3^-] = K_c \times P_{CO_2}$$
$$(0.307 \times P_{CO_2}) + [HCO_3^-] = [CO_2tot]$$

Equation 33

Although these two expressions are analogous to those for the weak acids, an important difference exists between the physiological effects: weak acids are usually large molecules (proteins, phosphates) and their concentration ([Atot]) in any tissue is influenced only by the water content—they do not move readily across cell membranes. Carbon dioxide, on the other hand, is produced in metabolism and moves rapidly from one compartment to another according to carbon dioxide pressure gradients. Thus, P_{CO_2} may be considered an independent variable in arterial plasma, being determined by alveolar ventilation; the system is "open" in this compartment. However, in tissues and venous blood, [CO_2tot] is the independent variable because it is influenced by carbon dioxide production, tissue blood flow, and carbon dioxide diffusion in a closed environment.

4. Water dissociation into H^+ and OH^- is determined by the ion product for water at any given temperature, as expressed by:

$$[H^+] \times [OH^-] = K_w$$

Equation 34

At 37°C, $K_w = 4.4 \times 10^{-14}$, which means that neutral pH ($[H^+] = [OH^-]$) occurs at an $[H^+]$ of 2.2×10^{-7} or a pH of approximately 6.8. Unlike the other variables, the total water content in a tissue does not influence $[H^+]$ directly, but changes in water influence the concentrations of the other variables; this becomes an important effect in heavy exercise, when muscle water increases by as much as 15 per cent and plasma water decreases in approximately equal proportion. The main reason for the intracellular shift of water appears to be the metabolic production of small osmotically active products, such as La^- and glucose phosphates from the larger glycogen molecule (Lindinger et al., 1995).

5. In all compartments, electrical neutrality is observed, as expressed in

$$[SID] - [HCO_3^-] - [A^-] + [H^+] - [OH^-] = 0$$

Equation 35

Use of these relationships shows that the separate contributions of changes in [SID], [Atot], and Pco_2 or $[CO_2tot]$ (the independent variables) on changes in $[H^+]$, $[HCO_3^-]$ and $[A^-]$ (the dependent variables) may be quantified for the fluid compartment in question (Jones, 1997). Large differences between tissues emerge in terms of the variables and their roles in homeostasis.

IN MUSCLE. Intracellular [SID] is large ($\simeq 110$ mEq/L), dominated by high $[K^+]$; $[Cl^-]$ is low, but PC^{2-} (30 mEq/L) acts as a strong acid (Hultman and Sahlin, 1980). During exercise, decreases in intramuscular SID, which tend to increase $[H^+]$, are mainly due to decreases in $[K^+]$ (by as much as 40 mEq/L) and to increases in $[La^-]$ (to as high as 50 mEq/L); large decreases in PC^{2-} increase [SID], thus tending to alkalinize, or attenuate potential increases in $[H^+]$. High protein and phosphate concentrations contribute to a weak acid concentration ([Atot]) ($\simeq 140$ mEq/L) that is seven to 10 times as high as in plasma, allowing them to act as important buffers ($A^- + H^+ \rightarrow AH$), with decreases in $[A^-]$ minimizing the effects of decreases in [SID]. Pco_2 in tissues is higher than in arterial blood at rest, and $[HCO_3^-]$ is less than half the plasma level, at approximately 10 mmol/L. During exercise, carbon dioxide production increases at a faster rate than that of its removal by blood flow, and total CO_2 content ($[CO_2tot]$) increases and acts as an independent variable; because [SID] tends to fall and $[H^+]$ rises, the result is a large increase in Pco_2 in muscle, aiding its diffusion into venous blood. Until recently, carbonic anhydrase was thought not to be present in muscle, and it was argued that during exercise this was an advantage because it slowed the formation of HCO_3^-, which would not move as rapidly out of muscle as carbon dioxide. However, because HCO_3^- is a dependent variable, its forma-

tion probably occurs only at low intensities of exercise when only small changes in [SID] occur. Finally, in heavy exercise, increases in intracellular water occur as a result of osmotic and hydrostatic forces that tend to reduce the concentration of ions and the other variables.

When these changes are considered in relation to exercise intensity, reductions occur in $[PC^{2-}]$ at low and moderate loads and mainly at the onset of exercise (Sahlin, 1978; Hultman and Sjöholm, 1986); $[La^-]$ increases logarithmically with increasing loads, and reductions in $[K^+]$ and increases in water occur mainly at high loads. The result is that increases in $[H^+]$ are not substantial except at high loads, and $[HCO_3^-]$ may show an increase at low and moderate loads, with a marked fall at high loads; this behavior partly accounts for the large increases in carbon dioxide output in heavy exercise. The interaction between changes in the acid-base systems means that muscle $[H^+]$ can increase from resting levels of 100 nEq/L (pH, 7.0) to as high as 400 nEq/L (pH, 6.4) in maximal sprint exercise (Hermansen and Osnes, 1972; Spriet et al., 1989; Jones and Heigenhauser, 1992).

IN PLASMA. The balance between the systems at rest is toward [SID] ($\simeq 40$ mEq/L), but large variations in $Paco_2$ may effect large and rapid changes in arterial $[H^+]$. Increases in $[H^+]$ during exercise are usually related to reductions in [SID] associated with increases in $[La^-]$ (to as high as 20 mEq/L) but are modulated by changes in inorganic strong ions, mainly Cl^-. Shifts in water between plasma and cells also modify the concentrations of strong ions and Atot. However, the buffering effect of Atot is limited, because the ratio of $[A^-]$ to [Atot] in plasma is only about 1/10 in the physiological pH range, and [Atot] is only 20 mEq/L.

These differences between fluid compartments emphasize (1) the importance of fluid and ion shifts between them in the acid-base perturbations occurring in exercise and (2) the fact that many more variables are involved in the ionic changes of exercise than merely the production of lactic acid. During exercise, many systems teleologically respond in a homeostatic manner, to maintain an ionic environment suitable for the muscle contraction and at the same time not to incur changes in blood plasma, such as large increases in $[K^+]$ and $[H^+]$, that might impair function of the brain and heart. These homeostatic mechanisms include increases in muscle blood flow effecting the removal of carbon dioxide and La^-, carbon dioxide excretion by the lungs, reuptake of K^+ into muscle, metabolism of lactate, and redistribution of water. However, when exercise is very intense, or if some or all of these mechanisms are impaired, muscle pH falls to levels at which flux-generating enzymes are inhibited, excitation-contraction coupling is impaired, and reduction in cross-bridge cycling occurs, all leading inevitably to muscle fatigue.

THE INTEGRATION BETWEEN MECHANISMS

In any description of the changes in individual mechanisms, there is a risk of overlooking the integrative aspects of exercise, which result in the total response being greater than can be supported by any of the individual contributions alone. Oxygen supply in an exercising athlete may increase to more than 20 times the resting oxygen consumption (from 0.25 to over 5.0 L/min). This increase is not brought about by a 20-fold increase in any one mechanism, but the demand is shared between mechanisms—the cardiac output may increase to about six times the resting value (from 5 to 30 L/min) and the arteriovenous oxygen difference, representing oxygen extraction from arterial blood, may increase to over three times the resting value (from 50 to over 150 mL/L). Oxygen transport depends on a series of linked mechanisms that influence oxygen in the transport fluids (air, blood) and tissues; this concept can be expressed in a flow scheme as follows:

Inspired oxygen (altitude)

↓

Pulmonary ventilation
(alveolar ventilation, distribution)

↓

Pulmonary gas exchange
(diffusion, ventilation-perfusion)

↓

Arterial oxygen
(oxygen capacity, saturation)

↓

Cardiac output
(stroke volume, cardiac frequency)

↓

Muscle blood flow
(peripheral vascular resistance)

↓

Oxygen extraction
(capillary-tissue diffusion)

↓

Muscle oxygen utilization←Oxygen stores
(respiratory enzymes)

↓

Venous oxygen

The interdependence of, and linkage between, mechanisms were brilliantly described by Sir Joseph Barcroft in his book *Features in the Architecture of Physiological Function* (1934), which contains three chapters entitled ''Every Adaptation Is an Integration.'' Although we may easily grasp the concept of integration, the precise implications that follow its application to normal and abnormal physiological responses to exercise are often difficult to understand. This is mainly because of the complexity of all the interactions that may occur. However, if we are to understand the physiological adaptations, particularly when one or more systems are functioning poorly, our approach to exercise testing has to include the interactions as well as the measurement of individual adaptations. Barcroft met this challenge by a graphical approach to oxygen transport that expressed the contributions of pulmonary diffusion, cardiac output, tissue oxygen extraction, and blood oxygen carriage. He credited Murray and Morgan (1925) with the first demonstration of the use of such a diagram. The graph enables the relative contribution of each mechanism to be appreciated at the visual level, through changes in shape, and at the mathematical level, through the rigorous application of the equations used to construct the diagram. Figure 2–13, which shows the graph, has been adapted from Barcroft's original example, with some changes in terms and units. It shows the relative contributions of the mechanisms to a 10-fold increase in oxygen uptake, from 0.24 to 2.4 L/min. We may appreciate, from the shape of the two rectangles (rest and exercise), the extent to which the mechanisms share in the adaptation and the extent to which each encroaches on its own capacity to respond. We should not allow the uncertainty regarding some of the variables depicted (diffusing capacity, diffusion pressure gradient) to detract from the beauty of this representation; indeed, the usefulness of the graph lies partly in helping us to place limits on the changes that must occur in such mechanisms that are difficult to measure.

Rodolfo Margaria, who made many contributions to the understanding of exercise physiology since his work at the Harvard Fatigue Laboratory in the mid-30s, took a similar approach to the expression of oxygen transport mechanisms. His diagram explores the interactions among several oxygen transport mechanisms—cardiac output, stroke volume and heart rate, and alveolar ventilation (Margaria, 1976). Figure 2–14 shows the diagram as constructed for rest and exercise; the 10-fold increase in oxygen intake is brought about by a doubling of heart rate and an increase in stroke volume, with a threefold increase in cardiac output; alveolar ventilation, on the other hand, increases 10-fold. The

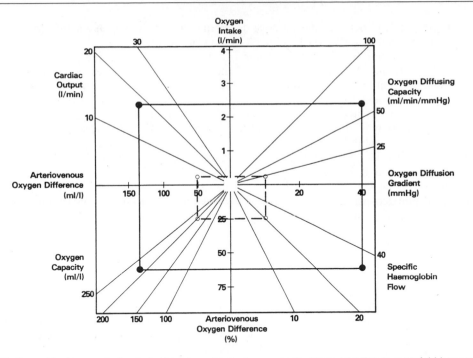

Figure 2–13. Barcroft's diagram to illustrate the integration between mechanisms adapting to a tenfold increase in O_2 intake (upper ordinate) from rest (-○-) to exercise (-●-), through increases in cardiac output and arteriovenous O_2 content difference (upper left quadrant); little change in blood O_2 capacity but increased venous desaturation (lower left quadrant); increased "specific hemoglobin flow"; and a combination of increased pulmonary O_2 diffusing capacity and increased mean alveolar-capillary O_2 pressure difference.

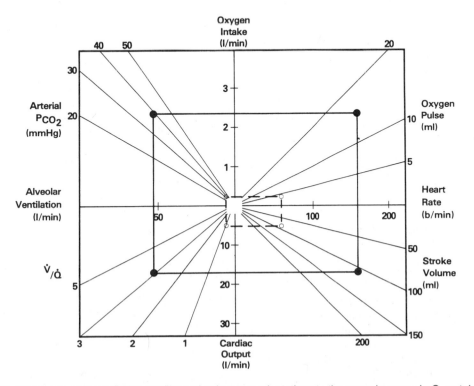

Figure 2–14. Margaria's diagram linking cardiac and pulmonary adaptations to the same increase in O_2 uptake shown in Figure 2–13 and using the same symbols.

relative sharing of the load between the lungs and heart ($\dot{V}$-$\dot{Q}$) increases from a 1:1 to a 3:1 ratio.

There are several reasons for dwelling in some detail on the Barcroft and Margaria approaches. First, they emphasize our debt to classic human physiology. Second, they emphasize an integrative approach to exercise that is not only illuminating but also based on variables that may be easily measured. Finally, they establish the pedigree of a similar approach applied to carbon dioxide transport, which we have found helpful; in addition to its value in expressing the integration between mechanisms, the approach has analytical value in that it is based on measurements that may be made easily during exercise, and it has proved to be a valuable teaching aid.

Consider carbon dioxide removal in a similar way to that described previously for oxygen delivery; carbon dioxide removal also depends on a series of linked mechanisms, as expressed in the following flow scheme:

CO_2 production (aerobic, anaerobic)

$\downarrow \rightarrow CO_2$ stores

Muscle blood flow

$\downarrow$

Venous CO_2

$\downarrow$

Venous return (cardiac output)

$\downarrow$

Pulmonary gas exchange
(ventilation-perfusion)

$\downarrow$

Pulmonary ventilation

$\downarrow$

Expired CO_2

Although several mechanisms are shared, the relative adaptive capacity of each to respond to either oxygen uptake or carbon dioxide removal may differ. For example, an impaired ventilatory response to exercise may result in a low arterial oxygen content; because ventilation is the start of the oxygen transport line, this defect may be counteracted by an increase in cardiac output, which maintains oxygen delivery. However, because ventilation is at the end of the carbon dioxide transport line, an adaptation of any other mechanism can have only a limited effect in maintaining carbon dioxide excretion. For this reason, studies of the integration between mechanisms removing carbon dioxide from tissues tend to complement information related to oxygen transport.

The carbon dioxide transport line just shown can be expressed as a series of equations and graphs linked to form a quadrantic diagram (Fig. 2–15) (McHardy et al., 1967). The construction of the diagram and its use in exercise tests are detailed in Chapter 11; I limit the present discussion to examining the adaptations to a 10-fold increase in carbon dioxide output. From the diagram (see Fig. 2–15) we see that the increase has been achieved without any change in arterial P_{CO_2}, through a sixfold increase in $\dot{V}_E$ (from 9 to 55 L/min) and by almost halving the V_D/V_T ratio (from .32 to .17). If the V_D/V_T ratio remained at resting level, either arterial P_{CO_2} would rise to about 54 mm Hg or $\dot{V}_E$ would increase to 70 L/min. Turning to the cardiac adaptation, we see that a 10-fold increase in $\dot{V}_{CO_2}$ is associated with a threefold increase in cardiac output (from 6 to 20 L/min) and a threefold increase in the venoarterial carbon dioxide content difference; as arterial P_{CO_2} shows little change, the oxygenated mixed venous P_{CO_2} increases from 50 to 70 mm Hg, implying an increase in carbon dioxide stored. The diagram shows that both cardiac output and the venoarterial carbon dioxide content difference have to increase. It also demonstrates that if carbon dioxide were not stored and mechanisms were geared to maintaining $P_{\bar{V}CO_2}$ at its resting value of 50 mm Hg, arterial P_{CO_2} would have to fall to 26 mm Hg, requiring an increase in $\dot{V}_E$ to over 80 L/min. In Chapter 11, the diagram will be used again to explore adaptation and maladaptation from a pathophysiological viewpoint.

Clinical Implications of Integration

The linkage between mechanisms has a number of implications for the way in which the total system behaves in different clinical situations and the ways in which limitation of exercise capacity may occur. Broadly, four types of effect may be identified.

1. *Adaptation.* The effect of a defective gas transfer process may be lessened by adaptive changes at other points in the system. For example, impaired oxygen delivery may be maintained in the face of a reduction in Sa_{O_2} owing to a pulmonary gas exchange disorder, by an increase in $\dot{Q}_{tot}$. If this adaptation is absent, for example, in a patient with chronic respiratory disease owing to the coexistence of pulmonary hypertension or ischemic heart disease, exercise capacity is even more seriously impaired. The adaptive interdependence is also particularly evident

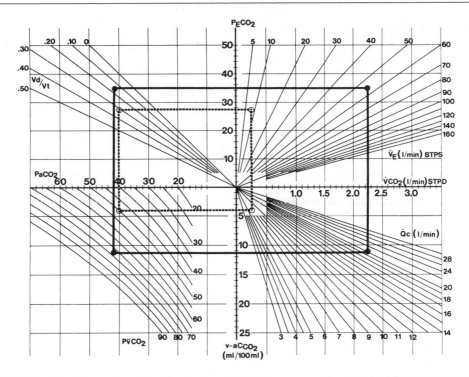

Figure 2–15. McHardy's diagram describing the changes in CO_2 transport mechanisms as CO_2 output increases by ten times the resting rate.

in the responses to endurance training, in which increases in muscle aerobic enzymes and greater utilization of fat as a fuel are accompanied by decrements in heart rate, increases in stroke volume, and reductions in systemic blood pressure. These improvements in oxygen delivery and muscle aerobic capacity and the fall in the metabolic respiratory quotient all contribute to a reduction in $\dot{V}CO_2$ for a given $\dot{V}O_2$. The associated fall in $\dot{V}E$ is the most dramatic physiological effect of training, being accompanied by reductions in respiratory muscle effort, and thus in dyspnea.

2. *Association.* The effect of an impaired gas transfer process may be associated with secondary effects that then become limiting. For example, an impaired $\dot{Q}tot$ response to exercise is often associated with lactate production, which in turn leads to increases in $\dot{V}CO_2$ and $\dot{V}E$. Thus, the patient with seriously impaired cardiac function may present with breathlessness and an apparent ventilatory limitation.

3. *Maladaptation.* When the main defect in exercise capacity lies in the muscle, as in a diffuse myopathy, there is little room for

adaptation in other mechanisms in order to maintain function. In this situation tachycardia and hyperventilation may be seen and may be misleading in the assessment and identification of the functional deficit.

4. *Equalization.* The linkage between mechanisms may lead in the long term to loss of function in several of the processes contributing to exercise performance. For example, the enforced inactivity imposed on a patient with a cardiac disorder may lead to a secondary fall in muscle aerobic capacity. If at this point the cardiac defect is remedied, as, for example, in coronary bypass surgery, muscle function rather than the heart may then limit exercise capacity.

FITNESS, TRAINING, AND DETRAINING

Several aspects of fitness have been alluded to already. Whether we define it in terms of the maximal $\dot{V}O_2$ or more generally in terms of the capacity to enjoy moderate endurance activity without discomfort (Bannister, 1969), the term implies an optimal usage of the oxygen transport mechanisms and muscle metabolism, which allow the exercising human to use his or her own stored energy resources and those of the environment to generate a power output without undue strain and effort. The superior performance of an athlete is achieved through such optimal usage. Performance depends partly on attributes that are distributed throughout the healthy population, such as stature, which influences size of the heart, lungs, and muscles; age, which mainly influences the number of muscle motor units and possibly maximal heart rate; and hemoglobin content, which influences the oxygen-carrying capacity of the central circulation.

Exercise training increases the effectiveness of these attributes by improving function in a number of ways, varying in their extent according to the type of training as well as its intensity, duration, and frequency. Two main contrasting types of exercise training are recognized, but often a combination forms part of the elite athlete's training program; "endurance" training involves exercise of relatively low intensity but maintained for long periods, and "strength" training involves the brief, intermittent development of high muscle tensions. Although the effects of training carried out by athletes are more or less specific to the activity, in less active individuals, there is considerable overlap. Studies of the effects of training in athletes involve subjects who start training from a vastly different state than that found in sedentary individuals or disabled patients. Thus, patients with cardiac and respiratory disorders who undergo strength training show marked improvements in endurance in addition to improvements in muscle strength (McCartney et al., 1991; Simpson et al., 1992; McKelvie et al., 1995; the same concept applies to elderly subjects (McCartney et al., 1995).

Endurance training typically leads to improvements in neuromuscular function (McComas, 1994) but to little change in muscle size or fiber distribution. There are increases in mitochondrial volume (Howald, 1985) and in the activity of enzymes regulating pyruvate and free fatty acid oxidation, particularly in oxidative fibers (Gollnick et al., 1973). Muscle stores of glycogen and fat (Howald, 1985) increase, and the rate of adipose tissue fat mobilization also increases. During exercise, carbon dioxide production is reduced and the respiratory exchange ratio is low, indicating a greater usage of fat as fuel and leading to sparing of muscle glycogen. Whereas blood lactate level increases at about 60 per cent of $\dot{V}O_2$max in untrained subjects, many endurance athletes are able to maintain a $\dot{V}O_2$ in excess of 80 per cent for long periods. Because $\dot{V}O_2$max in athletes may be twice that in untrained individuals, athletes may generate a power that exceeds the unfit person's $\dot{V}O_2$max by 50 per cent and may maintain it without any increase in blood lactate concentration. The metabolic changes are accompanied by improved efficiency of cardiorespiratory exercise responses: cardiac stroke volume and left ventricular ejection fraction are increased, systolic arterial pressure is lower, ventilation is lower, and pulmonary gas exchange variables (VD/VT ratio, venous admixture) are improved. The sum total of the changes is expressed in a higher $\dot{V}O_2$max and an ability to maintain a high exercise intensity for a longer period than untrained persons. These changes are accompanied by more rapid adaptations at the onset of exercise in the activation of oxidative enzymes and in the cardiovascular responses. In strength training, muscles undergo repetitive contraction—isometric, isotonic, and eccentric. Persons who take part in this type of training alone show increases in muscle size owing to increased cross-sectional area of fibers rather than increased number of fibers (MacDougall et al., 1977); although the fiber type distribution in muscles is not changed, the increase in area is greatest in the fast-twitch fibers. The mitochondria do not increase, the activity of myosin ATPase and glycolytic enzymes is increased, and muscle stores of creatine phosphate and glycogen also increase. The increases in muscle strength are not accompanied by cardiorespiratory changes, and typically weightlifters have the lowest $\dot{V}O_2$max of elite athletes. Many endurance athletes (e.g., rowers) generate large muscle tensions and tend to show a combination of changes with very high $\dot{V}O_2$max.

A comparison of excellent male and female athletes may contribute some insights into factors influencing elite performance. An analysis of the Swedish National teams in various events showed that the $\dot{V}O_2$max in male athletes, expressed per kilo of body weight, was about 20 per cent higher than in females in the same sport, except for swimming, in which the difference was only 10 per cent. However, body fat in the males constituted about 5 per cent of body weight, compared with 15 per cent in females; thus, when expressed per kilo of fat-free body mass, the difference became insignificant (Åstrand and Rodahl, 1977).

The effects of inactivity are as dramatic as those of training (Saltin and Rowell, 1980); reductions in $\dot{V}O_2$max are associated with structural and biochemical changes in muscle and with changes in cardiovascular function, of which reductions in cardiac stroke volume and maximal cardiac output are the most important.

However serious the effects of inactivity may be in otherwise healthy subjects, their importance may become critical in patients with heart or lung disease. Because reserves of cardiac and ventilatory capacity are smaller, they are more readily encroached on by inefficient usage. In the past, physicians have been guilty, through direct advice or implication, of unduly limiting their patients' activities, and in so doing they may have been responsible for a decline in their capacity for work. Training may be a valuable therapeutic tool when carefully used in such patients. In patients with coronary heart disease, training leads to a lower heart rate and to reduced myocardial oxygen requirements. Similar effects may be expected in patients with pulmonary disease; an improvement in the cardiovascular adaptation to exercise may induce lower lactate production, lower carbon dioxide output, and thus smaller changes in blood P_{CO_2} and pH. These changes reduce the demand on a limited ventilatory capacity and make the most of any improvements in ventilation and gas exchange brought about by other therapeutic measures. Although some years ago strength training was avoided in patients with cardiorespiratory disorders due to an unjustified fear of the possible ill effects (e.g., an increase in blood pressure), more recently, carefully prescribed strength training has been safely and successfully applied to these patients (McKelvie et al., 1995). Improvements in endurance and muscle oxidative capacity accompany increases in strength. This has proved to be a breakthrough in rehabilitation medicine because the classic endurance exercise training is often difficult for patients; with strength training, improvements are readily demonstrated in a short time, leading to improved compliance and reduced effort in daily activities (McKelvie et al., 1995).

THE DEVELOPMENT OF EXERCISE CAPACITY IN MALES AND FEMALES

The factors that influence changes in exercise performance in growing children have been of great interest to exercise physiologists for several reasons. First, growth may be used to test hypotheses related to the integration between systems in exercise and so help to decide which factors limit performance. Second, an exploration of dimensional changes may identify attributes of potential elite athletes, or at least help to explain differences between persons, for example, differences in performance between males and females. Third, the more we understand the interplay between physical attributes, the better we are able to predict the expected response in a healthy person. The extent to which these aims are fulfilled by an examination of the studies of exercise in children may be hindered by a number of obvious limitations—the size of the sample and the extent to which it is representative of the population, the location of the study, the year it was carried out, and the relationship to other maturation changes, such as sexual development. Of these limitations, the most crucial may be the representativeness of the sample, particularly when predictive standards are being sought; it is likely that most studies have been of the more active members of the population, who are more likely to want to take part in such a study. This conclusion

is brought home in the study of Cumming (1977), who, in trying to establish normal standards for a test to be applied to children being investigated for cardiac disease, used data obtained in children referred to the clinic who were subsequently shown to be free of disease. The maximal power in these children, not surprisingly, was below published values obtained in other studies. For this application, in which it is important not to overdiagnose impairment, it is likely that the lower the published normal standards are, the more use they will be in a clinical application.

In taking a dimensional view of performance characteristics Åstrand and Rodahl (1977), in their classic text, develop the theoretical basis for the use of height as the main parameter of growth. Linear dimensions—length of bones and muscles, and thus of the levers used for muscular work—bear a linear relationship to height; put in another way, the ratio of changes during development are the same as the ratio of the change in height. Cross-sectional dimensions, for example, of muscles, airways, and blood vessels, are proportional to the square of changes in height. Volumetric dimensions—lung and heart volumes, blood volume—are proportional to the cube of height. Now, consider some aspects of muscle performance during development. The maximal force generated by muscle varies as its cross-sectional area, and thus the square of its linear dimension; thus, as a child's height increases, we expect strength to increase in the ratio of height squared. Recent measurements of maximal force generation in adults support this contention (Makrides et al., 1985). In terms of work performed (force × distance), as force is proportional to $(height)^2$ and distance to height, maximal work is a function of $(height)^3$. The time scale in this context has the dimension of $(length)^{-1}$; thus, power (work per unit time) is proportional to $(height)^2$.

Regarding variables that may contribute to maximal oxygen intake, increases in cardiac stroke volume and ventilatory tidal volume are proportional to $(height)^3$; maximal cardiac output and ventilation, on the other hand, are volumes per unit time and thus increase in proportion to $(height)^2$. Mass is proportional to $(height)^3$; thus, the time-related indices (maximum power, cardiac output, and ventilation) change in proportion to $(mass)^{2/3}$ and not in proportion to mass.

The maximal oxygen intake, being linearly related to maximal power, should be related to $(height)^2$ or $(mass)^{2/3}$; Åstrand and Rodahl (1977) point out that for athletes, this is actually the case, incidentally confirming the fallacy of expressing $\dot{V}_{O_2}max$ per unit mass ($\dot{V}_{O_2}max$ mL/kg).

We are now in a position to view exercise performance in children in relation to these dimensional factors. There have been many studies in children, and despite differences in geographical location and time, the agreement between them has generally been good. For example, the relationship between $\dot{V}O_2$max and height found in European males (Åstrand, 1952; Bink and Waffelbakker, 1968) is similar to that found in Californians (Cooper and Weiler-Ravell, 1984) and Canadians (Cunningham et al., 1984) studied 30 years later. However, the values are significantly higher than in some other studies (Adams et al., 1961; Cumming and Friesen, 1967; Gadhoke and Jones, 1969; Godfrey et al., 1971), possibly because of differences in subject recruitment. Also, values in California females (Cooper and Weiler-Ravell, 1984) are lower than those in Scandinavians (Åstrand, 1952). All studies have shown an increase with age in $\dot{V}O_2$max, with similar values in males and females up to age 13 to 14 years, but a divergence above this age, particularly when considered in relation to weight, and remaining even when considered in relation to height. This finding is not surprising in view of differences between postpubertal males and females in the dimensions of the heart and lungs and the volume of circulating hemoglobin.

In view of wide variability in the timing of the adolescent growth spurt, the study of Cunningham and associates (1984) has been of great importance. These authors recruited 62 males aged 9 to 10 years and observed them yearly for 6 years, allowing the investigators to identify the growth spurt and standardize age in relation to it (Blimkie et al., 1980). A linear increase in $\dot{V}O_2$max with height was found; between the ages of 10.8 and 14.8 years, height increased by 1.18, weight by 1.65, $\dot{V}O_2$max by 1.67, and cardiac stroke volume by 1.67. Thus, in this study, the increase in $\dot{V}O_2$max was proportional to (increase in height)^3 or 1.64. In females, the proportional change in $\dot{V}O_2$max approximates changes in height to the power 2.2 (Åstrand and Rodahl, 1977; Cooper and Weiler-Ravell, 1984). However, a comparison between studies shows a large range of variation; in a Scandinavian study, $\dot{V}O_2$max expressed in relation to height showed a $\dot{V}O_2$max in females of 160 cm in height to be only 15 per cent less than that in males, compared with 27 per cent less in the California study (Cooper and Weiler-Ravell, 1984).

The development of muscle size is under hormonal and local mechanical control, with muscle strength increasing linearly with age; as with many other functions, there is an accelerated increase in muscle length, cross-sectional area, and strength in males at the time of the growth spurt that is ascribed to the action of testosterone (McComas, 1977). Thus, in the postpubertal years, the strength of thigh muscles is related to the subject's height, but at a given height, males are about 25 per cent stronger than females; these differences are accounted for by differences in thigh muscle cross-sectional area (Davies, 1971; Makrides et al., 1985).

In comparisons of the contributions of other factors to $\dot{V}O_2$max in developing males and females, caution is needed if standardization is made to height rather than to height to a power function. This necessity is emphasized by a consideration of dimensions of the heart and lungs during development; at age 14 years, there is little difference in population averages of height, weight, vital capacity (Berglund et al., 1963), and heart volume (Simon et al., 1972); by age 16 years, relative differences between males and females are apparent, amounting to 1.10, 1.15, 1.25, and 1.26, respectively; at age 18 years, the differences have increased to 1.13, 1.28, 1.30, and 1.40, respectively. Thus, although the average 18-year-old male is only 13 per cent taller than the average 18-year-old female, vital capacity is 30 per cent higher and heart volume 40 per cent higher; the differences are in a ratio that is equal to the ratio of differences in height to the power of 2.0 to 3.0. These differences are maintained throughout adult life; as well as contributing to a difference in $\dot{V}O_2$max between the sexes, they also account for the lower tidal volume and higher frequency of breathing as well as lower stroke volume and higher heart rate at any given $\dot{V}O_2$ and height in females compared with males.

The topic of scaling the contributions of a number of variables to $\dot{V}O_2$max is of great interest in comparative physiology. Taylor and his colleagues have made many important contributions in this field; in a notable review of their work (Taylor et al., 1981), they concluded that although the metabolic power required by mammals for running at top speed should scale as length^2, or weight$^{0.67}$, measured $\dot{V}O_2$max is larger than this theoretical value and is proportional to weight$^{0.81}$. This conclusion is borne out by measurements in humans, which are discussed in Chapter 8.

Dimensions aside, studies of dizygotic and monozygotic twins have suggested a significant genetic influence on the development of $\dot{V}O_2$max (Klissouras, 1971), and in all studies in which activity data were collected, a significant effect may also be identified as explaining a small part of the population variance.

Variations between studies in different parts of the world may be accounted for in part by the growth patterns in different races, but they also receive contributions from differences in the extent of habitual activity (Miller et al., 1977). This conclusion is borne out by studies of young athletes, who show greater increases in vital capacity and heart volume as well as larger $\dot{V}O_2$max than their less active classmates (Engstrom et al., 1971). The results of these and other studies may tempt us to infer that the dimensions of the oxygen transport systems are dominant in $\dot{V}O_2$max, and certainly they do play a facilitative role. However, the finding that $\dot{V}O_2$max falls in young athletes once they stop training, in spite of their retaining their large lung and heart volumes (Eriksson et al., 1971), indicates a more important role for the aerobic metabolic potential of muscle in this regard. In studies of $\dot{V}O_2$max in which the level of leisure activity has been recorded, a significant influence of activity has invariably been found that is independent of body dimensions (Jones et al., 1985a).

The present discussion has obvious practical implications for the director of an exercise laboratory who is searching for standards to enable interpretation of maximal power or $\dot{V}O_2$max measured in children in a clinical context. This topic is discussed in Chapter 8.

THE EFFECTS OF AGING ON EXERCISE PERFORMANCE

An examination of aging provides another opportunity to look at the interrelationships between dimensions and functions contributing to exercise performance, to identify not only what lies behind the 30 per cent fall in $\dot{V}O_2$max between ages 20 and 60 years but also the explanation of the somewhat reassuring fact that an active 60-year-old may have $\dot{V}O_2$max values identical to those of an inactive 20-year-old. Contributing to our understanding have been the results of cross-sectional studies, a few longitudinal studies, studies of athletes and former athletes, and studies of the effects of training in inactive subjects, young and old.

Differences between the sexes in exercise responses, identified already in development, are largely maintained throughout adulthood. These include dimensional differences in height, lean body mass and muscle volume, lung volume and cardiac volume, and a lower hemoglobin content in females. The consensus is that such dimensional differences are capable of explaining all the differences between males and females in exercise variables, and that changes in function are much less important. Thus, although cardiac stroke volume is less in females, the maximum heart rate is similar to that of males; thus, maximum cardiac output is less in females in proportion to their smaller cardiac size. Declines in function with aging appear similar in the two sexes.

Rather than attempt a detailed review of aging changes, available elsewhere (Strandell, 1964; Smith and Serfass, 1981), only the relevant changes are listed, in order to identify those mechanisms capable of adaptation in the face of aging and those functions that deteriorate irrevocably.

All studies are in agreement that after reaching a peak at age 15 to 25 years, $\dot{V}O_2$max declines by almost 1 per cent per year, whether the subject is an athlete who keeps up a high level of activity or an untrained person (Åstrand and Rodahl, 1977; Jones et al., 1985a). The decline in power and $\dot{V}O_2$max approximately scales as a function of age$^{-0.5}$ (Jones et al., 1989). The $\dot{V}O_2$max of excellent athletes who stop training usually remains well above the average for the general population, possibly because of genetically determined factors. Also, short-term studies of training have shown that $\dot{V}O_2$max may be increased by as much as 40 per cent in both the young and the old (Makrides et al., 1986). Thus, although we may identify a steady deterioration with increasing age in many variables related to exercise, there is still room for considerable variability among persons at any given age. With increasing age, and particularly after age 60, there is a gradual decline in muscle volume and lean body mass associated with loss of muscle fibers, and a reduction in their size; these changes affect the FG muscle fiber type to a greater extent than they affect the FOG and SO types (Aniansson et al., 1981). The finding of Campbell and co-workers (1973) of a dramatic reduction in functioning motor units supplying the hand muscles after age 60 suggests that the muscle changes are neural in origin. In contrast to the structural changes, the metabolic potential of muscles, as shown by enzyme activity studies, appears to be well maintained into at least the eighth decade (Aniansson et al., 1981). The reduction in muscle size, particularly affecting fast-twitch fibers, is expressed most dramatically by a progressive reduction in muscle strength (Young et al., 1985) and short-term power output, which falls by about 6 per cent per decade (Makrides et al., 1985); in everyday terms, the reduction in strength is mainly reflected in such activities as stair climbing (Aniansson et al., 1981), activities requiring endurance being less affected. The age-related changes in muscle may be reversed by muscle training (Aniansson and Gustafsson, 1981).

Age-related structural changes in the respiratory system are associated with reductions in a number of physiological functions; between ages 20 and 60 years, vital capacity falls by 19 per cent (Morris et al., 1971), maximum airflow by 17 per cent, and FEV_1 by 30 per cent; these changes, together with reductions in respiratory muscle strength, lead to a fall in breathing capacity of about 30 per cent. Pulmonary vascular resistance doubles (Ehrsam et al., 1983), carbon monoxide transfer capacity falls by 40 per cent, and there is a 15–mm Hg reduction in resting arterial PO_2. The potential effects of these changes on $\dot{V}O_2$max are lessened by the large reserve capacity normally present in the lungs; although the fall in arterial PO_2 potentially reduces oxygen delivery to tissues, the change occurs on the flat part of the oxyhemoglobin dissociation curve, with little change occurring in oxygen content. During exercise, ventilation at a given oxygen intake is a little higher in the elderly, owing to a relative increase in carbon dioxide output and a higher V_D/V_T ratio; with reductions in respiratory muscle strength, these factors contribute to greater breathlessness.

Although heart size increases by about 10 per cent between ages 20 and 60 years, systolic ejection during exercise falls from about 80 per cent to 60 per cent; the normal exercise-related increase in ejection fraction is lost above age 60 years, probably indicating a decline in contractile reserve (Port et al., 1980). These changes account for a fall in maximum stroke volume in exercise of about 20 per cent during this time. Added to this is a reduction in maximum heart rate of about 10 per cent, at a rate of about six beats per decade, to account for a reduction in maximum cardiac output of about 30 per cent. The normal increase in systolic arterial pressure in exercise is magnified with increasing years; at age 20 years, the increase is about 15 mm Hg per L/min increase in $\dot{V}O_2$, but at age 60 years, it amounts to about 35 mm Hg. The mechanisms that underlie the age-related changes in cardiovascular function remain topics for active research; vanBrummelen and colleagues (1981) demonstrated reductions in beta-adrenoceptor responsiveness in both heart (rate and contractility) and peripheral vessels (vasodilation) that may provide a unifying hypothesis for the age-related changes in maximum heart rate, contractility, and blood pressure. Endurance training in elderly subjects is associated with increases in stroke volume and reductions in arterial pressure (Makrides et al., 1986). These changes, occurring over relatively short periods of time and paralleled by increases in muscle size and strength, provide an argument for the dominance of reductions in muscle activity and function in the age-related fall in $\dot{V}O_2$max. In terms of standards for the results of exercise tests, results may be adequately predicted on the basis of age, sex, and height, if necessary, supplemented by information on habitual activity and measurements of lean body mass or thigh muscle volume, as detailed in Chapter 8.

"NORMAL" RESPONSES TO EXERCISE

As with many other physiological techniques, standards in exercise testing have to be examined from a number of divergent standpoints to answer a series of questions. First, is the racial makeup of the population appropriate to the referral population? At first, this question may seem important, but differences between races appear small once stature has been normalized (Miller et al., 1977). Second, is the population as representative of the local population as other laboratory standards, such as for pulmonary function measurements? Often, the subjects of normal population studies have been volunteers or drawn from groups who are particularly active; the results of these studies may be ideal for assessing fitness but may have shortcomings in the assessment of children with cardiac disease, whose $\dot{V}O_2$max may be appropriate to their level of activity and appear low, even in the absence of a cardiac defect. Thus, for clinical applications, there are arguments for the use of the lowest standards, or for making an allowance for the effects of inactivity. Third, to what extent may a regression equation relating $\dot{V}O_2$max to some dimensional independent variable be used as a predictor in a given patient? The point here is that an equation relating $\dot{V}O_2$max to, say, height may have been derived in a population having a skewed distribution of height; thus, it may be used fairly precisely for a subject who is 160 cm tall but may be seriously in error for a subject whose height is 120 cm. Also, as pointed out earlier, there are theoretical arguments against some of the simple linear functions between dimensions and performance characteristics, even when it may be statistically impossible to show that variance is reduced in the population by a more complex function. Unfortunately, the sample size may have been too small to differentiate between such functions. Finally, which independent variable is to be used for the prediction? Of the simple dimensions, height is preferred to weight, but lean body mass (Cotes, 1975; Cunningham et al., 1984) or total hemoglobin content (Ericksson et al., 1971) may be preferable to both; whether the additional expense in making these measurements is justified by the improvement in predictive precision is a question for the clinician and physiologist to answer together. We have taken the view that serious errors are unlikely to be made from the simple relationships, as outlined in Chapter 8.

Studies of submaximal exercise in children have shown that most variables change similarly to those of adults, once allowance has been made for differences in size and the subject's level of activity. Thus, although cardiac output at a given oxygen intake is about 1.0 L/min less in children (Eriksson, 1971), the slope of the relationship is the same as in adults, and the intercept is a function of height (Godfrey et al., 1971); cardiac stroke volume is less, in proportion to (height)^3, and thus heart rate is higher, having an inverse relationship to height (Gadhoke and Jones, 1969; Godfrey et al., 1971); maximum heart rate is higher than in adults. Ventilation increases linearly to oxygen intake, as in adults, the "anaerobic threshold" being reached at an oxygen intake that is related to height (Cooper and Weiler-Ravell, 1984). As in adults, tidal volume and tidal dead-space volume are related to vital capacity (Godfrey et al., 1971) and thus scale to height[3].

WHAT LIMITS EXERCISE?

Up to now, I have studiously avoided this important question. Much has been written on the topic, and arguments have been made, at one time or another, for limitation at some point in the oxygen transport line (heart, lungs, peripheral circulation), in oxygen utilization (muscle biochemistry), in neuromuscular function ("central" and "peripheral" muscle fatigue), or in the control of hydrogen ion concentration in muscle or blood. A case may be made for failure in any of these diverse mechanisms in different exercise conditions, but such is the extent of cooperation and linkage between mechanisms that it is usually impossible to define which is *the* one mechanism that is to blame in limiting an athlete or a patient from going on for any longer. For these reasons, I take an easier path out of this controversial maze and suggest that we need to understand the factors that contribute to limiting symptoms rather than to failure of muscle contraction. When a symptom reaches an unacceptable intensity, the person stops exercising, usually short of catastrophe. In this light, the protective role of symptoms is emphasized; one would have to question the wisdom of the body if we did exercise to the point of respiratory muscle failure, for example! Of course, the extent to which symptoms are tolerated depends on motivation, personality, and other attributes, in addition to the physiological mechanisms considered in this chapter.

The most common symptoms that are identified by both healthy subjects and patients are extreme effort of the limb muscles ("fatigue" or "weakness") or of the respiratory muscles ("dyspnea" or "breathlessness"). These symptoms are analyzed further in Chapter 3, mainly to emphasize the importance of quantifying them routinely by psychophysical techniques during exercise tests. Other symptoms assume importance in certain clinical conditions—chest pain in coronary artery disease, leg pain in arteriosclerosis—and still others in less common situations—faintness in cardiac arrhythmias and other causes of hypotension, focal weakness in neurological disorders.

Rather than dismissing symptoms as subjective and, by implication, worthless, it is better to quantify them whenever possible so that they may be considered in relation to all the other objective measurements that we all accept as important in exercise evaluation.

REFERENCES

Adams FH, Linde LM, Miyake H. The physical working capacity of normal schoolchildren: I. California. Pediatrics 1961;28:55–64.

Ahlborg G, Felig P, Hagenfeldt L, et al. Substrate turnover during prolonged exercise in man. J Clin Invest 1974;53:1080–1090.

Aickin CC, Thomas RC. An investigation of the ionic mechanism of intracellular pH regulation in mouse soleus muscle fibres. J Physiol 1977;273:295–316.

Andersen P, Saltin B. Maximal perfusion of skeletal muscle in man. J Physiol 1985;366:233–249.

Aniansson A, Grimby G, Hedberg M, et al. Muscle morphology, enzyme activity and muscle strength in elderly men and women. Clin Physiol 1981;1:73–86.

Aniansson A, Gustafsson E. Physical training in elderly men with special reference to quadriceps muscle strength and morphology. Clin Physiol 1981;1:87–98.

Åstrand P-O. Experimental Studies of Physical Working Capacity in Relation to Sex and Age. Copenhagen: Munksgaard; 1952.

Åstrand P-O, Hallback I, Hedman R, et al. Blood lactates after prolonged severe exercise. J Appl Physiol 1963;7:218.

Åstrand P-O, Rodahl K. Textbook of Work Physiology, 2nd ed. New York: McGraw-Hill; 1977.

Bannister R. The meaning of physical fitness. Proc R Soc Med 1969;62:1159.

Barcroft H. Circulation in skeletal muscle. In: Hamilton WF, editor. Handbook of Physiology, Vol. 2, Circulation Section II. Washington, DC: American Physiological Society; 1963.

Barcroft J. Features in the Architecture of Physiological Function. London: Cambridge University Press; 1934.

Berglund E, Birath G, Grimby G, et al. Spirometric studies in normal subjects: I. Forced expirograms in subjects between 7 and 70 years of age. Acta Med Scand 1963;173:185–191.

Bergström J, Hermansen L, Hultman E, et al. Diet, muscle glucogen and physical performance. Acta Physiol Scand 1967;71:140–150.

Bessman SP, Carpenter CL. The creatine-creatine phosphate energy shuttle. Annu Rev Biochem 1985;54:831–862.

Bevegård S, Holmgren A, Jonsson B. The effect of body position on the circulation at rest and during exercise with special reference to the influence on the stroke volume. Acta Physiol Scand 1960;49:279–298.

Bevegård S, Holmgren A, Jonsson B. Circulatory studies in well-trained athletes at rest and during heavy exercise with special references to stroke volume and the influence of body position. Acta Physiol Scand 1963;57:26–56.

Bink B, Waffelbakker F. Physical working capacity, at maximum levels of work, of boys 12–18 years of age. Nederlands Instituut voor Praeventieve Geneeskunde, 1968.

Black LF, Hyatt RE. Maximal respiratory pressures: Normal values and relationship to age and sex. Am Rev Respir Dis 1969;99:696–702.

Blimkie CJR, Cunningham DA, Nichol PM. Gas transport capacity and echocardiographically determined cardiac size in children. J Appl Physiol 1980;49:994–999.

Bloom SR, Johnson RH, Park DM, et al. Differences in the metabolic and hormonal response to exercise between racing cyclist and untrained individuals. J Physiol 1976;258:1–18.

Bohr C. Ueber die Lungenathmung. Skand Arch Physiol 1889;2:236–268.

Brooke MH, Kaiser KK. Muscle fiber types: How many and what kind? Arch Neurol 1970;23:369–379.

Brooks GA. The lactate shuttle during exercise and recovery. Med Sci Sports Exerc 1986;18:355–364.

Brooks GA, Mercier J. Balance of carbohydrate and lipid utilization during exercise: The crossover concept. J Appl Physiol 1994;76:2253–2261.

Brown SE, Weiner S, Brown RA. Exercise performance following a carbohydrate load in chronic airflow obstruction. J Appl Physiol 1985;58:1340–1346.

Buick FJ, Gledhill N, Froese AB, et al. Effect of induced erythrocythemia on aerobic work capacity. J Appl Physiol 1980;48:636–642.

Caiozzo VJ, Davis JA, Ellis JF, et al. A comparison of gas exchange indices used to detect the anaerobic threshold. J Appl Physiol 1982;53:1184–1189.

Campbell MJ, McComas AJ, Petito F. Physiological changes in ageing muscles. J Neurol Neurosurg Psychiatry 1973;36:174–182.

Carlson LA, Ekelund L-G, Fröberg SO. Concentration of triglycerides, phospholipids and glycogen in skeletal muscle and of free fatty acids and B-hydroxybutyric acid in blood in man in response to exercise. Eur J Clin Invest 1971;1:248–254.

Cherniack NS, Longobardo GS. Oxygen and carbon dioxide gas stores of the body. Physiol Rev 1970;50:196–243.

Clark TJH, Freedman S, Campbell EJM, et al. The ventilatory capacity of patients with chronic airway obstruction. Clin Sci 1969;36:307–316.

Clode M, Campbell EJM. The relationship between gas exchange and changes in blood lactate concentrations in exercise. Clin Sci 1969;37:263–272.

Connett RJ, Gayeski TEJ, Honig CR. Lactate efflux is unrelated to intracellular PO_2 in a working red muscle in situ. J Appl Physiol 1986;61:402–408.

Cooper DM, Weiler-Ravell D. Gas exchange response to exercise in children. Am Rev Respir Dis 1984;129:S47–S48.

Cotes JE. Lung Function, 3rd ed. Oxford: Blackwell Scientific Publications, 1975, p. 198.

Cumming GR. Hemodynamics of supine bicycle exercise in "normal" children. Am Heart J 1977;93:617–622.

Cumming GR, Friesen W. Bicycle ergometer measurement of maximal oxygen uptake in children. Can J Physiol Pharmacol 1967;45:937–946.

Cunningham DA, Paterson DH, Blimkie CJR, Donner AP. Development of cardiorespiratory function in circumpubertal boys: A longitudinal study. J Appl Physiol 1984;56:302–307.

Cunningham DJC. Some quantitative aspects of the regulation of human respiration in exercise. Br Med Bull 1963;19:25–30.

Davies CTM. Human power output in exercise of short duration in relation to body size and composition. Ergonomics 1971;14:245–256.

Dawson MJ. Energetics and mechanics of skeletal muscle. In: Roussos C, Macklem PT, editors. The Thorax. New York: Marcel Dekker, 1985, pp. 3–43.

Edgerton VR, Roy RR, Gregor RJ, Rugg S. Morphological basis of skeletal muscle power output. In: Jones NL, McCartney N, McComas AJ, editors. Human Muscle Power. Champaign, IL: Human Kinetics Publishers; 1986.

Edhag O, Zetterquist S. Peripheral circulatory adaptation to exercise in restricted cardiac output. Scand J Clin Lab Invest 1968;21:123–135.

Edwards RHT. Human muscle function and fatigue. Ciba Found Symp 1981;82:1–18.

Edwards RHT. Physiological and metabolic studies of the contractile machinery of human muscle in health and disease. Phys Med Biol 1979;24:237–249.

Ehrsam RE, Perruchoud A, Oberholzer M, et al. Influence of age on pulmonary haemodynamics at rest and during supine exercise. Clin Sci 1983;65:653–660.

Ekblom B, Goldbarg AN, Gullbring B. Response to exercise after blood loss and infusion. J Appl Physiol 1972;33:175–180.

Ekblom B, Huot R. Response to submaximal and maximal exercise at different levels of carboxyhemoglobin. Acta Physiol Scand 1972;86:474–482.

Engstrom I, Eriksson BO, Karlberg P, et al. Preliminary report on the development of lung volumes in young girl swimmers. Acta Paediatr Suppl 1971;217:73–76.

Eriksson BO. Cardiac output during exercise in pubertal boys. Acta Paediatr Suppl 1971;217:53–55.

Eriksson BO, Engstrom I, Karlberg P, et al. A physiological analysis of former girl swimmers. Acta Paediatr Suppl 1971;217:68–72.

Farhi LE. Ventilation-perfusion relationship and its role in alveolar gas exchange. In: Caro CG, editor. Advances in Respiratory Physiology. London: Edward Arnold Publishers; 1966, pp. 148–197.

Farhi LE, Rahn H. Dynamics of changes in carbon dioxide stores. Anesthesiology 1960;21:604–614.

Faulkner JA, Heigenhauser GF, Shork A. The cardiac output–oxygen uptake relationship of men during graded bicycle ergometry. Med Science Sport 1977;9:143–147.

Felig P, Wahren J. Amino acid metabolism in exercising man. J Clin Invest 1971;50:2703–2725.

Fitch S, McComas AJ. Influence of human muscle length on fatigue. J Physiol 1985;362:205–213.

Fitting JW, Chartrand DA, Bradley TD, et al. Effect of thoracoabdominal breathing patterns on inspiratory effort sensation. J Appl Physiol 1987;62:1665–1670.

Fitts RH. Cellular mechanisms of muscle fatigue. Physiol Rev 1994;74:49–94.

Fowle ASE, Matthews CME, Campbell EJM. The rapid distribution of ^3H_2O and $^{11}CO_2$ in the body in relation to the immediate carbon dioxide storage capacity. Clin Sci 1964;27:51–65.

Freedman S. Sustained maximum voluntary ventilation. Respir Physiol 1970;8:230–244.

Gadhoke S, Jones NL. The responses to exercise in boys aged 9 to 15. Clin Sci 1969;37:789–801.

Galbo H, Christensen NJ, Holst JJ. Catecholamines and pancreatic hormones during autonomic blockade in exercising man. Acta Phys Scand 1977;101:428–437.

Gayeski TE, Connett RJ, Honig CR. Minimum intracellular PO_2 for maximum cytochrome turnover in red muscle in situ. Am J Physiol 1987;252:H906–H915.

Gladden LB, Yates JW, Stremel RW, Stamford RA. Gas exchange and lactate anaerobic thresholds: Inter- and intraevaluator agreement. J Appl Physiol 1985;58:2082–2089.

Godfrey S, Davies CTM, Wozniak E, et al. Cardio-respiratory response to exercise in normal children. Clin Sci 1971;40:419–431.

Gollnick PD, Armstrong GRB, Saltin B, et al. Effect of training on enzyme activity and fiber composition of human skeletal muscle. J Appl Physiol 1973;34:107–111.

Gordon AM, Huxley AF, Julian FJ. The variation in isometric tension with sarcomere length in vertebrate muscle fibres. J Physiol 1966;184:170–192.

Grimby G, Saltin B, Wilhelmsen L. Pulmonary flow-volume and pressure-volume relationship during submaximal and maximal exercise in young well-trained men. Bull Physiopath Respir 1971;7:157–168.

Grimby G, Stiksa J. Flow-volume curves and breathing patterns during exercise in patients with obstructive lung disease. Scand J Clin Lab Invest 1970;25:303–313.

Groom AC, Ellis CG, Potter RF. Microvascular geometry in relation to modeling oxygen transport in contracted skeletal muscle. Am Rev Respir Dis 1984;129(Suppl S):6–9.

Guz A, Noble MIM, Eisele JH, et al. Experimental results of vagal block in cardiopulmonary disease. In: Porter R, editor. Breathing: Hering-Breuer Centenary Symposium. London: J & A Churchill; 1970.

Hamilton AL, Killian KJ, Summers E, Jones NL. Muscle strength, symptom intensity, and exercise capacity in patients with cardiorespiratory disorders. Am J Respir Crit Care Med 1995;152:2021–2031.

Hansen JE, Sue DY, Wasserman K. Predicted values for clinical exercise testing. Am Rev Respir Dis 1984;129(Suppl S):49–55.

Harris EA, Seelye ER, Whitlock RML. Gas exchange during exercise in healthy people. Clin Sci 1976;51:335–344.

Harris P. Lactic acid and the phlogiston debt. Cardiovasc Res 1969;3:381–390.

Havel RJ. Some influences of the sympathetic nervous system and insulin on mobilization of fat from adipose tissues. Studies of the turnover rates of free fatty acids and glycerol. Ann NY Acad Sci 1965;131:91–101.

Havel RJ, Naimark A, Borchgrevink CF. Turnover rate and oxidation of free fatty acids of blood plasma in man during exercise; studies during continuous infusion of palmitate-I-C^{14}. J Clin Invest 1963;42:1054–1063.

Havel RJ, Pernow B, Jones NL. Uptake and release of free fatty acids and other metabolites in the legs of exercising men. J Appl Physiol 1967;23:90–96.

Henneman E, Somjen G, Carpenter DO. Functional significance of cell size in spinal motoneurons. J Neurophysiol 1965;28:560–580.

Hermansen L, Osnes JB. Blood and muscle pH after maximal exercise in man. J Appl Physiol 1972;32:304–308.

Hesser CM, Matell G. Effect of light and moderate exercise on alveolar-arterial O_2 tension difference in man. Acta Physiol Scand 1965;63:247–256.

Holmgren A. Circulatory changes during muscular work in man. Scand J Clin Lab Invest 1956;8(Suppl 24):1–97.

Honig CR, Odoroff CL, Frierson JL. Capillary recruitment in exercise: Rate, extent, uniformity and relation to blood flow. Am J Physiol 1980;238:H31–42.

Howald H. Malleability of the motor system: Training for maximizing power output. J Exp Biol 1985;115:365–373.

Hultman E, Bergström J, McLennan Anderson N. Breakdown and resynthesis of phosphorylcreatine and adenosine triphosphate in connection with muscular work in man. Scand J Clin Lab Invest 1967;19:56–66.

Hultman E, Sahlin K. Acid-base balance during exercise. Exerc Sport Sci Rev 1980;8:41–127.

Hultman E, Sjöholm HY. Biochemical causes of fatigue. In: Jones NL, McCartney N, McComas AJ, editors. Human Muscle Power. Champaign, IL: Human Kinetics Publishers, 1986, pp. 215–238.

Huxley HE. The crossbridge mechanism of muscular contraction and its implications. J Exp Biol 1985;115:17–30.

Inman MD. The Role of Expiratory Muscle Activity in Ventilation During Exercise. Hamilton, Ontario: McMaster University; 1992, Ph.D. Thesis.

Jones GL, Killian KJ, Summers E, Jones NL. Inspiratory muscle forces and endurance in maximal resistive loading. J Appl Physiol 1985;58:1608–1615.

Jones NL. Hydrogen ion balance during exercise. Clin Sci 1980;59:85–91.

Jones NL. Pulmonary Gas Exchange During Exercise. London: London University; 1964, M.D. Thesis.

Jones NL. Pulmonary gas exchange during exercise in patients with chronic airway obstruction. Clin Sci 1966;31:39–50.

Jones NL. Acid-base physiology. In: Crystal RG, West JB, Barnes PJ, Weibel ER, editors. The Lung: Scientific Foundations. New York: Lippincott-Raven Press; 1997, pp. 1657–1672.

Jones NL, Ehrsam R. The anaerobic threshold. In Terjung RL, editor. Exercise and Sports Science Reviews, Vol. 10. Philadelphia: Franklin Institute; 1982, pp. 49–83.

Jones NL, Goodwin JF. Respiratory function in pulmonary thromboembolic disorders. BMJ 1965;1:1089–1093.

Jones NL, Haddon RWT. Effect of a meal on cardiopulmonary and metabolic changes during exercise. Can J Physiol Pharmacol 1973;51:445–450.

Jones NL, Heigenhauser GJF. Effects of hydrogen ions on metabolism during exercise. In: Lamb DR, Gisolfi CV, editors. Energy Metabolism in Exercise and Sport. Dubuque, IA: Brown and Benchmark, 1992, pp. 107–148.

Jones NL, Heigenhauser GJF, Kuksis A, et al. Fat metabolism in heavy exercise. Clin Sci 1980;59:469–478.

Jones NL, Jones G, Edwards RHT. Exercise tolerance in chronic airway obstruction. Am Rev Respir Dis 1971;103:477–491.

Jones NL, Jurkowski JE. Body carbon dioxide storage capacity in exercise. J Appl Physiol 1979;46:811–815.

Jones NL, Makrides L, Hitchcock C, et al: Normal standards for an incremental progressive cycle ergometer test. Am Rev Respir Dis 1985a;131:700–708.

Jones NL, McCartney N, Graham T, et al. Muscle performance and metabolism in maximal isokinetic cycling at slow and fast speeds. J Appl Physiol 1985b;59:132–136.

Jones NL, McHardy GJR, Naimark A, et al. Physiological dead space and alveolar-arterial gas pressure differences during exercise. Clin Sci 1966;31:19–29.

Jones NL, Rebuck AS. Tidal volume during exercise in patients with diffuse fibrosing alveolitis. Bull Eur Physiopathol Respir 1979;15:321–327.

Jones NL, Summers E, Killian KJ. Influence of age and stature on exercise capacity during incremental cycle ergometry in men and women. Am Rev Respir Dis 1989;140:1373–1380.

Jones NL, Sutton JR, Taylor R, et al. Effect of pH on cardiorespiratory and metabolic responses to exercise. J Appl Physiol 1977;43:959–964.

Jurkowski JE, Jones NL, Walker WC, et al. Ovarian hormonal responses to exercise. J Appl Physiol 1978;44:109–114.

Karlsson J. Lactate and phosphagen concentration in working muscle of man. Acta Physiol Scand Suppl 1971;358:1–72.

Killian KJ, Jones NL. Mechanisms of exertional dyspnea. Clin Chest Med 1994;15:247–257.

Klissouras V. Heritability of adaptive variation. J Appl Physiol 1971;31:338–344.

Kushmerick MJ. Energy balance in muscle contraction: a biochemical approach. Curr Top Bioenerg 1977;6:1–37.

Lange-Anderson K, Shephard RJ, Denolin H, et al. Fundamentals of Exercise Testing. Geneva: World Health Organization; 1971.

Larsson L, Grimby G, Karlsson J. Muscle strength and speed of movement in relation to age and muscle morphology. J Appl Physiol 1979;46:451–456.

LeBlanc J, Nadeau A, Boulay M, et al. Effects of physical training and adiposity on glucose metabolism and ^{125}I-insulin binding. J Appl Physiol 1979;46:235–239.

Lemon PWR, Mullen JP. Effect of initial muscle glycogen levels on protein catabolism during exercise. J Appl Physiol 1980;48:624–629.

Lemon PWR, Nagle FJ. Effects of exercise on protein and amino acid metabolism. Med Sci Sports Exerc 1981;13:141–149.

Lenfant C, Ways P, Aucutt C, et al. Effect of chronic hypoxic hypoxia on the O_2-Hb dissociation curve and respiratory gas transport in man. Respir Physiol 1969;7:7–29.

Levine G, Housley E, MacLeod P, et al. Gas exchange abnormalities in mild bronchitis and asymptomatic asthma. N Engl J Med 1970;282:1277–1282.

Lindinger MI. Origins of $[H^+]$ changes in exercising skeletal muscle. Can J Appl Physiol 1995;20:357–368.

Lindinger MI, McKelvie RS, Heigenhauser GJF. K^+ and Lac^- distribution in humans during and after high-intensity exercise: Role in muscle fatigue attenuation? J Appl Physiol 1995;78:765–777.

MacDougall JD, Ward GR, Sale DG, Sutton JR. Biochemical adaptation of human skeletal muscle to heavy resistance training and immobilization. J Appl Physiol 1977;43:700–703.

Makrides L, Heigenhauser GJF, McCartney N, et al. Maximal short term exercise capacity in healthy subjects aged 15–70 years. Clin Sci 1985;69:197–205.

Makrides L, Heigenhauser GJF, McCartney N, Jones NL. Physical training in young and older healthy subjects. In: Sports Medicine for the Mature Athlete. Indianapolis: Benchmark Press, 1986, pp. 363–372.

Mancini DM. Pulmonary factors limiting exercise capacity in patients with heart failure. Prog Cardiovasc Dis 1995;37:347–370.

Margaria R. Biomechanics and Energetics of Muscular Exercise. Oxford: Clarendon Press; 1976.

Maughan RJ, Watson JS, and Weir J. Strength and cross-sectional area of human skeletal muscle. J Physiol 1983;338:37–49.

McCartney N, Heigenhauser GJF, Jones NL. Power output and

fatigue of human muscle in maximal cycling exercise. J Appl Physiol 1983;55:218–224.

McCartney N, Hicks AL, Martin J, Webber CE. Long-term resistance training in the elderly: Effects on dynamic strength, exercise capacity, muscle, and bone. J Gerontol 1995;50A:B97–B104.

McCartney N, McKelvie RS, Haslam DRS, Jones NL. Usefulness of weightlifting training in improving strength and maximal power in coronary artery disease. Am J Cardiol 1991;67:939–945.

McComas AJ. Human neuromuscular adaptations that accompany changes in activity. Med Sci Sports Exerc 1994;26:1498–1509.

McComas AJ. Neuromuscular Function and Disorders. London: Butterworth, 1977.

McGilvery RW. Biochemistry and Functional Approach, 2nd ed. Philadelphia: WB Saunders Co., 1979.

McHardy GJR. Diffusing capacity and pulmonary gas exchange. Br J Dis Chest 1972;66:1–20.

McHardy GJR, Jones NL, Campbell EJM. Graphical analysis of carbon dioxide transport during exercise. Clin Sci 1967;32:289–298.

McKelvie RS, Lindinger MI, Jones NL, Heigenhauser GJF. Erythrocyte ion regulation across inactive muscle during leg exercise. Can J Physiol Pharmacol 1992;70:1625–1633.

McKelvie RS, Teo KK, McCartney N, et al. Effects of exercise training in patients with congestive heart failure: A critical review. J Am Coll Cardiol 1995;25:789–796.

McParland C, Krishnan B, Wang Y, Gallagher CG. Inspiratory muscle weakness and dyspnea in chronic heart failure. Am Rev Respir Dis 1992;146:467–472.

Miller GJ, Saunders MJ, Gilson RJC, et al. Lung function in healthy boys and girls in Jamaica in relation to ethnic composition, test exercise performance, and habitual physical activity. Thorax 1977;32:486–496.

Molé PA. Exercise metabolism. In: Exercise Medicine: Physiological Principles and Clinical Application. Orlando, FL: Academic Press; 1983, pp. 43–88.

Morris JF, Koski A, Johnson LC. Spirometric standards for healthy non-smoking adults. Am Rev Respir Dis 1971; 103:57–67.

Murray CE, Morgan J. Oxygen exchange, blood, and the circulation: A co-ordinated treatment of the factors involved in oxygen supply on the basis of the diffusion theory. J Biol Chem 1925;65:419–444.

Newsholme EA, Start C. Regulation in Metabolism, 2nd ed. London: John Wiley & Sons; 1977.

Opie LH, Owen P, Thomas M, et al. Coronary sinus lactate measurements in assessment of myocardial ischemia. Am J Cardiol 1973;32:295–305.

Owles WH. Alterations in the lactic acid content of the blood as a result of light exercise and associated changes in the CO_2-combining power of the blood and in the alveolar CO_2 pressure. J Physiol 1930;69:214–237.

Parker JO. The hemodynamic response to exercise in patients with healed myocardial infarction without angina: With observations on the effects of nitroglycerin. Circulation 1967; 36:734–751.

Peachey LD. Excitation-contraction coupling: The link between the surface and the interior of a muscle cell. J Exp Biol 1985;115:91–98.

Pernow B, Havel RJ, Jennings DB. The second wind phenomenon in McArdle's syndrome. Acta Med Scand 1967; 472(Suppl):294–307.

Pernow B, Wahren J, Zetterquist S. Studies on the peripheral circulation and metabolism in man. IV. Oxygen utilization and lactate formation in the legs of healthy young men during strenuous exercise. Acta Physiol Scand 1965;64:289–298.

Peter JB, Barnard RJ, Edgerton VR, et al. Metabolic profiles of three fibre types of skeletal muscle in guinea pigs and rabbits. Biochemistry 1972;77:2626–2633.

Petté D. Metabolic heterogeneity of muscle fibres. J Exp Biol 1985;115:179–189.

Port S, Cobb FR, Coleman E, et al. Effect of age on the response of the left ventricular ejection to exercise. N Engl J Med 1980;303:1133–1137.

Piiper J. Measurement of the gas-exchanging function of the lung. Revision of concepts, quantities and units in gas-exchange physiology. Proc R Soc Med 1973;66:971–980.

Pruett EDR. Plasma insulin concentrations during prolonged work at near maximal oxygen uptake. J Appl Physiol 1970;29:155–158.

Putman CT, Jones NL, Lands LC, et al. Skeletal muscle pyruvate dehydrogenase activity during maximal exercise in humans. Am J Physiol 1995; 269:E458–E468.

Rebuck AS, Jones NL, Campbell EJM. Ventilatory response to exercise and to CO_2 rebreathing in normal subjects. Clin Sci 1973;43:861–867.

Redwood DR, Rosing DR, Epstein SE. Circulatory and symptomatic effects of physical training in patients with coronary-artery disease and angina pectoris. N Engl J Med 1972; 286:959–991.

Rennie MJ, Edwards RHT, Davies CTM, et al. Protein and amino acid turnover during and after exercise. Biochem Soc Trans 1980;8:499–501.

Riley RL, Cournand A. "Ideal" alveolar air and the analysis of ventilation-perfusion relationships in the lungs. J Appl Physiol 1949;1:825–847.

Riley RL, Cournand A. Analysis of factors affecting partial pressures of oxygen and carbon dioxide in gas and blood of lungs: Theory. J Appl Physiol 1951;4:77–101.

Roth DA, Brooks GA. Lactate and pyruvate transport is dominated by a pH gradient-sensitive carrier in rat skeletal muscle sarcolemmal vesicles. Arch Biochem Biophys 1990a;279:386–394.

Roth DA, Brooks GA. Lactate transport is mediated by a membrane-bound carrier in rat skeletal muscle sarcolemmal vesicles. Arch Biochem Biophys 1990b;279:377–385.

Rowell LB. Human cardiovascular adjustments to exercise and thermal stress. Physiol Rev 1974;54:75–159.

Rowell LB. Human Cardiovascular Control. Oxford: Oxford University Press; 1993, pp. 1–500.

Sahlin K. Intracellular pH and energy metabolism in skeletal muscle of man. Acta Physiol Scand 1978;455(Suppl):1–56.

Sale DG. Testing strength and power. In: MacDougall JD, Wenger HA, Green HJ, editors. Physiological Testing of the High-Performance Athlete. Champaign, IL: Human Kinetics Publishers, 1991, pp. 21–106.

Saltin B. Design and performance of muscular systems: Malleability of the system in overcoming limitations: Functional elements. J Exp Biol 1985;115:345–354.

Saltin B, Blomquist B, Mitchell JH, et al. Response to submaximal and maximal exercise after bed rest and training. Circulation 1968;38:Suppl 7.

Saltin B, Rowell LB. Functional adaptations to physical activity and inactivity. Fed Proc 1980;39:1506–1513.

Sannerstedt R, Schroder G, Werkö L. Clinical pharmacology and short-term treatment. Haemodynamic analysis of some principles applied in the treatment of arterial hypertension. In: Gross FL, editor. Antihypertensive Therapy: Principles and Practice. Berlin: Springer-Verlag; 1966.

Schantz P, Billeter R, Henriksson J, Jansson E. Training-induced increase in myofibrillar ATPase intermediate fibers in human skeletal muscle. Muscle Nerve 1982;5:628–636.

Segel N, Hudson WA, Harris P, et al. The circulatory effects of electrically induced changes in ventricular rate at rest and during exercise in complete heart block. J Clin Invest 1964;43:1541–1550.

Shapell SD, Murray JA, Nasser MG, et al. Acute change in hemoglobin affinity for oxygen during angina pectoris. N Engl J Med 1970;282:1219–1224.

Shephard RJ. Oxygen cost of breathing during vigorous exercise. Q J Exp Physiol 1966;51:336–350.

Simon G, Reid L, Tanner JM, et al. Growth of radiologically determined heart diameter, lung width, and lung length from 5–19 years, with standards for clinical use. Arch Dis Child 1972;47:373–381.

Simpson K, Killian KJ, McCartney N, et al. Randomized controlled trial of weightlifting exercise in patients with chronic airflow limitation. Thorax 1992;47:70–75.

Smith EL, Serfass RC, editors. Exercise and Aging. New Jersey: Enslow Publishers; 1981.

Sonnenblick EH, Braunwald E, Williams JF, et al. Effects of exercise on myocardial force-velocity relations in intact unanesthetized man: relative roles of changes in heart rate, sympathetic activity, and ventricular dimensions. J Clin Invest 1965;44:2051–2062.

Spriet LL, Heigenhauser GJF, Jones NL. Endogenous triacylglycerol utilization by rat skeletal muscle during heavy exercise. J Appl Physiol 1986;60:410–415.

Spriet LL, Lindinger MI, McKelvie RS, et al. Muscle glycogenolysis and H^+ concentration during maximal intermittent cycling. J Appl Physiol 1989;66:8–13.

Stewart PA. How to Understand Acid-Base: A Quantitative Acid-Base Primer for Biology and Medicine. New York: Elsevier North-Holland, 1981.

Strandell T. Heart rate, arterial blood lactate concentration and oxygen uptake during exercise in old men compared with young men. Acta Physiol Scand 1964;60:197–216.

Stubbing DG, Pengelly LD, Morse JLC, Jones NL. Pulmonary mechanics during exercise in normal males. J Appl Physiol 1980a;49:506–510.

Stubbing DG, Pengelly LD, Morse JLC, Jones NL. Pulmonary mechanics during exercise in subjects with chronic airflow obstruction. J Appl Physiol 1980b;49:511–515.

Sullivan MJ, Green HJ, Cobb FR. Altered skeletal muscle metabolic response to exercise in chronic heart failure. Relation to skeletal muscle aerobic enzyme activity. Circulation 1991;84:1597–1607.

Sullivan MJ, Green IIJ, Cobb FR. Skeletal muscle biochemistry and histology in ambulatory patients with long-term heart failure. Circulation 1990;81:518–527.

Sutton J, Lazarus L. Growth hormone in exercise: Comparison of physiological and pharmacological stimuli. J Appl Physiol 1976;41:523–527.

Sutton JR, Jones NL, Toews CJ. Growth hormone secretion in acid-base alterations at rest and during exercise. Clin Sci Molec Med 1976;50:241–247.

Taylor CR, Maloiy GMO, Weibel ER, et al. Design of the mammalian respiratory system: III. Scaling maximum aerobic capacity to body mass: Wild and domestic mammals. Respir Physiol 1981;44:25–37.

Tartulier M, Bourret M, Deyrieus F. Pulmonary arterial pressures in normal subjects: Effects of age and exercise. Bull Physiopath Resp 1972;8:1295–1321.

Terjung R. Endocrine responses to exercise. Exerc Sports Sci Rev 1979;7:153–180.

Tharp GD. The role of glucocorticoids in exercise. Med Sci Sports 1975;7:6–11.

Thorstensson A, Larsson L, Tesch P, Karlsson J. Muscle strength and fiber composition in athletes and sedentary men. Med Sci Sports 1977;9:26–30.

Torre-Bueno JR, Wagner PD, Saltzman HA, et al. Diffusion limitation in normal humans during exercise at sea level and simulated altitude. J Appl Physiol 1985;58:989–995.

Trivedi B, Danforth WH. Effect of pH on the kinetics of frog muscle phosphofructokinase. J Biol Chem 1966;241:4110–4114.

vanBrummelen P, Buhler FR, Kiowski W, Amann FW. Age-related changes in cardiac and peripheral vascular responsiveness to isoprenaline: Studies in normal subjects. Clin Sci 1981;60:571–577.

Wade OL, Bishop JM. Cardiac Output and Regional Blood Flow. Oxford: Blackwell Scientific; 1962.

Ward GR, MacDougall JD, Sutton JR, et al. Activation of human muscle pyruvate dehydrogenase with activity and immobilization. Clin Sci 1986;70:207–210.

Wasserman K. The anaerobic threshold measurement to evaluate exercise performance. Am Rev Respir Dis 1984;129:S35–S40.

Wasserman K, Whipp BJ, Koyal SN, et al. Anaerobic threshold and respiratory gas exchange during exercise. J Appl Physiol 1973;35:236–243.

Werkö L. Mitral Valvular Disease. Haemodynamic Studies of the Consequences for the Circulation. Baltimore: Williams & Wilkins, 1964.

West JB. Distribution of gas and blood in the normal lung. Br Med Bull 1963;19:53–58.

Whalen RG. Myosin isoenzymes as molecular markers for muscle physiology. J Exp Biol 1985;115:43–53.

Wilhelmsen L, Selander S, Söderholm B, et al. Recurrent pulmonary embolism. Medicine 1963;42:335–355.

Wilkie DR. Man as a source of mechanical power. Ergonomics 1960;3:1–18.

Wilkie DR. Equations describing power input by humans as a function of duration of exercise. In: Cerretelli P, Whipp BJ, editors. Exercise Bioenergetics and Gas Exchange. New York: Elsevier North-Holland; 1980, pp. 75–80.

Yeh MP, Gardner RM, Adams TD, et al. "Anaerobic threshold": Problems of determination and validation. J Appl Physiol 1983;55:1178–1186.

Young A, Stokes M, Crowe M. The size and strength of the quadriceps muscles of old and young men. Clin Physiol 1985;5:145–154.

Young DR, Shapira J, Forrest R, et al. Model for evaluation of fatty acid metabolism for man during prolonged exercise. J Appl Physiol 1967;23:716–725.

3

Sensory Aspects of Exercise

For many years, exercise physiologists were interested only in the motor aspects of exercise—the ability to generate power, the changes in all the support systems, and the factors contributing to muscular fatigue. Traditionally, exercise capacity and the limiting factors have been assessed physiologically and clinically by measurement of maximal oxygen intake, observation of maximal values of heart rate ("cardiovascular limitation") and ventilatory capacity ("ventilatory limitation"), and measurement of indicators of lactic acid production ("limitation of oxygen delivery"). Interest in the sensations experienced during exercise, and in their intensity, has been recent. In some ways, this is surprising because we all experience a variety of sensations that progressively increase in intensity as we exercise harder. Exercise being a voluntary activity, we stop when the intensity of the sensations becomes unacceptable. For this reason, the intensity of the sensations experienced in exercise becomes interesting in its own right. Of course, in other ways, the lack of interest by physiologists in the sensations is not surprising, because the sensations are often considered to be subjective and by implication subject to bias and not amenable to measurement. The relatively young discipline of psychophysics has developed very rapidly, and it is now clear that sensory intensity may be measured with considerable precision, even in completely naive subjects. Our own experience has led us to adopt sensory measurements as a routine in exercise testing, and they have become a cornerstone in the assessment of capacity and limiting factors. Furthermore, they have uncovered several previously unappreciated factors contributing to disability and handicap in patients with cardiorespiratory disorders. Whereas before investigators were concerned with which system was limiting for maximal exercise, the factors that contribute to the intensity of the limiting symptoms are now sought, and often, a quite different conclusion is reached. For these reasons, this topic was thought to deserve a chapter to itself in this edition.

The measurement of sensory intensity owes much to S.S. Stevens, who through the 1940s to 1970s carried out many studies at Harvard and championed the application of mathematics to sensory events, in spite of considerable opposition from skeptics (Stevens, 1975). In a wider field, the problem reflected the philosophical debate that occupied Wittgenstein and others regarding the question of whether language can be used to describe sensation so as to decide "is A feeling the same sensation as B?" The fundamental process involved in making any measurement is the matching of one continuum (number continuum being one example) to another while conforming to preset rules. The rules and the independent continuum define a "scale." If matching is invariant, reproducible, and responsive and obeys the preset rules, then the scale is valid. The scale may be nominal (able to distinguish one event from another), ordinal (able to rank observations in order of magnitude), interval (able to determine the magnitude of differences between observations, while preserving rank order), and ratio (able to establish relationships between observations in terms of ratios). No theoretical reason exists why any of these direct measurements cannot be applied to any sensation.

By studying a variety of sensations, mainly those evoked by stimuli whose intensity could be accurately measured, such as lifted weights, and the intensities of light and sound, Stevens showed that the sensory intensity evoked by most stimuli did not follow a linear relationship but involved a power function. The sensation magnitude (ψ) was related to the stimulus magnitude (ϕ) raised by an exponent (β) that was unique to the sensory process under study and expressed in what came to be termed "Stevens' Power Law":

$$\psi = \kappa\phi^\beta$$

(the constant κ "depends on units of measurement and is not very interesting" [Stevens, 1975]). For some sensations, the intensity increased exponentially with increasing stimulus; an example is the sensation of effort associated with the lifting of weights. For example, the perception of a lifted weight increases threefold when the physical intensity increases twofold; in this example, $\beta = 1.6$. Stevens and later experimenters validated his psychophysical law and the method of open magnitude scaling he introduced, showing that subjects could reproduce the same ratio relationships when they were asked to adjust the stimulus (open magnitude production) and that the same ratio relationships were consistent across matching continua (cross-modality matching) when they were corrected for their known ratio properties (transitivity). Systematic errors and variability between individuals were identified, but in most circumstances, these factors could be avoided by modification of the experimental design (Stevens, 1971). Although open magnitude scaling was useful, it became apparent that its utility was limited to the study of stimulus parameters within the same individuals. For estimating absolute sensory intensity and for comparing absolute intensity across individuals, open magnitude scaling was of less use.

Category scaling techniques were pragmatically used to achieve these ends before they were understood theoretically. Such scales had defined categories such as slight, mild, moderate, and severe; or numbers from zero to 5, zero to 7, or zero to 10; or a simple line with an infinite number of intervals (visual analogue scale). The use of these scales is based on the premise that sensory intensity varies from the threshold of detection to a functionally defined maximum. Any given intensity lying between these extremes has a locality that can be defined by a point on the line, a number, or a category. In essence, the sensory range is partitioned, but for a given proportional change in physical magnitude, the increase in perceived magnitude is systematically less than that expected (Stevens and Galanter, 1957). Although visual analogue scaling (a type of cross-modality matching) (Mador and Kufel, 1992) is currently popular, its validity in measuring absolute sensory intensity through its ratio properties is severely limited.

Stevens' work was applied to the perception of effort in exercise by the Swedish psychologist Gunnar Borg, who beginning in the late 1950s and through the 1970s progressively developed scaling methods based on a rigorous application of quantitative semantics. He began by applying open magnitude scaling to the sensation of perceived exertion (Borg and Dahlstrom, 1959). As work intensity doubled, the perceived intensity increased threefold, in keeping with Stevens' power law; in this instance

$$\psi = \kappa \, \text{Work}^{1.6}$$

For comparisons of perceived exertion across individuals and across time in the same individual, a scale was required that incorporated absolute magnitude, ranging from zero to maximum, with valid ratio properties. If physical magnitude (work intensity) doubled, perceptual magnitude should increase threefold, in keeping with the known and validated power law. Knowing that both the perceptual range and the physical range were finite, and knowing the ratio properties of the perception, Borg reasoned that it must be possible to construct a valid scale by describing sensory intensity in simple descriptive terms that are universally used, such as "slight," "moderate," and "severe." He empirically studied these properties by defining the average locality in the range of stimulus magnitude from zero to maximum that subjects matched to these sensory descriptors and by establishing the ratio properties of these descriptive terms relative to each other, suspecting that their addition would add a sense of absolute and relative magnitude. Borg then specifically tagged the descriptors to numbers in order to preserve both the absolute intensities and the ratio properties, reasoning that the numbers would be used in a different way from a scale in which the numbers were used on their own (Borg, 1985). Thus, quasi-valid ratio properties could be crudely preserved, an index of absolute magnitude was obtained, and the resulting exponent approximated the exponent found with open magnitude scaling.

The pinnacle of Borg's work (Borg, 1980) was a category scale in which verbal descriptions of intensity were linked to a scale of numbers from zero (no sense of effort) to 10 (maximal effort) (Fig. 3–1). Regardless of whether "valid" ratio properties or properties of absolute intensity were preserved, the power of this scale was in the choice of the numbers related to intensity, which provided ratio properties; an intensity of "4" described as "somewhat severe" represented twice the intensity of "2" or "slight," thus complying with Stevens' law. Some bias, possibly related to previous experi-

0	Nothing at all	
0.5	Very, very slight	(just noticeable)
1	Very slight	
2	Slight	
3	Moderate	
4	Somewhat severe	
5	Severe	
6		
7	Very severe	
8		
9	Very, very severe	(almost maximal)
10	Maximal	

Figure 3–1. The Borg psychophysical scale for measurement of sensory intensity in exercise.

ence or to psychological factors, may influence differences between two individuals, but such differences are small; for example, Borg and his associates have shown that individuals with type A personality scale symptoms less in relation to physiological variables than do those with type B personality (Hassmén et al., 1993). Our own experience with the Borg scale in a cardiac exercise rehabilitation program has shown that some individuals underrate or deny symptom intensity. However, the scale has proved remarkably easy to use in practice and is readily understood by people from a variety of educational and language backgrounds. Although other scaling methods, such as visual analogue scaling, have their supporters, the Borg scale remains the most powerful because of its ratio properties. Its link to the verbal descriptions is also an advantage, in that "moderately severe" effort has a more generally understood meaning than does "7 cm" of effort, for example. Furthermore, the linear scales are unable to provide the ratio properties that Stevens' psychophysical law demands.

SENSATIONS EXPERIENCED DURING EXERCISE

It comes as no surprise that in view of the number of changes occurring at many sites during exercise, many sensory neurons are stimulated and give rise to consciously appreciated sensations or symptoms. Many sensations may be discriminated and reproducibly scaled, but the most useful are those that represent the summation of several mechanisms and are experienced as a sense of effort arising in the active skeletal muscles, of effort in breathing, and of pain (e.g., claudication and angina).

Skeletal Muscle

The conscious initiation of physical exertion activates a motor program, consisting of the activation of motor units and repetitive muscle contraction. The associated increases in muscle metabolism result in increases in oxygen consumption and carbon dioxide and lactic acid production to an extent that is dependent on the achieved power. "Kinesthetic" sensations arising in the moving muscles, tendons, and joints give rise to muscular sensations (McCloskey, 1978), and both central and peripheral mechanisms play roles in the muscle senses. By having subjects match the magnitude of perceived weight using the paired upper limbs, Gandevia and McCloskey (1977b) demonstrated that a weight lifted by a nonfatigued arm was matched to a smaller weight lifted by the fatigued arm. Reasoning that the descending motor commands would vary inversely with the size of the reflexly driven component of the contraction, they also demonstrated that the heaviness of a lifted weight decreased when

vibration reflexes were induced in the agonist and increased with vibration of the antagonist (Gandevia and McCloskey, 1977b). Finally, they went on to show that partial neuromuscular blockade increased the perceived heaviness of lifted weights (Gandevia and McCloskey, 1977a). These studies firmly established the sense of innervation arising from the stimulation of Golgi tendon organs, muscle spindles, and joint receptors and appreciated as sensations of tension, power, and movement.

A more subtle factor involves the responsiveness of the alpha motor neurons to central activation, which may be facilitated by afferent activity from muscle spindles but inhibited by afferent activity from Golgi tendon organs (Matthews, 1982). Also, the stimulation of free nerve endings between the muscle fibers that results from the release of mediators during high-intensity metabolic activity may be an important source of afferent inhibition of the alpha motor neurons (Fock and Mense, 1976). With continued high-intensity activity, the responses of the muscle to alpha motor neuron activity decline, and associated with falls in the intracellular pH (Cooke et al., 1988) and reductions in calcium release are reductions in cross-bridge cycling and impaired motor unit activation (Fuchs et al., 1970). The result is a reduction in the responsiveness of the alpha motor neurons, coupled with a reduction in muscle activation. For the maintenance of power, an increase is required in the central motor command, leading to the addition of a centrally arising sense of effort to the peripherally arising senses of tension and movement (McCloskey et al., 1974).

The sense of effort, representing the conscious awareness of the magnitude of the willed motor command, originated as a philosophical concept but fell out of favor after the recognition of muscular sensory receptors. However, by the 1970s, the sense of effort had re-emerged, with experimental psychophysical studies showing that awareness of the central motor command was essential to explain all the sensations generated by muscular activity. Thus, the activation of the motor program initiated by volition was considered to stimulate small central neurons, acting as central sensory receptors and mediating a conscious sense of effort (Roland, 1978). Through these mechanisms, the sense of effort represents the interplay between many factors—the power developed by the active muscles in relation to their strength, the expression of force-velocity and length-tension characteristics, and the development of impaired neuromuscular function, which prevents the development of the expected or needed contraction: the definition of "fatigue" (Edwards, 1981).

Exertional discomfort appears to be an inherent sensory component of the sense of muscle effort. Discomfort closely follows the sense of effort but is variably related to tension and movement, and maximal effort is experienced with both intense muscular shortening and intense muscular tension. The magnitudes of both shortening and tension depend on the intensity of the motor command and on the nature of the forces opposing shortening. If the forces opposing muscle contraction are substantial, the tension generated is large and muscle shortening is small; if the forces opposing muscle contraction are minimal, the tension generated is small but muscle shortening is large. Although exertional discomfort occurs in both situations, the subject can easily distinguish differences in the sensory consequence, in terms of rate and extent of contraction, with effort being sensed independently of both.

Breathing

Dynamic exercise involving large muscle groups, such as in cycling, is accompanied by large increases in muscle oxygen consumption, carbon dioxide production, and hydrogen ion (H^+) concentration. Reflexes result in respiratory and circulatory increases to meet these homeostatic demands. Although the homeostatic responses are essentially nonvolitional and most are unaccompanied by any sensation (e.g., the peripheral vascular changes), the motor activation of the respiratory muscles results in increases in the frequency, velocity, and extent of their contraction, all of which are consciously sensed. Respiratory muscle tension stimulates Golgi tendon organs, providing a conscious sense of tension. Respiratory muscular contraction stimulates muscle spindles and joint receptors, providing a conscious sense of movement related to breathing volume and flow. Stretch receptor stimulation may lead to a sense of chest tightness. Finally, when chemoreceptor activity increases as a result of increases in P_{CO_2} or decreases in P_{O_2}, an unpleasant urge to breathe occurs, with a sense of satisfaction or satiation when breathing is appropriate to the neurochemical drive (Banzett et al., 1990).

Over the past 30 years, experimental studies have clearly shown that humans can consciously recognize, discriminate, and scale the magnitude of respired volume (Gliner et al., 1981; Stubbing et al., 1981; Wolkove et al., 1982), ventilation, and respiratory pressures (Bakers and Tenney, 1970; Stubbing et al., 1983). They can also accurately sense the magnitude of external (Killian et al., 1981) and internal loads imposed on breathing (Rubinfeld and Pain, 1976; Burdon et al., 1982). These sensations do not require chemoreceptor stimulation and appear to result from the stimulation of muscular receptors and perhaps other mechanisms, such as stretch receptors in the lungs. A contemporary view of dyspnea (Killian and Jones, 1994) incorporates these closely linked mechanisms. As discussed in relation to skeletal muscle, the sense of respiratory effort represents the summation of several effects that are expressed in the central respiratory motor command.

Muscle and Chest Pain

In the early part of this century, Hough (1901) distinguished two types of muscle pain related to exercise, one occurring at the time of exercise and another occurring after a delay and associated with soreness. Pain is experienced in the exercising skeletal muscle in heavy exercise, particularly shortly after heavy work begins, but in incremental exercise, it is not as prominent as the sense of effort, except in clinical (e.g., claudication) and experimental (e.g., vascular occlusion) situations in which muscle blood flow is severely impaired and marked changes occur in intramuscular metabolite and ion concentrations. It is then accompanied by a profound sensation of fatigue. Release of mediators, such as bradykinin and adenosine, and changes in the ionic composition of interstitial fluid with high $[H^+]$ and $[K^+]$ presumably stimulate free nerve endings that mediate pain sensation. This type of pain resolves rapidly when the metabolic and ionic changes resolve. The occurrence of anginal chest pain associated with electrocardiographic and angiographic evidence of impaired coronary blood flow and with rapid clearing when exercise stops suggests that similar mechanisms are active in the myocardium.

The delayed pain and soreness may follow pain experienced at the time of exercise, but it often does not. Asmussen (1956) realized that it was more likely to occur after muscle contractions occurring at the same time that the muscle lengthens—for example, after a mountain descent rather than a climb. Later investigators showed that ultrastructural changes occurred and proposed that mechanical tearing of the sarcolemma and sarcomeres allows calcium, proteases, free radicals, and other toxic metabolic products to injure the muscle (for review, see Armstrong, 1984). This type of muscle pain is not considered further here.

SENSE OF SKELETAL MUSCLE EFFORT

Many studies of perceived effort, assessed by the Borg scale, have been conducted in healthy subjects (Killian, 1992b) (Fig. 3–2). When the measured (Borg) intensity is normalized to the predicted maximum exercise capacity (Wmax), no sense of effort occurs until 20 per cent of Wmax is reached, but at higher loads, a progressive increase in intensity occurs, to a Borg rating of 5 to 9 (''severe'' to ''very, very severe'') at maximum exercise. During incremental cycle ergometric exercise in which the extent of muscle contraction and the pedaling fre-

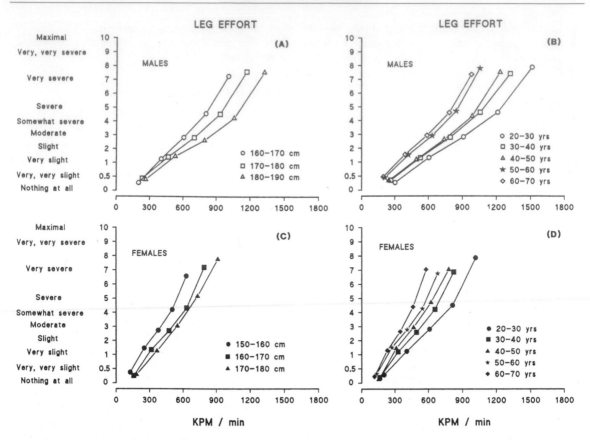

Figure 3–2. Borg rating of leg muscle effort during progressive cycle ergometer exercise to capacity in a large population of normal subjects, males *(top panels)* and females *(lower panels)*, showing influence of height *(A and C)* and age *(B and D)*. (From Killian KJ. Symptoms limiting exercise. In: Jones NL, Killian KJ, editors. Breathlessness. The Campbell Symposium. Burlington, Canada: Boehringer-Ingelheim; 1992b, pp. 132–142.)

quency are held constant, the dominant variables are the tension developed (workload) and muscle strength; as the subject approaches maximum exercise, the changes in muscle ionic state are associated with increasing effort, implying that greater central command is being exerted to produce the given power. A recent study by Hamilton (1995) found that the Borg score was related by power functions to these variables.

$$\text{Effort (Borg)} = 0.0014 \times \%\text{Wmax}^{1.86}$$

The influence of muscle strength on the intensity of effort experienced at any level of exercise was expressed by

$$\text{Effort} = 0.0051 \times W^{1.31} \times QS^{-0.56} \ (r^2 = 0.59)$$

where W is expressed in kilopond-meters per minute and quadriceps strength (QS) in kilograms (Fig. 3–3). Here, a doubling of muscle strength is associated with a 30 per cent reduction in effort. When a given exercise power output is maintained, an in-

crease in effort occurs that shows a power function relationship to time (Kearon et al., 1991) (Fig. 3–4).

$$\text{Effort} = k \times \%\text{Wmax}^{2.13} \times t^{0.39}$$

where k is a constant that varies among individuals, and t is time in minutes.

Thus, the higher the muscle power output, the more rapidly effort increases as exercise is continued. The equation implies that a doubling of power is associated with a 4.4-fold increase in effort and that a doubling of the duration is associated with a 1.3-fold increase.

Not surprisingly, trained individuals show a large shift of the effort-power curve to the right; although the difference between trained and untrained individuals appears small, when expressed in ratio terms, the difference is dramatic. At a power of 50 per cent of predicted exercise capacity, the trained subject experiences half the effort felt by the untrained. This may be explained by higher strength, less lactate and carbon dioxide accumulation, and less change in the ionic state in muscle in trained subjects at any given exercise intensity.

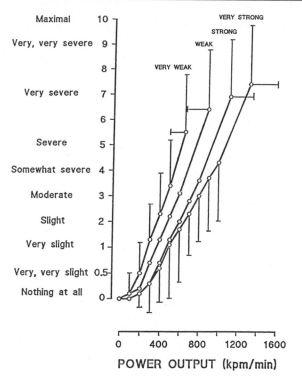

Figure 3–3. Effect of muscle strength on Borg rating of leg muscle effort during progressive exercise in a group of healthy male subjects. (From Hamilton AL. Sensory Limitations to Voluntary Muscular Performance. Hamilton, Ontario: McMaster University; 1995, Ph.D. Thesis.)

Neuromuscular disorders and other conditions associated with muscle weakness lead to an increase in the effort experienced during incremental exercise. Reductions in muscle strength are often found in patients with cardiorespiratory disorders, presum-

ably reflecting the inactivity that usually coexists (Sargeant et al., 1977) and contributing to disability and an increase in effort experienced during daily activities. The prospective measurement of muscle strength in all patients referred for exercise tests in our laboratory allowed Killian to demonstrate that patients with respiratory and cardiac disorders experienced an increase in leg muscle effort compared with that of control subjects that was related to reductions in muscle strength and contributed to reductions in exercise capacity. In patients with respiratory impairment, 30 per cent experienced an intensity of leg muscle effort that was greater than the intensity of breathlessness; this phenomenon provided the reason for stopping further exercise (Killian et al., 1992). In a large group of patients with respiratory impairment, reductions in quadriceps strength contributed to the sensation of effort:

$$\text{Effort} = 0.0040 \times W^{1.28} \times QS^{-0.39} \ (r^2 = 0.59)$$

The clinical importance of these findings was highlighted by trials of specific muscle strengthening exercises, which led to reductions in effort and increases in capacity in patients with respiratory (Simpson et al., 1992) and cardiac disorders (McCartney et al., 1991). These studies have been of great importance, not least for dispelling pejorative attitudes toward many patients who stop exercise at a level that is below that expected by clinicians. Usually, in the past, where a subject undergoing a treadmill cardiac stress test stopped exercising at below the "target" heart rate, the test was termed "submaximal" and thus nondiagnostic or useless, with the implication that insufficient effort had been exerted. Measurement of patients' perception of effort would have shown that to them,

Figure 3–4. Change in sensation of leg muscle fatigue with time, during exercise of constant intensity (four levels corresponding to 33% of maximum exercise capacity *(A)*, 40% *(B)*, 63% *(C)*, and 84% *(D)*. (From Kearon MC, Summers E, Jones NL, Campbell EJM. Effort and dyspnea during work of varying intensity and duration. Eur Respir J 1991;4:917–925.)

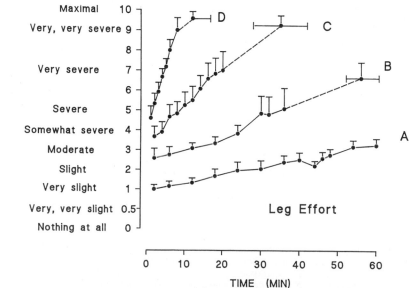

at least, the test was not submaximal. Similarly, in patients being assessed for occupational respiratory disorders, the attainment of a load associated with a ventilation that was less than that expected from spirometry would similarly be judged submaximal, often unfairly.

In cardiac disorders, the net cardiac output may be sustained, but a characteristic feature of increasing cardiac impairment is a reduction in muscular perfusion during exercise (Wilson et al., 1984). Flow to any muscle is dependent on the driving pressure and the resistance of the feeding vessels. Resistance to flow is increased and reductions in systemic pressure also impair ability to autoregulate blood flow relative to the metabolic demands. The reduction in perfusion reduces the responsiveness of the muscles to motor neural stimulation, leading to increased effort, and may be common to both active skeletal muscle and the respiratory muscles. Associated increases in lactate formation may not be related to impaired oxygen supply but to impaired function of muscle oxidative enzymes (Sullivan et al., 1991). Thus, the sense of increased effort in cardiac patients is the result of many factors, not

all of which can be ascribed to impaired cardiac function alone (Wilson and Mancini, 1993; Wilson et al., 1993).

From this discussion, it may be appreciated that the measurement of muscle effort during a clinical exercise test, with comparison to appropriate reference values, provides important information and may reveal limiting factors that were previously unsuspected. A higher effort than expected may then be interpreted in terms of muscle strength; evidence of lactate formation; poor adaptation of muscle gas exchange mechanisms, such as inadequate muscle perfusion; and even muscle metabolic derangements. Examples appear in Chapter 13.

SENSE OF BREATHING EFFORT (DYSPNEA OR BREATHLESSNESS)

Because dyspnea is mainly related to respiratory muscle activity, it might be thought that the factors underlying the effort of breathing are merely the same as those underlying the effort experienced with any other skeletal muscle. Similarly, a measurement of the Borg scale during incremental exer-

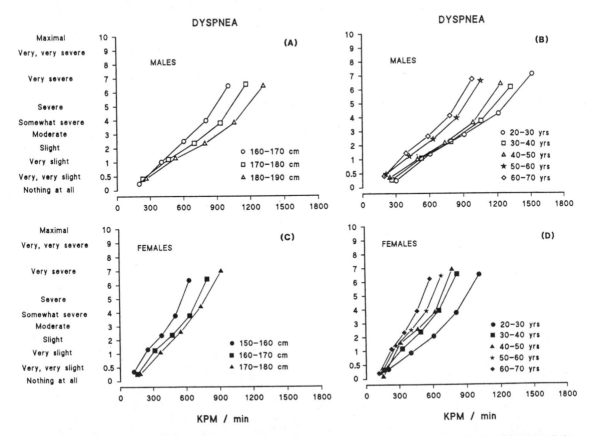

Figure 3–5. Borg rating of effort experienced in breathing during progressive exercise to capacity in a large population of normal subjects, showing effects of height *(A and B)* and age *(B and D)* in males *(upper panels)* and females *(lower panels)*. (From Killian KJ. Symptoms limiting exercise. In: Jones NL, Killian KJ, editors. Breathlessness. The Campbell Symposium. Burlington, Canada: Boehringer-Ingelheim; 1992b, pp. 132–142.)

cise would appear to be sufficient for quantification of the effects of different factors. However, the situation is more complex, which may account for some of the difficulties in explaining dyspnea; indeed, only a few years ago, the difficulties in understanding dyspnea were reviewed in an editorial entitled "The enigma of breathlessness" (1986). First, in contrast to skeletal muscle, respiratory muscle activity is an involuntary response to the metabolic demands of exercise and of reflexes activated by changes in blood and the exercising muscle. Ventilation is further modified by the pattern (frequency and tidal volume) of breathing that may be adopted in response to elastic and resistive impedances to breathing and by the gas exchange efficiency of the lungs, which influences the degree of dead space ventilation and decreases in arterial P_{O_2}. There is a wide range in the tidal volume (reflecting the extent of muscle contraction), the inspiratory flow rate (reflecting the velocity of contraction), and the breathing frequency (reflecting changes in the muscle duty cycle and frequency of contraction); and the end-expiratory volume may vary (reflecting the initial length of the diaphragm). All these factors act through the length-tension and force-velocity characteristics of inspiratory muscles (Grassino, 1992) to influence the force output that accompanies a given central command. To these factors are added the increases in respiratory muscle tension, geared to overcome increases in the impedance to breathing (elastic and flow resistive), and the effects of respiratory muscle weakness.

In progressive cycle ergometer exercise in normal subjects, breathing effort measured by the Borg scale shows a threshold at about 25 per cent of maximal exercise capacity (Wmax), with a steady increase with increasing work up to a Borg scale rating of 6 to 8 (Fig. 3–5), as expressed in the equation

$$\text{Dyspnea} = 0.0058 \times \%\text{Wmax}^{1.44}$$

Within this response, subjects with weaker respiratory muscles report higher ratings for a given power output and ventilation (Fig. 3–6). The interaction between these factors may be expressed by

$$\text{Dyspnea} = 0.0098 \times \text{W}^{1.24} \times \text{MIP}^{-0.58}$$
$$(r = 0.70)$$

where W is in kilopond-meters per minute, and maximal inspiratory pressure (MIP), measured with an occluded airway at functional residual capacity (FRC) (Black and Hyatt, 1969), is in centimeters of water. As with the sense of leg muscle effort, dyspnea increases with the duration as well as the intensity of sustained exercise (Kearon et al., 1991):

$$\text{Dyspnea} = \text{k} \times \%\text{Wmax}^{2.41} \times \text{t}^{0.47}$$

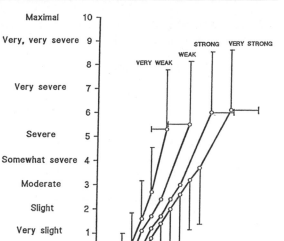

Figure 3–6. Effect of respiratory muscle strength (assessed by maximal inspiratory pressure) on Borg rating of leg muscle effort during progressive exercise in a group of healthy male subjects. (From Hamilton AL. Sensory Limitations to Voluntary Muscular Performance. Hamilton, Ontario: McMaster University; 1995, Ph.D. Thesis.)

Subjects asked to breathe through external resistive and elastic loads show increases in effort that are related both to the higher tension generated in the inspiratory muscles and to changes in the pattern of breathing, which generally appear to be adopted in order to minimize dyspnea (Jones et al., 1984; El-Manshawi et al., 1986).

In cardiac or pulmonary diseases, factors contributing to the effort of breathing include the strength of the inspiratory muscles, the resistance (pressure-flow) and elastance (pressure-volume) opposing the action of the inspiratory muscles, the magnitude of ventilation required to achieve appropriate gas exchange, and often the factors contributing to an excessive ventilation in terms of increases in carbon dioxide production and additional drives to breathe, such as hypoxia or acidemia.

Dyspnea in Respiratory Disorders

Approaches based on an understanding of the physiological principles outlined above have amply demonstrated the contributions of increased impedance to breathing, inefficient ventilatory responses, and reductions in respiratory muscle strength to the intensity of dyspnea experienced by patients with respiratory disorders (Killian, 1992a).

METABOLISM. Patients with severe resistive or elastic loads to breathing show a modest increase in oxygen intake and carbon dioxide output (Jones, 1966), and the latter may also increase as a result of unfitness or a recent meal, thereby contributing to dyspnea in patients who are very limited in their exercise capacity (Brown et al., 1985).

INCREASED VENTILATION. Impaired pulmonary gas exchange with ventilation-perfusion mismatching often increases the V_D/V_T ratio and leads to decreases in arterial P_{O_2} (Jones, 1966), both effects tending to increase $\dot{V}_E$ at a given $\dot{V}_{CO_2}$.

The contributions of an increased V_D/V_T ratio and decreasing P_{O_2} during exercise to the dyspnea of patients with chronic air flow limitation have been demonstrated in numerous studies (Jones et al., 1971; Jones and Berman, 1984; O'Donnell and Webb, 1992). Also, the adaptation to increased loading may include a reduction in tidal volume and an increase in breathing frequency, with an inevitable increase in V_D/V_T and $\dot{V}_E$.

INCREASED AIR FLOW RESISTANCE (Fig. 3–7). Increases in expiratory resistance are associated with prolonged expiratory time and in-

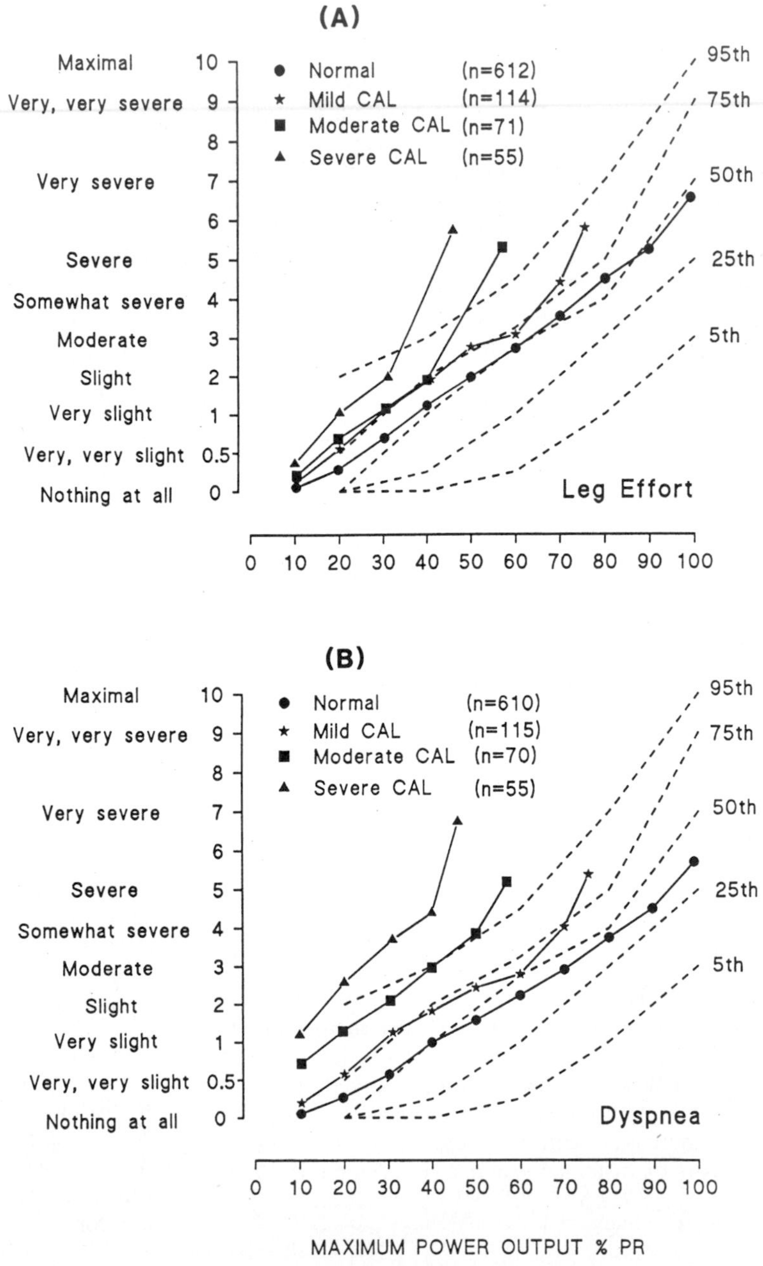

Figure 3–7. Intensity of dyspnea and leg muscle effort in patients with air flow limitation plotted as a function of predicted exercise capacity, showing increases in dyspnea related to reductions in FEV_1. (Mild CAL: FEV_1 of 60–80%; moderate CAL: 40–60%; severe CAL: <40% predicted.) Leg muscle effort is also increased. Also shown are the percentiles of responses in normal individuals. CAL = chronic air flow limitation; PR = predicted. (From Killian KJ. Symptoms limiting exercise. In: Jones NL, Killian KJ, editors. Breathlessness. The Campbell Symposium. Burlington, Canada: Boehringer-Ingelheim; 1992b, pp. 132–142.)

creased end-expiratory lung volume; the first leads to increases in inspiratory flow, and the second, to breathing at a high lung volume and thus to shortened diaphragmatic length. The effort in breathing increases as a result of the generation of higher tensions by the inspiratory muscles and because of higher velocities of contraction and the reductions in muscle length (Killian et al., 1984; Leblanc et al., 1988).

INCREASED ELASTANCE. Patients with stiff lungs or chest cage abnormalities have to generate higher tension for a given VT, and they breathe with a reduced VT and an increased frequency (Burdon et al., 1983). Ventilation is often grossly increased because of inefficient gas exchange, leading to a high VD/VT ratio and a hypoxic drive.

REDUCTION IN RESPIRATORY MUSCLE STRENGTH (Fig. 3–8). The respiratory muscles may be weak because of reductions in static strength, but also because they are contracting at a high lung volume (shortened initial length) with a higher velocity and a greater frequency than that in healthy subjects. Prolonged increases in respiratory muscle work also lead to diaphragmatic fatigue, expressed through an increased respiratory effort at a given V̇E (Gandevia et al., 1981).

INTERACTION BETWEEN DIFFERENT FACTORS. Each of the factors outlined above may contribute to dyspnea in a given patient and to varying extents in different patients. The interaction is complex because some variations in breathing pattern are adopted in order to minimize respiratory muscle tension, and thus dyspnea, even though in comparison with a normal individual, these patients tend to increase the intensity of effort (Jones and Killian, 1991). The validation of psychophysical methods for the measurement of the intensity of dyspnea opened the way for quantitative approaches to the factors contributing to the symptom (Killian, 1985).

In patients with impaired pulmonary function,

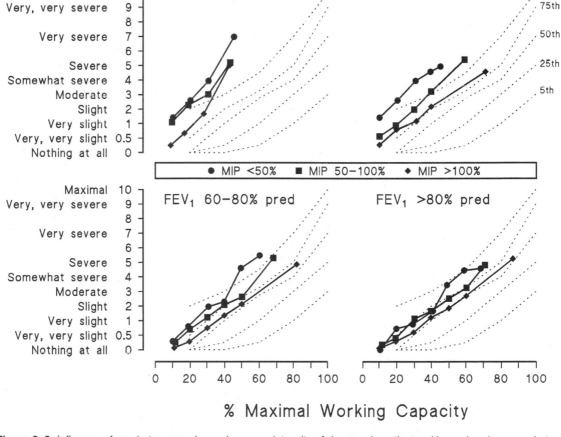

Figure 3–8. Influence of respiratory muscle weakness on intensity of dyspnea in patients with varying degrees of air flow limitation (assessed in terms of FEV₁). MIP = maximum inspiratory pressure; FEV₁ = forced expiratory volume in 1 second; pred = predicted. (From Jones NL. Christie, Meakins and exercise intolerance in chronic airflow limitation. Can Respir J 1996;3:227–234.)

Leblanc and colleagues (1986) were able to quantify dyspnea as a function of increases in respiratory muscle tension (P_{pl}), expressed as a fraction of muscle strength (maximum static inspiratory pressure [MIP]); inspiratory flow ($\dot{V}I$), reflecting the velocity of muscle shortening; tidal volume (V_T) as a ratio of vital capacity (VC), representing the extent of muscle shortening; breathing frequency (f_b); and muscle duty cycle (T_I/T_{tot}). The relationships were of the form

$$\text{Dyspnea (Borg)} = k_1 P_{pl}/\text{MIP} + k_2 \dot{V}I + k_3 V_T/\text{VC} + k_4 f_b + k_5 T_I/T_{tot} + k_6$$

All these factors are well assessed by standard techniques that can be included as part of a routine exercise assessment.

Dyspnea in Patients with Cardiac Disorders

The factors contributing to dyspnea in respiratory patients are relatively well understood compared with those contributing to dyspnea in patients with cardiac disorders. In cardiac disease, dyspnea appears disproportionate to any coexisting respiratory impairment, as reflected in spirometric indices and abnormal blood gas status. Cardiac patients are dyspneic during exercise, even though pulmonary resistance and elastance are often only minimally impaired. However, when studied during exercise, low cardiac output and muscle blood flow are associated with lactate production and large increases in central venous P_{CO_2} and pulmonary carbon dioxide output (Rubin and Brown, 1984). Increases in carbon dioxide output during exercise correlate well with functional classifications of cardiac impairment (Weber et al., 1982) and are associated with large increases in ventilation (Weber et al., 1984), which may be three to four times that in a healthy individual at a comparable workload. These increases are mainly related to increases in carbon dioxide output and an acidemic drive to breathe.

Although spirometry measurements are often little impaired in cardiac patients, such small reductions may be associated with weakness of the respiratory muscles; this weakness contributes to dyspnea (Mancini et al., 1994). Furthermore, the magnitude of inspiratory effort is dependent on the responsiveness of the respiratory muscles to central motor command; reductions in blood flow to the respiratory muscles may lead to fatigue related to the accumulation of metabolic end products. The importance of respiratory muscle weakness in the dyspnea experienced by patients with cardiac failure is highlighted by studies showing a reduction in dyspnea after respiratory muscle strength training (Mancini et al., 1995).

Fluid retention with pulmonary edema and pleu-ral effusions may play a prominent role in cardiac dyspnea as a result of the accompanying changes in the mechanical state of the lungs. In patients with cardiac impairment, pulmonary artery wedge pressure increases during exercise, but the evolution of frank pulmonary edema has not been clearly demonstrated during exercise, although these factors are often cited as the cause of dyspnea (Weber et al., 1984). In pulmonary embolic disease and pulmonary hypertension, a well-recognized inverse relationship exists between alveolar hyperventilation and pulmonary vascular resistance (Jones and Goodwin, 1965), which with an increase in the V_D/V_T ratio leads to a total ventilation that may be as much as three times that expected at a comparable workload. Janicki and colleagues (1982) demonstrated that the increase of $\dot{V}E$ to $\dot{V}CO_2$ during exercise correlates closely with the increase in resting pulmonary vascular resistance in such patients. The additional drives to breathe in pulmonary vascular disorders may include intravascular receptor stimulation (juxtacapillary receptors/c receptors), which is characterized by alveolar hyperventilation.

Although some aspects of dyspnea in cardiorespiratory diseases remain unclear or controversial, many of the contributing factors have been identified. As long ago as 1938, Christie summarized the position as follows: "Though the conditions under which dyspnea occurs are various and manifold, giving rise to an impression of complexity, the fundamental causes are few and relatively simple." We would add that the measurement of dyspnea in routine exercise testing is also relatively simple but helpful in identifying the causes.

INTENSITY OF MUSCLE AND ANGINAL CHEST PAIN

Measurement of pain intensity is difficult because verbal descriptions of pain intensity are less easily anchored to a scale that spans from zero to maximum, and validation by comparison to a physical measurement, such as pressure, is difficult (Edwards, 1981). Within these constraints, the measurement of perceived pain in incremental exercise with the Borg scale shows several interesting features that appear to be consistent between subjects. Perceived muscle pain intensity increases as a power function of 1.67 to the work intensity in cycling exercise; this behavior is similar to perceived effort, but the two sensations are discriminable, and their behavior during constant work rate exercise differs, with pain being more prominent than effort early in exercise. The application of the Borg scale to angina appears to work satisfactorily and was applied by Borg and Linderholm (Borg and Linderholm, 1970) during exercise in patients with coronary artery disease, in whom the severity of pain at a given relative workload could be related to the extent of electrocardiographic changes. Given these findings, the Borg scale applied to chest pain and leg pain is a simple and practical addition to routine exercise testing for angina and claudication.

REFERENCES

Armstrong RB. Mechanisms of exercise-induced delayed onset muscular soreness: A brief review. Med Sci Sports Exerc 1984;16:529–538.

Asmussen E. Observations on experimental muscular soreness. Acta Rheum Scand 1956;2:109–116.

Bakers JHCM, Tenney SM. Perception of some sensations associated with breathing. Respir Physiol 1970;10:85–92.

Banzett RB, Lansing RW, Brown R, et al. 'Air hunger' from increased PCO2 persists after complete neuromuscular block in humans. Respir Physiol 1990;81:1–18.

Black LF, Hyatt RE. Maximal respiratory pressures: Normal values and relationship to age and sex. Am Rev Respir Dis 1969;99:696–702.

Borg G. Psychophysical studies of effort and exertion: Some historical, theoretical and empirical aspects. In: Borg G, Ottoson D, editors. The Perception of Physical Exertion in Physical Work. Proceedings of an International Symposium held at the Wenner-Gren Centre, Stockholm. London: Macmillan Press; 1985, pp. 3–12.

Borg GAV. A category scale with ratio properties for intermodal and interindividual comparisons. In: Geissler HG, Petzold P, editors. Psychophysical Judgment and the Process of Perception. Proceedings of the 22nd International Congress of Psychology. Amsterdam: North-Holland Publishing Co.; 1980, pp. 25–34.

Borg GAV, Dahlstrom H. The perception of muscular work. Nord Med 1959;62:1383–1386.

Borg GAV, Linderholm H. Exercise performance and perceived exertion in patients with coronary insufficiency, arterial hypertension, and vasoregulatory asthenia. Acta Med Scand 1970;187:17–26.

Brown SE, Weiner S, Brown RA. Exercise performance following a carbohydrate load in chronic airflow obstruction. J Appl Physiol 1985;58:1340–1346.

Burdon JGW, Juniper EF, Killian KJ, et al. Perception of breathlessness in asthma. Am Rev Respir Dis 1982;126:825–828.

Burdon JGW, Killian KJ, Jones NL. Pattern of breathing during exercise in patients with interstitial lung disease. Thorax 1983;38:778–784.

Christie R. Dyspnea. Q J Med 1938;7:421–454.

Cooke R, Franks K, Luciani GB, Pate E. The inhibition of rabbit skeletal muscle contraction by hydrogen ions and phosphate. J Physiol (Lond) 1988;395:77–97.

Editorial. The enigma of breathlessness. Lancet 1986;1:891–892.

Edwards RHT. Human muscle function and fatigue. In: Porter R, Whelan J, editors. Human Muscle Fatigue: Physiological Mechanisms. London: Pitman Medical Publishing Co.; 1981, pp. 1 18.

El-Manshawi A, Killian KJ, Summers E, Jones NL. Breathlessness during exercise with and without resistive loading. J Appl Physiol 1986;61:896–905.

Fock S, Mense S. Excitatory effects of 5-hydroxytryptamine, histamine and potassium ions on muscular group IV afferent units: A comparison with bradykinin. Brain Res 1976; 105:459–469.

Fuchs F, Reddy Y, Briggs FN. The interaction of cations with the calcium-binding site of troponin. Biochim Biophys Acta 1970;221:407–409.

Gandevia SC, Killian KJ, Campbell EJM. The effect of respira-

tory muscle fatigue on respiratory sensations. Clin Sci 1981;60:463–466.

Gandevia SC, McCloskey DI. Changes in motor commands, as shown by changes in perceived heaviness, during partial curarization and peripheral muscle anaesthesia in man. J Physiol (Lond) 1977a;272:673–689.

Gandevia SC, McCloskey DI. Sensation of heaviness. Brain 1977b;100:345–354.

Gliner JA, Folinsbee LJ, Horvath SM. Accuracy and precision of matching inspired lung volume. Percept Psychophysics 1981;29:511–515.

Grassino AE. Limits of maximal inspiratory muscle function. In: Jones NL, Killian KJ, editors. Breathlessness. The Campbell Symposium. Burlington, Canada: Boehringer-Ingelheim; 1992, pp. 27–33.

Hamilton AL. Sensory Limitations to Voluntary Muscular Performance. Hamilton, Ontario: McMaster University; 1995, Ph.D. Thesis.

Hassmén P, Stähl R, Borg G. Psychophysiological responses to exercise in type A/B men. Psychosom Med 1993;55:178–184.

Hough T. Ergographic studies in muscular soreness. Am J Physiol 1901;7:76–92.

Janicki JS, Weber KT, Likoff MJ, et al. Exercise pulmonary pressure-flow relations in pulmonary arterial or venous hypertension. Circulation 1982;66:11–48.

Jones GL, Killian KJ, Summers E, et al. Abstract: The sense of effort, oxygen cost and pattern of breathing associated with progressive elastic loading to fatigue. Fed Proc 1984;42:1420.

Jones NL. Pulmonary gas exchange during exercise in patients with chronic airflow obstruction. Clin Sci 1966;31:39 50.

Jones NL, Berman LB. Gas exchange in chronic airflow obstruction. Am Rev Respir Dis 1984;129:S81–S83.

Jones NL, Goodwin JF. Respiratory function in pulmonary thromboembolic disorders. BMJ 1965;1:1089–1093.

Jones NL, Jones G, Edwards RHT. Exercise tolerance in chronic airway obstruction. Am Rev Respir Dis 1971;193:477–491.

Jones NL, Killian KJ. Limitation of exercise in chronic airway obstruction. In: Cherniack NS, editor. Chronic Obstructive Pulmonary Disease. Philadelphia: WB Saunders Co.; 1991, pp.196–206.

Kearon MC, Summers E, Jones NL, Campbell EJM. Effort and dyspnea during work of varying intensity and duration. Eur Respir J 1991;4:917–925.

Killian KJ. The objective measurement of breathlessness. Chest 1985;88:84S–90S.

Killian KJ. The nature of breathlessness and its measurement. In: Jones NL, Killian KJ, editors. Breathlessness. The Campbell Symposium. Burlington, Canada: Boehringer-Ingelheim; 1992a, pp. 74–87.

Killian KJ. Symptoms limiting exercise. In: Jones NL, Killian KJ, editors. Breathlessness. The Campbell Symposium. Burlington, Canada: Boehringer-Ingelheim; 1992b, pp. 132–142.

Killian KJ, Gandevia SC, Summers E, Campbell EJM. Effect of increased lung volume on perception of breathlessness, effort, and tension. J Appl Physiol 1984;57:686–691.

Killian KJ, Jones NL. Mechanisms of exertional dyspnea. Clin Chest Med 1994;15:247–257.

Killian KJ, Mahutte CK, Campbell EJM. Magnitude scaling of externally added loads to breathing. Am Rev Respir Dis 1981;123:12–15.

Killian KJ, Summers E, Jones NL, Campbell EJM. Dyspnea and leg effort during incremental cycle ergometry. Am Rev Respir Dis 1992;145:1339–1345.

Leblanc P, Bowie DM, Summers E, et al. Breathlessness and exercise in patients with cardiorespiratory disease. Am Rev Respir Dis 1986;133:21–25.

Leblanc P, Summers E, Inman MD, et al. Inspiratory muscles during exercise: A problem of supply and demand. J Appl Physiol 1988;64:2482–2489.

Mador MJ, Kufel TJ. Reproducibility of visual analogue scale measurements of dyspnea in patients with chronic obstructive pulmonary disease. Am Rev Respir Dis 1992;146:82–87.

Mancini DM, Henson D, Lamanca J, et al. Benefit of selective respiratory muscle training on exercise capacity in patients with chronic congestive heart failure. Circulation 1995; 91:320–329.

Mancini DM, Henson D, Lamanca J, Levine S. Evidence of reduced respiratory muscle endurance in patients with heart failure. J Am Coll Cardiol 1994;24:972–981.

Matthews PBC. Where does Sherrington's "muscular sense" originate? Muscles, joints, corollary discharges? Annu Rev Neurosci 1982;5:189–218.

McCartney N, McKelvie RS, Haslam DRS, Jones NL. Usefulness of weightlifting training in improving strength and maximal power in coronary artery disease. Am J Cardiol 1991;67:939–945.

McCloskey DI. Kinesthetic sensibility. Physiol Rev 1978; 58:763–820.

McCloskey DI, Ebeling P, Goodwin GM. Estimation of weights and tensions and apparent involvement of a "sense of effort." Exp Neurol 1974;42:220–232.

O'Donnell DE, Webb KA. Breathlessness in patients with severe chronic airflow limitation: Physiologic correlations. Chest 1992;102:824–831.

Roland PE. Sensory feedback to the cerebral cortex during voluntary movement in man. Behav Brain Sci 1978;1:129–171.

Rubin SA, Brown HV. Ventilation and gas exchange during exercise in severe chronic heart failure. Am Rev Respir Dis 1984;129:S63–4.

Rubinfeld AR, Pain MCF. Perception of asthma. Lancet 1976;22:882–884.

Sargeant AJ, Davies CTM, Edwards RHT, et al. Functional and structural changes after disuse of human muscle. Clin Sci Mol Med 1977;52:337–342.

Simpson K, Killian KJ, McCartney N, et al. Randomized controlled trial of weightlifting exercise in patients with chronic airflow limitation. Thorax 1992;47:70–75.

Stevens SS. Issues in psychophysical measurement. Psychol Rev 1971;78:426–450.

Stevens SS. Psychophysics: Introduction to Its Perceptual, Neural, and Social Prospects. New York: John Wiley & Sons; 1975.

Stevens SS, Galanter EH. Ratio scales and category scales for a dozen perceptual continua. J Exp Psychol 1957;54:377–411.

Stubbing DG, Killian KJ, Campbell EJM. The quantification of respiratory sensations by normal subjects. Respir Physiol 1981;44:251–260.

Stubbing DG, Ramsdale EH, Killian KJ, Campbell EJM. Psychophysics of inspiratory muscle force. J Appl Physiol 1983;54:1216–1221.

Sullivan MJ, Green HJ, Cobb FR. Altered skeletal muscle metabolic response to exercise in chronic heart failure: Relation to skeletal muscle aerobic enzyme activity. Circulation 1991;84:1597–1607.

Weber KT, Kinasewitz GT, Janicki JS, Fishman AP. Oxygen utilization and ventilation during exercise in patients with chronic cardiac failure. Circulation 1982;65:1213–1223.

Weber KT, Wilson JR, Janicki JS, Likoff MJ. Exercise testing in the evaluation of the patient with chronic cardiac failure. Am Rev Respir Dis 1984;129:S60–S62.

Wilson JR, Mancini DM. Factors contributing to the exercise limitation of heart-failure. J Am Coll Cardiol 1993;22:A93–A98.

Wilson JR, Mancini DM, Dunkman WB. Exertional fatigue due to skeletal muscle dysfunction in patients with heart failure. Circulation 1993;87:470–475.

Wilson JR, Martin JL, Schwartz D, Ferraro N. Exercise intolerance in patients with chronic heart failure: Role of impaired nutritive flow to skeletal muscle. Circulation 1984;69:1079–1087.

Wolkove N, Altose MD, Kelsen SG, et al. Perception of lung volume and Weber's Law. J Appl Physiol 1982;52:1679–1680.

4

Clinical Uses of Exercise Testing

In Chapter 1, some of the main clinical applications of exercise testing were reviewed—the objective measurement of exercise capacity; the observation of exercise-related symptoms; the measurement of reserve in the systems brought into play by exercise; the identification of diagnostic patterns of response; the exclusion of a previously suspected disorder; the detection of a previously undiagnosed disorder; and the measurement of change occurring over a period of time, either spontaneously or as the result of an intervention. This chapter expands on these applications in various fields of medicine, reviewing the experience that has been gained in the past two or three decades, and sets the scene for later discussions of guidelines for test procedures and measurements.

Until a few years ago, for many clinical conditions, an exercise test evaluated one or two functions that were thought to be responsible for disability, for example, electrocardiographic evidence of myocardial ischemia in coronary artery disease, evidence of lactic acid production as an indication of impaired tissue oxygen delivery in chronic heart failure, and arterial hypoxemia in pulmonary infiltrative disorders. In the past decade, an integrative approach to impaired exercise performance has at last become appreciated. With the realization that exercise involves many systems, exercise tests that provide information related to all the systems have been increasingly applied (Weber et al., 1988; Swedberg, 1994), leading to a great leap in our understanding of the contributing factors. Whereas left ventricular function and oxygen delivery used to be the emphasis in chronic heart failure, for example, we now know that loss of muscle size (Miyagi et al., 1994) and strength (Magnusson et al., 1994), reduction of mitochondrial oxidative enzyme capacity (Wilson, 1995) and other metabolic factors (Arnolda et al., 1990), loss of muscle potassium (Barlow et al., 1994), impairment in the control of the microcirculation (Nakamura et al., 1995), inefficient pulmonary gas exchange (Puri et al., 1995), and weakness in respiratory muscles (Mancini et al., 1994a) may contribute to varying degrees. As well as increasing the value of exercise testing in clinical decision making (Wasserman and Sue, 1991), the new knowledge has led to an in-

creasing use of treatment modalities that a few years ago would have been laughed at, such as weight training (McKelvie et al., 1995) and respiratory muscle training (Mancini et al., 1995), both of which are successfully used in the patient with chronic heart failure. A similar story could be told about patients with chronic obstructive pulmonary disorders, once called ''respiratory cripples''; we now know that they are crippled by more than just severe airway obstruction.

This chapter affords an opportunity to discuss the clinical utility of exercise testing, which is an important consideration in the decision of whether an exercise test is performed in a given clinical situation. As with any investigational technique, it is often difficult to decide on the true value of exercise testing in clinical assessment. Exercise has been applied to many clinical conditions in order to provide information on the pathophysiology, but whether this information is needed for the making of clinical decisions is a question that can be answered only in the context of individual requirements. Ideally, the information should be of direct clinical relevance and should not be readily available from other techniques applied at rest. In this chapter, I try to indicate the value of exercise in these terms, to assist the reader in determining whether exercise might be helpful as well as interesting from a purely physiological point of view. Often, the evidence consists of correlations between the exercise responses and other features of the disease, such as symptom severity or an accepted measurement of impairment. Examples of such correlations are those between maximum exercise capacity and the New York Heart Association grading of disability in heart disease (Weber et al., 1984), or the forced expiratory volume (FEV_1) in chronic airway obstruction (Jones et al., 1971). However, such correlations usually have a large residual variance; sometimes, the value of exercise measurements is in providing explanations for the variability.

OBJECTIVE MEASUREMENT OF EXERCISE CAPACITY

The maximal power and maximal oxygen uptake achieved both reflect the integrated response of all the systems involved in exercise. As such, they are probably the most important measurements obtained from an exercise test. This statement has many implications. First, wherever possible, exercise tests should be performed to a symptom-limited maximal level, or to a point where all the required information has been obtained. Second, the type of test chosen has to be appropriate for the systems under examination; for example, a short test may assess only the muscle component and may not stress oxygen delivery mechanisms. Third, arbitrary definitions of a maximum test are to be avoided; for example, sometimes tests are termed "submaximal" if a predicted maximum heart rate is not reached, even though the patient does not consider it submaximal! Fourth, the assessment of exercise capacity requires adequate standards that enable the responses in a given patient to be compared with those expected were the patient completely healthy; this may be a tall order, but it is dealt with in Chapter 8.

There has been a reluctance to use the maximum achieved power output (Wmax) as a variable reflecting exercise capacity, in some respects because of difficulties inherent in its measurement during exercise involving running or walking, even when the activity is carried out on a treadmill. However, during cycling, exercise power may be calculated with great precision and thus may be used to define capacity; its close relationship to oxygen intake also provides a ready check of gas analysis methods. An emphasis has been placed on maximal oxygen uptake in the past, and sometimes a distinction has been drawn between the maximal oxygen uptake during an incremental exercise test, or "peak" $\dot{V}O_2$, and "true" $\dot{V}O_2max$; this implies that such an entity as maximal $\dot{V}O_2$ exists that presumably represents a value limited by maximal capacity of mechanisms in the oxygen transport line. However, it has become increasingly apparent that the maximal value is very dependent on several factors, including the type of exercise and its duration, the contraction characteristics of the muscles involved (velocity, extent, and duty cycle of contraction), and the extent to which different mechanisms have been recruited. For these reasons, it is preferable to consider the maximal $\dot{V}O_2$ as a variable, the $\dot{V}O_2$ observed under given conditions associated with maximal effort, rather than a limiting value, carrying connotations for what actually limits exercise. However, because of the close relationship between power and $\dot{V}O_2$, the peak $\dot{V}O_2$ is an excellent surrogate for power when power is not precisely known, as, for example, in treadmill exercise.

Maximal oxygen uptake ($\dot{V}O_2max$) may be analyzed in terms of the mechanisms contributing to the oxygen transport line, as outlined in Chapter 2. The finding of a $\dot{V}O_2max$ that is within the normal range predicted for the patient suggests that there is no serious impairment in pulmonary ventilatory and gas exchange mechanisms, in cardiac output and its distribution, or in muscle function. Reductions in $\dot{V}O_2max$ parallel reductions in these functional capacities fairly closely. For example, in patients with myocardial impairment, Weber and associates (1982b) found that a reduction in $\dot{V}O_2max$ to 16 mL/kg/min, or about half of the expected value of 35 mL/kg/min, was associated with a maximum cardiac output of about 14 L/min; further reductions in $\dot{V}O_2max$ to 12 and 8 mL/kg/min were associated with cardiac outputs of 8 and 5.5 L/min, respectively. Thus, in these patients with chronic cardiac failure, the measurement of $\dot{V}O_2max$ provided an accurate indication of the reduction in cardiac capacity.

Another example is afforded by a large study of patients with respiratory disease that was conducted by Killian (1985); multiple correlation analysis showed that significant contributions to reductions in maximum power were made by severity of airflow obstruction and reductions in respiratory muscle strength and pulmonary gas transfer capacity. In this group of patients, exercise capacity assessed the combined effects of impairment in several pulmonary mechanisms.

Measurements of Wmax and $\dot{V}O_2max$ correlate fairly closely with symptomatic limitations in cardiac and respiratory disorders, although a large variability may be encountered in severely disabled subjects. In part, this variability is an expression of the steep left portion of the function curve shown in Figure 1–1.

It is clear that in many conditions, the relationship between reductions in maximal exercise capacity and oxygen uptake and other indices of impairment, such as FEV_1 in airway obstruction or cardiac ejection fraction in heart disease, may be extremely variable. Sometimes this has been interpreted as a weakness of exercise testing, but we would rather use it as an argument for exercise testing's yielding additional information about the total system, which may or may not respond to an impairment by a number of adaptations. Also, because exercise capacity depends on the integrated function between many mechanisms, its measurement may afford an indication of the body's overall capacity to respond to stress. For example, in patients being assessed for major surgery, it may be important to know that the respiratory and cardiac systems are capable of responding normally to exercise (Rigg and Jones, 1978). Smith and colleagues (1984) demonstrated that patients who experienced increased postthoracotomy morbidity also showed a preoperative exercise capacity that was half that found in the patients who experienced no complications.

OBJECTIVE ASSESSMENT OF EXERCISE-RELATED SYMPTOMS

Exercise intolerance is a common complaint that may be difficult to quantify, owing to the many factors that influence the reporting of symptoms by patients. Exercise testing provides an opportunity to observe patients performing a standardized amount of exercise and to obtain their assessment of symptom intensity. It is often held that this is the most unreliable part of an exercise test and that patients "cannot be trusted" in their reporting of symptoms; however, to the patient, the symptom is the most important expression of the strain imposed both by an illness and by the test. Our experience has been that if care is taken to obtain a rating of symptom intensity while the test is going on, the information is made more reliable. The importance of limiting symptoms in exercise and of their measurement (Stevens, 1971) is reviewed in Chapter 3, and is only briefly reiterated here.

In healthy subjects, Borg scale ratings (Borg, 1982) for dyspnea and leg effort during incremental cycle ergometry show a threshold at 20 to 30 per cent of maximum power, followed by a linear increase in the numerical rating for intensity of both symptoms. Leg effort usually leads dyspnea by one point on the scale; at maximum exercise, most healthy subjects rate leg effort at 7 to 10 and dyspnea at 6 to 8. In respiratory patients, the reverse is the case; with increasing respiratory impairment, the threshold for dyspnea is lost and the slope increases; at maximum exercise, dyspnea may be rated at 6 to 10, and leg effort may be as low as 2 to 5. The Borg ratings obtained during an exercise test may be compared with normal standards expressed in relation to the percentage of predicted maximum power.

MUSCLE EFFORT. The physiological basis for relating the sense of effort to the force achieved in muscle contraction has been well established by studies in healthy subjects during exercise (Ekblom and Goldbarg, 1971) and undergoing local anesthesia or partial curarization (Gandevia and McCloskey, 1977). Because weakness is defined as difficulty or failure to generate a force, and fatigue as difficulty or failure to maintain a given force, the underlying mechanisms may be situated anywhere between the brain and the muscle mitochondrium or may be related to impaired oxygen or substrate supply. Surprisingly, until recently, there was little attempt to quantify the sensation and the accompanying reductions in functional capacity as part of clinical evaluation. However, an objective measurement of maximum exercise capacity and the associated sense of muscle effort help to identify patients who may require further investigation and to iden-

tify the contributory mechanisms. A reduced maximum power, together with a high rating for muscle effort, suggests that muscle is the site of the final breakdown in the exercise responses. If there are no indications of a cardiorespiratory limitation, a primary neuromuscular disorder should be considered. Measurements of muscle size and strength and studies of short-term power output and electrically stimulated contractions are informative in this type of problem (Edwards, 1982).

The measurement of power and effort in exercise is helpful for follow-up of a patient undergoing treatment for a neuromuscular disorder (Edwards, 1982) or for a patient undergoing occupational assessments (Garg and Saxena, 1979).

DYSPNEA. If there is one absolute indication for exercise testing, it is to quantify and elucidate the mechanisms contributing to dyspnea. Pulmonary function tests carried out at rest are notoriously disappointing in explaining dyspnea, leading to the concept of "inappropriate" dyspnea (Burns and Howell, 1969), in which a major contributory factor is taken to be the patient's psychological status. Exercise testing reduces the number of inappropriate responses and may be helpful in formulating a clinical approach; a valuable benefit is the explanation to the patient of the factors contributing to the sensation, which, in our experience, are seldom purely psychogenic.

Dyspnea may be most usefully defined as an increased sense of respiratory effort (Means, 1924; Killian, 1985). In the past, attempts have been made to explain dyspnea in terms of the respiratory muscle work or the oxygen consumption of respiratory muscles. Both of these concepts are inadequate because no account is taken of respiratory muscle strength and of the effects of the extent and rate of contraction on the muscles' capacity to accomplish work or increase oxygen consumption. If, instead, dyspnea is defined in terms of respiratory muscle effort, the sensation may be considered analogous to the sense of effort in other skeletal muscles and may be analyzed in terms of the tension generated in relation to the maximum tension-generating capacity. A similar approach may then be taken to both sensations, with the inspiratory muscles being considered as a special case. Similar methods may be used to rate the perception of effort, an approach established on the basis of several studies in healthy subjects exercising with respiratory loads (Killian, 1985) and in patients (Leblanc et al., 1986).

The analysis of the exercise responses in dyspneic patients may be more complex than that in patients who present with muscle fatigue because in most patients, several factors contribute to the sense of respiratory effort (Killian and Jones, 1984). Given a patient who stops exercise at a reduced power output with a high rating for respiratory effort, the following factors can be systematically examined.

1. *Ventilatory demands of exercise.* Ventilation in exercise is the end result of several processes—metabolic carbon dioxide production, both aerobic and anaerobic; respiratory control mechanisms (Jones, 1976), which influence alveolar ventilation; and pulmonary gas exchange, which influences the dead space–tidal volume ratio. Thus, in many patients with cardiac and pulmonary disorders, an increase in pulmonary ventilation at a given exercise level is a major contributing factor to dyspnea.

2. *Impedance to breathing.* Elastic and resistive components that impede the ability to achieve the required ventilation during exercise may be assessed through measurements of the mechanics of breathing. However, in terms of their effect on exercise performance, the vital capacity—representing the capacity to generate a tidal volume—and maximal inspiratory flow—representing the capacity to shorten the inspiratory time—are usually sufficient for identifying the situations in which the ventilatory capacity is encroached on by the ventilatory demands of exercise. The part played by these factors in pulmonary disorders is usually fairly obvious; in cardiac disease it may be subtler, but a small tidal volume during exercise may be an indication of subclinical pulmonary edema. In a small number of problem patients, measurement of esophageal pressures for the quantification of impedance may be justified.

3. *Strength of the inspiratory muscles.* Although inspiratory muscle strength may be easily assessed by the measurement of the maximum inspiratory pressure generated against an occluded airway, the operating characteristics of the respiratory muscles also have to be considered in terms of their length-tension and force-velocity properties. As in any skeletal muscle, the maximum tension that may be generated falls with increasing shortening (larger tidal volume) and increasing velocity of contraction (increasing inspiratory flow rates). Whereas we may control these characteristics for skeletal muscles during a test by standardizing pedal frequency and saddle height on a cycle ergometer, for respiratory muscles, they are set by the patient and thus need to be taken into account.

4. *Pattern of breathing.* The pattern of breathing in terms of tidal volume, frequency, inspiratory time, and the duty cycle (T_I/T_{tot}) all contribute to defining the operating characteristics of the respiratory muscles. Thus V_T is an index of respiratory shortening; f_b, of frequency of contraction; T_I, of contraction duration; V_T/T_I, of the contraction velocity; and T_I/T_{tot}, of the duty cycle of the inspiratory muscles. These measures are easily made during an exercise test and may be shown to contribute significantly to the sensation of dyspnea in patients with a wide variety of disorders (Killian, 1985).

The linkage between these factors often leads to several contributions to dyspnea (Leblanc et al., 1986); the most severely dyspneic patients usually have an increased $\dot{V}_E$ during exercise, an increased impedance to breathing, and weak respiratory muscles. This setting reinforces the need to take an integrative approach to the interpretation of exercise test results in order to identify all the contributing factors. Although these factors are most obvious in patients with respiratory disorders, patients with cardiovascular or neuromuscular disorders are often referred for the investigation of dyspnea; an analysis of the exercise responses is usually helpful in resolving what may be a confusing clinical problem. A number of the clinical examples presented in Chapter 13 illustrate this general principle.

CHEST PAIN. In terms of total number of exercise tests carried out in clinical investigation, chest pain exceeds all other indications by several orders of magnitude. This huge clinical usage is paralleled by the volume of published literature on the use of exercise testing in diagnosing and assessing the severity of coronary artery disease. Even a limited review of this work is liable to leave the reader confused by the polar extremes of the conclusions that have been drawn—that exercise tests are so insensitive and nonspecific as to be clinically useless, through to claims of virtual 100 per cent sensitivity and specificity (Hollenberg et al., 1985). The wide spectrum of conclusions may be explained by a number of factors. First, the independent measure of disease in the best designed studies has been the arterial caliber by coronary angiography; this is subject to variation and observer error and is only variably related to coronary arterial flow. Second, the selection of subjects for study has not been uniform; the differences in prevalence of disease in the study populations have to be considered. Third, the diagnostic criteria have varied. Finally, several new approaches, advocated for improving diagnostic accuracy, have not been compared with the current best alternatives. Agreement has not been reached in the cardiological literature (Sheffield, 1985), but a statement by the American Heart Association presents a consensus (Fletcher et al., 1995).

The clinical characteristics of anginal pain are well known, and its observation and quantitation during a progressive symptom-limited exercise test add to the diagnostic information. Borg and his colleagues have used his scale successfully for this purpose (Borg and Linderholm, 1970; Sylven et al., 1991), and the information may be used for many purposes, including the assessment of disease severity, indications for intervention, and measures of outcome and prognosis (Mark et al., 1991).

The electrocardiographic criteria and interpretation are discussed in Chapter 7. The recent statement from a working party of the American Heart Association provides a useful summary of the use of exercise testing in cardiological investigation (Fletcher et al., 1995). It is clear that a number of factors related to the testing procedure are important if valid clinical information is to be obtained: the exercise must involve large muscle groups; power output must be incremented gradually; the test stops when a symptom-limited maximum output is reached or when the observer decides either that it is unsafe to continue or that all the necessary information has been obtained; a quantitative measure of maximum power is obtained ($\dot{V}O_2max$, maximal cycle ergometer output, or treadmill speed and grade) (Hollenberg et al., 1980); and observations of heart rate, electrocardiogram, blood pressure, and chest pain intensity are regularly obtained during the test.

In the same way that a quantitative assessment of dyspnea and muscle effort during the test is helpful in evaluating other exercise-related symptoms, a grading scale for angina may be helpful in quantifying severity and classifying chest pain into typical angina, probable angina, and nonanginal categories. The Borg scale may be used for this purpose (Borg and Linderholm, 1970).

EVALUATION OF CARDIAC FUNCTION

An adequate clinical assessment of cardiac function cannot be made at rest; the evaluation of symptoms, signs, and resting investigations, however invasive, leaves much to be desired in any but the most impaired functional state (Franciosa et al., 1981). The information gained from a progressive incremental exercise test conducted to a symptom-limited maximum level is precise, reproducible, and easily obtained. Even simple noninvasive measurements afford quantitative insights into ventricular performance, valve adequacy, structural defects, and control of cardiac rate and peripheral vascular function. Basic measurements are those of maximum power and oxygen intake, defined as a percentage of that expected for the age, sex, size, and activity of the person, and the responses (through increasing exercise intensity) of heart rate and rhythm and systemic arterial pressure, electrocardiographic parameters, and ventilation. These measurements may be supplemented, where necessary, with more complex measurements of cardiac output and ventricular volumes that are made in steady-state exercise at a known proportion of the previously established maximum capacity.

MAXIMUM CARDIAC OUTPUT, STROKE VOLUME, AND VENTRICULAR FUNCTION.

There are many clinical situations in which objective measurements of cardiac reserve may be helpful in establishing a diagnosis, assessing severity of disease, deciding the place of therapeutic measures, and generally in advising patients regarding occupational and work-related stress. Cardiac reserve is used in this context to denote the ability of the cardiac output to increase from rest values to meet the oxygen demands of exercise.

The variables influencing oxygen delivery to muscles may be expressed in terms of the Fick equation:

Oxygen uptake = cardiac output × arteriovenous O_2 difference

$$\dot{V}O_2 = \dot{Q} \times (CaO_2 - C\bar{v}O_2)$$

Because cardiac output is the product of stroke volume and cardiac frequency, the equation may also be written as follows:

$$\dot{V}O_2 = (V_S \times f_c)(CaO_2 - C\bar{v}O_2)$$

Thus, the maximum ability to supply exercising muscles with oxygen depends on maximum values for stroke volume and cardiac frequency and maximum extraction of oxygen by tissues.

It might be expected that low stroke volume or low cardiac frequency is always associated with a low cardiac output at any given oxygen uptake. However, for several reasons, cardiac output at a given oxygen intake is seldom grossly reduced in patients with cardiac disease. First, an increase in heart rate may compensate for a limited stroke volume if venous return and the mean circulatory pressure are maintained (Smith et al., 1976). Second, given a healthy myocardium, an increase in stroke volume may compensate for a low frequency, as a result of, for example, complete heart block.

Third, there is a limit to which an increase in the arteriovenous oxygen difference may compensate for a low cardiac output, owing to the necessity to perfuse organs such as brain, liver, and kidneys, which are high-flow, low-oxygen-extraction systems. Because normal subjects during exercise are capable of extracting a large proportion of the oxygen delivered to muscle, it is difficult for a cardiac patient to adapt much more by increasing extraction. Therefore, the limits imposed on frequency or stroke volume adaptations mean that the *maximum* cardiac output is characteristically reduced by cardiac disease and thus limits maximum oxygen uptake.

An example illustrates these points. In a patient whose maximum cardiac output is 10 L/min and who requires a flow of 4 L/min to nonmuscular essential tissues, only 6 L/min is available to supply extra oxygen to muscle in exercise. Even if we assume a maximum extraction of oxygen from blood flowing through muscle of 200 mL/L (the oxygen capacity of arterial blood), an oxygen uptake of only 1200 mL/min of oxygen above resting values, or about 1400 mL/min in total, is possible. Because the lower limit of the normal cardiac output at an oxygen intake of 1400 mL/min is 10.4 L/min, the cardiac output in the patient is only marginally low. However, because 10 L/min is the patient's *maximum* cardiac output, as opposed to 25 or more liters per minute in a normal subject, there is considerable impairment in cardiac reserve.

This reasoning, based on Fick's principle, lies behind the use of exercise in testing cardiac reserve in any cardiac disease. Significant cardiac disease reduces maximum oxygen uptake and maximum cardiac output but may not reduce the cardiac output much at a given submaximal oxygen uptake.

A number of conclusions follow. First, a patient who achieves a normal maximum oxygen uptake with a normal cardiac frequency response also has a normal cardiac output and stroke volume. Second, measurement of the cardiac frequency response to increasing oxygen uptake yields information on the stroke volume. By the Fick principle

$$\dot{V}_{O_2} \div f_c = V_s \times (CaO_2 - C\bar{v}O_2).$$

Thus, for a given value of $\dot{V}_{O_2}/f_c$ (the "oxygen pulse"), limits may be set for V_s by assuming a value for the arteriovenous oxygen difference. Finally, in many clinical situations, it is possible to obtain a measure of the cardiac reserve without measuring cardiac output directly.

Clinically useful information regarding cardiac reserve may be obtained through exercise testing in most categories of cardiac disease and is briefly reviewed below.

If myocardial contractility is impaired, as in congestive cardiomyopathy or complicating coronary artery disease, low stroke volume is the rule, and sometimes impaired cardiac rates are found, leading to a severe impairment of exercise capacity. A limited cardiac output response is associated with a reduction in maximal oxygen uptake, usually accompanied by evidence of muscle anaerobic metabolism, which can be recognized through an increase in blood lactate concentration or, indirectly, through an increase in carbon dioxide output and ventilation (see below). This is one reason for the measurement of ventilation in all exercise tests.

Poor myocardial function, in addition to reducing maximum cardiac output and stroke volume, also usually impairs the systolic arterial pressure response to exercise. Because arterial pressure at a given exercise level increases with increasing age, measurements need to be normalized for this effect, but once this revision has been carried out, the peak pressure may be used as one index of contractility (Bruce, 1977). The techniques of nuclear angiography (Jones RH et al., 1981) and echocardiography (Sugushita et al., 1983) have been used to measure ejection fraction and stroke volume in a number of conditions; although at first sight these measurements are more "direct" reflections of ventricular function, the technical demands are great and the information content is similar to that obtained from maximal oxygen intake, heart rate, and arterial pressure.

ANAEROBIC THRESHOLD. Conceptually, the anaerobic threshold is the exercise intensity at which the body's oxygen requirements cannot be met by the oxygen transport systems. Practically, it is measured by identifying the oxygen intake at which the first evidence of lactate accumulation appears, either by measuring plasma lactate or ventilation during an incremental exercise test (Caiozzo et al., 1982). Although one may criticize the overliteral interpretation of an anaerobic threshold, and although there is argument regarding the precision of its measurement (Jones and Ehrsam, 1982), some authors have enthusiastically endorsed its use in the functional assessment of cardiac reserve (Matsumara et al., 1983; Lipkin et al., 1985; Weber and Janicki, 1985). Because the prediction of the threshold in normal subjects is much less precise than that of maximal oxygen intake (see Chapter 8), the two measurements should be considered complementary to each other. Certainly it is helpful to identify whether lactate production has occurred in a patient whose $\dot{V}_{O_2}$max is low and in whom other conventional indications of a maximal cardiac adaptation, such as a maximal heart rate, have not been identified (Powles et al., 1979). However, there is mounting evidence that the appearance of the lactate threshold at a low workload does not imply cardiovascular dysfunction. Studies using the technique of magnetic resonance spectroscopy to measure myoglobin-bound oxygen content in working muscle demonstrated that lactate production may occur without any evidence of oxygen lack in patients with heart failure (Mancini et al., 1994b; Yamabe et al., 1994). The recent demonstration of changes in muscle mass, strength, and metabolic function is an indication of the importance of evaluating muscle function in such patients (Sullivan et al., 1990; Minotti et al., 1991; Wilson, 1995).

CARDIAC RATE. Up to this point, we have viewed cardiac frequency as a mechanism for increasing cardiac output and maintaining cardiac output in the face of a limited stroke volume. Primary impairment of cardiac rate may occur in a number of conditions—ischemic heart disease (Ellestad and Wan, 1975; Powles et al., 1979), complete heart block (Segel et al., 1964), and impaired function of the autonomic nervous system. The impairment of cardiac frequency control is well reflected in the response of cardiac rate to increasing exercise. Exercise may also be helpful in assessing the extent to which cardiac rate is inhibited by beta blockade. The overall response to exercise in the patient with a low-frequency response chiefly depends on the extent to which ventricular volumes and myocardial contractility adapt to increase stroke volume. In a young subject with congenital heart block, stroke volume may rise to well above 200 mL, and cardiac output is maintained (Segel et al., 1964). In a patient with chronotropic incompetence owing to ischemic heart disease, stroke volume may not be able to increase much because of poor myocardial function, and a low cardiac rate contributes to a low cardiac output.

CARDIAC ACCELERATION. To be able to meet the demands of heavy exercise that begins suddenly—for example, in climbing stairs—the cardiac rate has to increase rapidly, or an oxygen deficit occurs. Patients with ischemic and valvular heart disease may not be able to achieve this increase, even though cardiac output is adequate if the high-intensity exercise is approached slowly enough for the adaptation to be completed. Studies of the transient responses at the onset of exercise have shown that patients may adapt very slowly (Auchincloss et al., 1974); sometimes, studies of this type may help to explain breathlessness that is experienced in short-duration, high-level activity alone (Zimmerman et al., 1982). In a standardized incremental cycle ergometer exercise test, such delays are evidenced by a smaller increment in $\dot{V}o_2$ than is expected for the increments in power (Sietsema et al., 1994; Cross and Higginbotham, 1995) and are accompanied often by a greater than expected $\dot{V}co_2$.

CARDIAC RHYTHM. Exercise may be used to provoke and study some cardiac arrhythmias, the most common being ventricular ectopic beats. Crawford and associates (1974) compared the incidence of ventricular premature beats during exercise testing with that during ambulatory monitoring over a period of 10 to 12 hours and showed that exercise testing had a predictive value of 84 per cent. A lesser predictive value was obtained by Ryan and colleagues (1975), who used 24-hour monitoring for arrhythmia detection. Exercise testing is helpful in the Wolff-Parkinson-White syndrome in that it can identify patients at risk of paroxysmal tachycardia (Levy et al., 1979). Examples of other exercise-related arrhythmias are given in Chapter 7.

PERIPHERAL VASCULAR FUNCTION. Delivery of arterial blood to exercising muscle depends on efficient peripheral distribution mediated by a decrease in the resistance of muscle blood vessels and by an increase in systemic arterial pressure. Patients with cardiac disease, particularly if myocardial function is depressed, may be unable to increase arterial pressure and thus adequately perfuse active muscles in heavy exercise. In addition, a number of clinical conditions may interfere with the peripheral vasculature, and exercise may be an important tool in the assessment of muscle flow. Patients with congestive heart failure exhibit abnormalities in the autonomic regulation of peripheral vasodilation during exercise (Nakamura et al., 1995).

Also, the maintenance of normal left ventricular function is in part dependent on a well-maintained ventricular afterload. Thus, patients who are unable to control vascular resistance effectively are in double jeopardy from poor distribution of blood flow and low stroke volume; vasoregulatory asthenia (Levander-Lindgren and Ek, 1962) and diabetic neuropathy are two of many conditions in which this may occur (Thulesius, 1976). Where there is also a neuropathic defect of heart rate regulation, as in the Shy-Drager syndrome, the reduction in exercise capacity is devastating. In all these conditions, an exercise assessment is an essential part of the clinical work-up.

PULMONARY FUNCTION DURING EXERCISE IN CARDIAC DISORDERS. The strain imposed on the lungs by the combination of increased metabolic demands, poor pulmonary blood flow distribution, and increased pulmonary vascular pressures in patients with cardiac disease has been recognized for many years (Harrison and Pilcher, 1930) and is one reason why measurement of the respiratory responses to exercise may be helpful in their assessment (Mancini, 1995). There is an increased ventilatory response, shown as an increase in the slope of $\dot{V}E/\dot{V}O_2$ and $\dot{V}E/\dot{V}CO_2$ with progressive cardiac impairment (Weber et al., 1984; Sullivan et al., 1988), together with a reduction in alveolar-capillary diffusing capacity. Reductions in lung compliance (Evans et al., 1995) and respiratory muscle weakness (Hammond et al., 1990; McParland et al., 1992; Mancini et al., 1995) may also contribute to dyspnea in cardiac patients.

MUSCLE FUNCTION IN CARDIAC DISORDERS. In any chronic condition associated with exercise-induced symptoms, a progressive decrease in skeletal muscle mass, strength, capillary density, and metabolic function occurs. In cardiac patients, these changes are reflected in a reduction in muscle strength (Jones and McCartney, 1986; Magnusson et al., 1994), evidence of lactate production at low work loads (Yamabe et al., 1994), and an increase in muscle effort. There is evidence of muscle underperfusion (Wilson et al., 1989) and impaired metabolic function (Minotti et al., 1992; Mancini et al., 1994b). Such abnormalities are worth looking for because they may be reversed by prescribed muscle training (Stratton et al., 1994; McKelvie et al., 1995).

Applications in Cardiac Disorders

Coronary Artery Disease

As well as being of clinical value in a diagnostic sense, exercise testing can provide information that may be of great help in the treatment of patients with coronary artery disease. These wider uses for exercise testing have been clearly argued in the past few years (Bruce, 1977), and studies have shown its utility in the assessment of ventricular function, in prediction of outcome, in prescription of activity and exercise programs, in preoperative and operative evaluation, and in establishment of the efficacy of many therapeutic measures.

MYOCARDIAL FUNCTION. Ventricular function is impaired by even mild coronary artery stenosis. Newman and associates (1980) used nuclear angiography to show that in contrast to normal subjects, who increased left ventricular ejection fraction from 69 per cent at rest to 75 per cent in exercise, patients with one-vessel stenosis showed a fall from 62 to 57 per cent, and those with three-vessel disease, from 57 to 47 per cent. These results are consistent with those of many studies that have shown a progressive fall in exercise capacity with increasing extent of disease. Patients with severe ventricular dysfunction exhibit a fall in stroke volume with increasing exercise, contributing to a marked reduction in maximum cardiac output and an inability to maintain effective muscle perfusion pressure. These abnormalities are common in pa-

tients studied after myocardial infarction (Bruce et al., 1974). The frequency of radionuclide angiographic abnormalities in mild coronary artery disease may suggest that this technique is of value in diagnosis, but this question has not been resolved. However, measurements of maximal oxygen intake, heart rate, and blood pressure, all viewed in relation to age, have an established value in the overall assessment of functional reserve in coronary disease.

DIAGNOSIS OF HIGH-RISK CORONARY ARTERY DISEASE. "High risk" means left main or three-vessel disease; Weiner and associates (1980) and Chaitman and co-workers (1981) showed that these types of disease were associated with more marked ST changes; their data indicate that the posttest likelihood of high-risk disease may be estimated from prevalence values that are one third those of coronary artery disease in toto; thus, the likelihood of high-risk disease in the example above may be obtained by starting with a pretest likelihood of 1.9 per cent instead of 5.8 per cent and using the same likelihood ratio (LR) values in the rest of the calculation; the probability of high-risk disease is about 65 per cent. Other techniques have also been used to identify this subgroup of patients (see below).

In view of the ability of exercise testing to identify multivessel coronary disease (Hung et al., 1985; Okin et al., 1985; Bobbio et al., 1992), it is not surprising that the severity of exercise-related abnormalities may also predict outcome. Subjects showing ST depression in exercise have a 10- to 15-fold greater risk of developing other clinical events in the next 3 to 6 years (Froelicher et al., 1973; Aronow and Cassidy, 1975; Cumming et al., 1975), including sudden death (Bruce, 1977); both the extent of ST depression and the level of exercise at which it occurs are significantly related to outcome (Ellestad and Wan, 1975; Weiner et al., 1983), although whether ST depression is accompanied by angina does not influence outcome (Dagenais et al., 1988). Other exercise variables increase the predictive power of ST changes; McNeer and colleagues (1978) showed that only 63 per cent of patients with low maximum power or heart rate survived 4 years, compared with 93 per cent of those with normal exercise results. Ellestad and Wan (1975) also showed that exercise bradycardia is strongly predictive of future coronary events even in the absence of ST changes. In patients with established coronary artery disease, Bruce and colleagues (1974) identified three important prognostic factors: cardiomegaly, maximal oxygen intake of less than about 50 per cent, and maximum systolic pressure of less than 130 mm Hg. Absence of all three was associated with a 98 per cent 2-year survival, but mortality increased to 10 per cent, 25 per cent, and 88 per cent if one, two, or all three were present, respectively. Put in another way, the likelihood ratio for death in 2 years increased from 0.5 to 2, 8, and 160, respectively. Several studies have emphasized the prognostic importance of a fall in blood pressure during exercise (Thomson and Kelemen, 1975; Dubach et al., 1988). A prospective study in more than 12,000 subjects indicated that an abnormal exercise test result identified a group that may benefit from a preventive program designed to reduce risk factors for coronary disease (MRFIT Research Group, 1985). Another prospective study concluded that an exercise test score, consisting of exercise capacity, extent of ST-segment depression, and intensity of angina, provided a better 2-year outcome prediction than did a clinical assessment (Mark et al., 1991).

Following the findings of Théroux and colleagues (1979) that ST changes in a predischarge exercise test after myocardial infarction were associated with a 1-year mortality of 27 per cent, many investigators have confirmed the prognostic value of this application of testing (Weiner, 1982). The true value of the results of these studies is difficult to establish because of the selection of patients; thus, the patients with greatest disease severity may not even come to exercise testing and have the poorest prognosis (DeBusk et al., 1983; Deckers et al., 1987). As in other applications of testing to coronary patients, addition of other variables to ST depression, such as maximum heart rate, blood pressure, and exercise capacity, improves predictive accuracy (Weiner et al., 1983). The addition of thallium scintigraphy is helpful in assessing outlook after infarction (Gibson et al., 1983). Exercise testing after myocardial infarction may be useful in reassuring the patient that exercise can be safely undertaken, in prescribing or proscribing activity in convalescence, and in making therapeutic decisions about beta blockade or calcium channel blockers. An obvious use of exercise testing is in the prescription of activity in everyday life or in a cardiac rehabilitation program. In this application, the objective is to identify a level of exertion, recognizable for the patient on the basis of heart rate or a rating of perceived effort, that optimizes the desired exercise intensity to disability. Generally, a level is prescribed that is not associated with severe arrhythmia or ST depression, fall in blood pressure, or lactate accumulation (see below).

Beta adrenergic and calcium channel blocking drugs are now widely used in the management of angina and postinfarction, in addition to vasodilators. Sometimes, the wide variability in responsiveness and the frequency of undesirable side effects lead to difficulty in achieving optimal dosage of such agents. Exercise may be an ideal tool to monitor the efficacy of treatment, particularly if an improvement in exercise tolerance is one of the therapeutic objectives. Although much is known about the effects of such agents on exercise function (Silke et al., 1985), this use of exercise testing has not been widely adopted clinically. It is probably not feasible to test all patients, but an exercise test may be helpful in a patient who, for example, has not experienced a symptomatic benefit and may require a higher dose. The opposite clinical situation is also not uncommon; an exercise test carried out in a patient complaining of unaccustomed fatigue during treatment with a beta blocker may show that maximum oxygen intake is reduced and maximum heart rate is much lower than expected, indicating a higher-than-optimal dose. Because the test can be made simple for this application, there is scope for serial exercise testing as a guide to efficacy, particularly in complex situations.

Another obvious use of exercise is in the assessment of coronary artery surgery; increases in exercise capacity and reductions in ST depression parallel improvements in coronary flow (Lapin et al., 1973; Hollenberg et al., 1983; Dubach et al., 1989). Similar conclusions may be drawn regarding the value of exercise testing after angioplasty (Laarman et al., 1990).

The value of exercise testing in coronary artery disease has been well established; for some applications, it may be considered complementary to other, more expensive or invasive techniques, and in such situations, it makes good sense to use a simple noninvasive test as a screening procedure, or to place the results of other tests in the context of the maximal exercise capacity. Also, it may be asking too much of an exercise test to reflect the functional capacity of one mechanism, such as ventricular contractility; always the integrative nature of exercise needs to be borne in mind. In this way, clues may be obtained regarding the interplay between impaired mechanisms. For example, early after myocardial infarction, a central limitation of cardiac output may be recognized; several months later, exercise capacity may remain impaired, but the problem now is poor muscle performance secondary to inactivity (Jones and McCartney, 1986).

Valvular Disease

Early studies of mitral valve disease demonstrated the power of exercise studies in evaluating the severity of stenosis or incompetence and impairment of cardiac function (Holmgren et al., 1958; Werko, 1964; Blackmon et al., 1967). Bishop and Wade (1963) established relationships between reduced maximal oxygen intake and cardiac output, and the secondary effects on pulmonary vascular pressures in mitral stenosis. These studies and others have established the pattern of response to increasing severity of disease—a high heart rate with limited stroke volume; increasing impairment of cardiac output at first along the lower normal $\dot{Q}/\dot{V}_{O_2}$ relationship but in severe disease below it (Gazetopoulos et al., 1966); lactate production at progressively lower power outputs (Donald et al., 1954; Holmgren and Strom, 1959); and increased ventilation (Gazetopoulos et al., 1966) with congested lungs contributing to increasing dyspnea (Reed et al., 1978). Useful information has been obtained also in studies evaluating the response to valvulotomy and valve replacement (Rhodes et al., 1985), and more recent studies have confirmed the value of noninvasive exercise testing (Areskog, 1984; Vacek et al., 1986; Weber et al., 1986). A similar evolution in exercise responses has been found in aortic valve disease, although the reduction in exercise capacity is not as dramatic as that in mitral valve disease (Areskog, 1984; Weber et al., 1986). This is mainly due to the adaptive response of left ventricular structure and function; myocardial hypertrophy and maintained left ventricular preload act to maintain stroke volume and left ventricular ejection fraction. Thus, increases in heart rate are less dramatic than in mitral disease, and maximal oxygen intake, cardiac output, and systemic arterial pressure are reduced only in severe stenosis (Lee et al., 1970; Aronow and Harris, 1975). The adaptive responses of the left ventricle are particularly impressive in aortic regurgitation (Weber et al., 1986; Misra et al., 1987); radionuclide angiography may be used to measure ejection fraction in exercise and thus establish the degree of left ventricular adaptation (Shen et al., 1985). Simple noninvasive testing provides adequate indications for operative treatment and the assessment of response (Hossack and Neilson, 1979).

Changes in the electrocardiogram ST segment during exercise are common in aortic stenosis and reflect the balance between myocardial work and blood flow (the oxygen supply-demand ratio) (Kveselis et al., 1985). Although this may lead to difficulty in diagnosing coexisting coronary artery narrowing, Linderholm and co-workers (1985) showed that if ST depression is quantified and divided by the percentage of predicted maximum power, a high diagnostic accuracy may be obtained even in this difficult clinical situation. Effort syncope is a relatively common occurrence in aortic stenosis; if it is identified in the patient's history, precautions should be taken to carefully monitor the responses to exercise and prevent serious left ventricular overload (Fletcher et al., 1995).

Congenital Heart Disease

Although there are good theoretical arguments for the use of exercise tests in children with heart murmurs and clinically diagnosed heart disease (Godfrey, 1970), the huge experience of Cumming in their routine use led him to identify a number of problems that lessened their clinical utility (Cumming, 1978). The first is the identification of a valid "normal" population for use in comparison with patients; he proposed that clinic patients without disease be used for this purpose. Having established this data base, he found that only severe defects were associated with definite impairment in exercise function, and later studies have borne out this conclusion.

In congenital aortic and pulmonary stenosis, normal exercise capacity and cardiac output are maintained in all but the severest stenoses (< 0.5 cm^2/m^2 in area) when appreciable peak systolic pressure gradients (> 50 mm Hg) have developed (Ikkos et al., 1966; Moller et al., 1972; Cumming, 1978). As reported by Gazetopoulos and associates (1966), in 27 patients with isolated pulmonary stenosis in whom exercise capacity was severely impaired, the cardiac output in exercise was below the normal range in half of the patients.

In ventricular septal defects of small or moderate size (< 1 cm in diameter), there is no increase in left-to-right shunt flow in exercise, and a normal stroke volume and maximum oxygen intake is maintained (Bendien et al., 1984); only when the pulmonary to systemic flow ratio exceeds 2 or pulmonary hypertension is established is exercise capacity impaired (Cumming, 1978; Otterstad et al., 1985). This is also true for atrial septal defects (Davies and Gazetopoulos, 1966).

In cyanotic heart disease, exercise capacity is reduced in relation to the degree of arterial oxygen desaturation (Cumming, 1978). Most patients show progressive desaturation in exercise with increasing pulmonary vascular resistance. In such conditions, the oxygen saturation in exercise, expressed in relation to $\dot{V}_{O_2}$max as a percentage of predicted, is a reliable indication of the extent of right-to-left intracardiac shunting. Exercise testing is of interest in establishing the outcome after surgery, for example, after correction of atrial septal defects and the tetralogy of Fallot (Epstein et al., 1973).

Pulmonary Vascular Disease

Exercise testing may be of crucial importance in the detection of thromboembolic or obliterative pulmonary hypertension (Wilhelmsen et al., 1963). Patients may present with exercise limitation and dyspnea before clinical, electrocardiographic, or radiological abnormalities are apparent; however, during exercise the reduced pulmonary flow capacity is associated with a reduced maximal oxygen intake and low stroke volume. Lactate production, increased carbon dioxide output, and high dead space ventilation all contribute to a gross increase in exercise ventilation (Jones and Goodwin, 1965; Gazetopoulos et al., 1974), which correlates well with the degree of pulmonary vascular resistance (Janicki et al., 1984). Simple exercise tests provide a reliable index of progression. A fall in maximal oxygen intake to below 50 per cent of that predicted for a healthy subject implies a maximum cardiac output of less than 8 L/min and a pulmonary artery systolic pressure in excess of 100 mm Hg. Pulmonary hypertension and cardiac failure contribute to disability in severe pulmonary disorders and should be considered in any patient whose exercise impairment is out of proportion to impairment in pulmonary function. However, such patients usually exhibit severe defects in pulmonary gas exchange, with marked oxygen desaturation in exercise, and in this situation, the cardiac component may be difficult to separate from the pulmonary. Radionuclide angiography during exercise reveals abnormal right ventricular ejection fractions (Matthay et al., 1980), and in patients with overt cardiac failure, left ventricular ejection fractions are also low; this technique is helpful in evaluating the effectiveness of measures aimed at improving cardiac function (Mathur et al., 1985).

Cardiomyopathy, Cardiac Failure

Indices of resting cardiac function are notoriously poor for evaluating cardiac reserve in diffuse myocardial disorders (Franciosa et al., 1981), whereas changes in a number of exercise variables more or less accurately parallel overall symptomatic and clinical severity. Weber and colleagues (1984) make a strong case for exercise evaluation, showing a progressive fall in maximal cardiac output and stroke volume and increasing heart rate, with increasing clinical and hemodynamic impairment; a progressive increase in ventilation is also found with increasing disease severity (Weber et al., 1982a; Franciosa et al., 1984). Maximal oxygen intake and oxygen intake at the anaerobic threshold yield reliable measures of function that may be used to follow the clinical course or to evaluate therapy (Edwards et al., 1970). Exercise testing is used in the preoperative assessment of potential cardiac transplant recipients (Howard et al., 1994) but does not add to the assessment of outcome after major noncardiac surgery in patients who are not known to have coronary artery disease (Carliner et al., 1985).

Many studies of exercise in cardiac patients have demonstrated the value of a progressive incremental exercise test with relatively simple, noninvasive measurements: oxygen intake and carbon dioxide output, ventilation, heart rate, blood pressure, and electrocardiogram (Wilson et al., 1986). An assessment of cardiovascular function is obtained that may be applied in clinical management problems

and in the assessment of drug treatment (Sullivan et al., 1989). Also, the results may be used to select patients in whom other exercise techniques—radionuclide ventricular volumes, thallium scintigraphy, or cardiac catheterization—may be expected to add information for diagnostic or therapeutic decision making. The use of an integrative approach to exercise testing in cardiovascular disease was recently reviewed by Tjahja and colleagues (1994).

Peripheral Vascular Disease

The severity of intermittent claudication may be objectively assessed by treadmill walking or by other methods of dynamic calf exercise. If necessary, calf muscle blood flow is measured by the clearance of ^{133}Xe (Lassen and Kampp, 1965).

It is now possible to monitor Po_2 in exercising muscle (Holm and Bylund-Fellenius, 1981) in order to complement measurements of exercise function and claudication threshold, but these techniques are mainly applicable in research and specialized vascular clinics.

Cardiac Arrhythmias

The use of exercise testing in evaluating the functional effects and the prognostic importance of cardiac arrhythmias are discussed in Chapter 7.

Systemic Arterial Hypertension

Systolic arterial blood pressure increases with exercise, but diastolic pressure shows little change. Hypertensive responses during exercise were divided by Sannerstedt (1966) into three main groups. First, subjects with normal pressure at rest may show increases in systolic and diastolic pressures that are outside the 95 per cent confidence limits of the normal population. Although such subjects are considered to have "labile" or "reactive" hypertension, we do not know if this places them at any risk, if they may later develop hypertension at rest, or if there is anything to be gained from antihypertensive therapy. The finding of a closer correlation of left ventricular wall thickness to exercise blood pressure than to blood pressure at rest is another clue that exercise measurements may be helpful in assessing a patient with variable blood pressure at rest. Second is the group of patients with hypertension at rest in whom arterial pressure is raised to above-normal limits in exercise; such patients require treatment. The third group consists of patients with rest hypertension who do not show a further increase with exercise; this finding in a patient not undergoing antihypertensive therapy may indicate the early stage of left ventricular failure. The clinical value of exercise studies in hypertension remains to be established. It is possible that exercise testing may be helpful in assessing the need for treatment in borderline hypertension (Franz, 1985) and in establishing the response to treatment. The testing of children of hypertensive parents has been proposed as clinically justifiable (Radice et al., 1985), but another study suggests that exercise blood pressure has no advantage over resting measurements in predicting blood pressure trends in adolescents (Fixler et al., 1985).

Peripheral Vascular Control

The syndrome of vasoregulatory asthenia, well described in Scandinavian literature, consists of inadequate postural adjustment of blood pressure and impaired exercise performance—low maximal oxygen intake, high cardiac frequency, and lactic acid production (Holmgren and Strom, 1959). Oxygen extraction from blood flowing through exercising limbs is reduced, suggesting that distribution of muscle blood flow is poor. Improvement has been shown to follow exercise training (Levander-Lindgren and Ek, 1962). The group of patients with this syndrome may also include a number of subgroups that have not been completely separated—such as patients who show the effects of inactivity ("unfitness") (Saltin et al., 1968), those in whom activity of enzymes that limit aerobic metabolic fluxes is low, and those who have functional disturbances of the mitral valve (Devereux, 1979) in addition to poor vascular control. The diagnosis of this syndrome may be made only through exercise studies to demonstrate low exercise capacity, high heart rate response, and lactic acid production in the absence of organic heart disease.

Diseases of the autonomic nervous system, such as diabetic neuropathy and the Shy-Drager syndrome, are rare causes of severe effort intolerance owing to a combination of impaired blood pressure control and impaired cardiac rate; exercise studies provide one measure of the functional severity.

Cardiac "Nondisease"

The ability of an exercise test to exclude significant cardiac disease allows it to play a role in the rapid investigation of heart murmurs and chest pain syndromes, in which cardiac neurosis may dominate the symptoms. The demonstration of normal exercise performance may be used for reassurance and encouragement of patients with such disorders and, when the patients are children, of their parents (Bergman and Stamm, 1967).

EVALUATION OF RESPIRATORY FUNCTION

Just as in cardiovascular disorders, even complex investigations performed at rest are unable to quantify to any precise extent the impairment in respiratory reserve that accompanies pulmonary disorders. There are correlations between a variety of resting pulmonary function abnormalities and exercise capacity (Armstrong et al., 1966), but there is always a large residual variation that is not accounted for. The reason for the variability, as in cardiovascular diseases, is the interplay between many mechanisms that contribute to disability and exercise impairment. Thus, whereas resting functional characteristics, such as vital capacity, FEV_1, carbon monoxide transfer capacity, and strength of respiratory muscles, may all be shown to predict functional capacity, each may contribute independently to the impaired exercise capacity (Leblanc et al., 1986). To these factors may be added abnormalities of cardiac and skeletal muscle function. The power of exercise tests is in assessing the combined contributions of several impaired functions to the patient's overall disability (Jones, 1975a, 1975b).

Assessment of Pulmonary Reserve

We may use a series of Fick relationships to express the pulmonary responses to the metabolic demands of exercise, but we should bear in mind that in contrast to the cardiovascular system, the lungs are the first link in the oxygen transport chain but the last step in carbon dioxide transport. For this reason, impairment of pulmonary function may limit carbon dioxide excretion to a greater extent than it does oxygen uptake. This means that metabolic and acid-base changes during exercise may have an appreciable impact on exercise capacity in patients who may have a hard time clearing carbon dioxide because of impaired gas exchange, as well as limited ability to mount a ventilatory response in terms of increases in volume and flow, either because of the mechanical impedances to breathing or because of weakened respiratory muscles. Such factors have been shown to contribute quantitatively to dyspnea (Leblanc et al., 1986), which usually is the limiting symptom; however, in a surprisingly high proportion of respiratory patients, exercise capacity is actually limited by poor skeletal muscle function (Killian, 1992).

METABOLIC FACTORS. Because a diet that is high in carbohydrate generates more carbon dioxide for a given adenosine triphosphate (ATP) turnover than does fat utilization, patients with severe air flow limitation show a limited exercise capacity when given such a diet experimentally (Brown et al., 1985a). The postprandial surge of insulin inhibits free fatty acid usage and exerts a similar effect after a heavy meal (Brown et al., 1985b). Although lactate production is generally not increased during exercise in respiratory patients (Jones et al., 1971), the expected increase occurs if they undertake short-term heavy exercise (Sue et al., 1988), such as stair climbing, and if hypoxemia is severe or cardiac failure is also present. In addition, inactivity leads to reductions in aerobic muscle enzyme activity, which contributes to lactate formation in some respiratory patients. Lactate production may exert a substantial limiting effect because of a limited ability to respond acutely to the acid-base challenge and its contribution to dyspnea.

It has been argued on the basis of many studies that the increase in respiratory muscle work in pulmonary disorders is accompanied by an increase in oxygen consumption during exercise that might even exceed the increase in oxygen uptake achieved through the increase in ventilation (Otis, 1954). In healthy subjects loaded to the point of ventilatory failure, an increase of about 200 mL/min in $\dot{V}O_2$ is observed (Jones GL et al., 1985). This increase is similar to an increase in $\dot{V}O_2$ above that expected for the power output in patients with air flow limitation at maximum exercise (Jones et al., 1971); although this is small compared to $\dot{V}O_2max$ in healthy subjects, it may represent a relatively large proportion of the much reduced equivalent in such patients.

PULMONARY GAS EXCHANGE. The efficiency of gas exchange in the lung influences two key variables in exercise, the arterial oxygen saturation and the ventilatory response to carbon dioxide production, in more or less predictable ways. The equations below should not be taken as mathematically correct expressions but as conceptual relationships that identify the contributions of pulmonary mechanisms to exercise capacity and the variables that may be measured during exercise to quantify them.

Two main generic processes may be identified in oxygen intake ($\dot{V}O_2$) and carbon dioxide output ($\dot{V}CO_2$): alveolar ventilation ($\dot{V}A$) and alveolocapillary gas transfer (TL). We may express the ventilatory variables ("the pump") in a modified form of the alveolar ventilation equation (Eq. 18; Chapter 2) as follows:

$$\dot{V}CO_2 \sim \dot{V}E \ (1 \ - \ V_D/V_T) \ PaCO_2$$

where $\dot{V}E$ is the total ventilation, V_D/V_T is the dead space–tidal volume ratio, and $PaCO_2$ is the arterial PCO_2. This equation shows that meeting the increasing demands of $\dot{V}CO_2$ in exercise requires an adequate ventilatory reserve and low V_D/V_T if $PaCO_2$ is to be prevented from rising; if V_D/V_T is high, an increase in $\dot{V}E$ is required or $PaCO_2$ rises; and an intact respiratory control system is also seen as important.

The lungs' oxygen transfer capacity (TL; "the

exchanger") is only loosely defined but receives contributions from pulmonary capillary volume and flow (cardiac output), diffusion, and ventilation-perfusion matching. The efficiency of this function may be expressed by Fick's principle, as follows:

$$\dot{V}O_2 \sim TL \ (P_AO_2 \ - \ PaO_2)$$

or

$$TL \sim \dot{V}O_2/(P_AO_2 \ - \ PaO_2)$$

These equations show that impaired gas exchange leads to an increase in the alveoloarterial PO_2 difference and usually to a fall in PaO_2 in exercise. Relationships between reductions in carbon monoxide diffusing capacity and falls in arterial PO_2 were established by Bates and associates (1966), Johnson and co-workers (1965), and Fulmer and colleagues (1979). These studies showed that the changes in A-a PO_2 difference or in PaO_2 for a unit increase in $\dot{V}O_2$ provide clinically useful indices of gas exchange in pulmonary fibrotic conditions and emphysema.

The same relationship may be expressed in terms of oxygen saturation:

$$\dot{V}O_2 \sim TL \ (Sc'O_2 \ - \ SaO_2)$$

where $Sc'O_2$ and SaO_2 refer to the end-capillary and arterial oxygen saturations, respectively. The fall in SaO_2 with increasing $\dot{V}O_2$ is also a good index of gas exchange function and is probably to be preferred to the fall in PO_2 because it is less affected by the shape of the oxyhemoglobin dissociation curve. If we take 100 per cent as the "ideal" value for $Sc'O_2$ and redefine the equation in terms of $\dot{V}O_2$ percentage predicted, we obtain the following:

$$TL \sim \dot{V}O_2 \ \%/(100 \ - \ SaO_2)$$

As P_AO_2 and thus $Sc'O_2$ are determined mathematically by $PaCO_2$ at any given inspired PO_2, the relationship between $\dot{V}O_2$ and SaO_2 is a reflection of all the processes involved in pulmonary oxygen intake, including cardiac output, gas exchange (diffusion, ventilation-perfusion), and alveolar ventilation. Thus, in terms of the measurements in exercise tests, the $\dot{V}O_2max$ and SaO_2 are probably the most critical, and a simple index of overall function is provided by

$$(\dot{V}O_2 \ \% \ predicted) \ \times \ SaO_2$$

Any of the equations above may be used as indices of gas exchange function, but I would caution against too literal a use of them for two reasons. First, none of the variables included in the relationships may be considered as strictly independent; for example, a reduced cardiac output response to exercise may contribute to a low $\dot{V}O_2max$ and to a fall in arterial oxygen secondary to the effect of venous admixture of low venous oxygen content (wide arteriovenous oxygen difference). Second, we have no confidence that similar values for the indices actually "mean" similar gas exchange function; for example, in the last equation it seems unlikely that a patient who has an SaO_2 of 80 per cent at 80 per cent $\dot{V}O_2max$ has a gas exchange impairment similar to that in another patient whose SaO_2 is 90 per cent at 70 per cent $\dot{V}O_2max$. The value of both $\dot{V}O_2max$ and SaO_2 measurements is, however, based on solid evidence. Of course, to apportion the blame when $\dot{V}O_2max$ and SaO_2 are reduced, we may also need $\dot{V}E$, $\dot{V}CO_2$, and $PaCO_2$ and an assessment of the maximal ventilatory capacity (i.e., the capacity of the pump).

PULMONARY MECHANICS. Changes in the mechanical characteristics of the lungs and conducting airways tend to dominate the dyspnea that usually limits exercise in pulmonary patients. Increased elastance limits increases in tidal volume because a normal end-inspiratory lung volume cannot be reached; reduced elastic recoil in emphysema contributes to reductions in expiratory flow but also prevents the normal reduction in end-expiratory lung volume, which allows some unloading of inspiratory muscles (Leblanc et al., 1988). Breathing capacity is usually assessed by measurement of FEV_1, and expiratory air flow may be extremely limited in chronic air flow limitation; however, reductions in inspiratory flow that result from airway obstruction, when they occur, may limit ventilatory capacity during exercise to a greater relative extent than expiratory limitation and play a large role in dyspnea (Noseda et al., 1994). Furthermore, the work of the inspiratory muscles is greatly increased; this may be one factor contributing to the large increases in arterial PCO_2 that are sometimes seen in patients with chronic bronchitis (Jones, 1966). Thus, a flow-volume loop may be more helpful in assessing ventilatory capacity than may FEV_1 alone.

RESPIRATORY MUSCLE TENSION AND WORK. The respiratory muscles power the ventilatory pump; because most of the work is done on inspiration, the brunt of this work falls on the inspiratory muscles. Expiratory muscles play a small part by reducing end-expiratory lung volume, thereby lengthening the inspiratory muscles and placing them on a favorable part of their length-tension curve. Inspiratory and expiratory muscle strength are adequately assessed on a routine basis by measurement of the maximal pressures achieved against an occluded airway on inspiration (MIP) and expiration (MEP). In a large population of

patients with a variety of respiratory disorders, MIP was able to explain 50 per cent of the variance in dyspnea intensity (Hamilton et al., 1995). In addition, variables that are related to the velocity and extent of respiratory muscle shortening, the frequency of contraction, and the contraction duty cycle were shown to exert significant effects on dyspnea (Leblanc et al., 1986). Thus, measurement of resting maximal flow and volume, MIP, and MEP, together with changes in the pattern of breathing and tidal volume, usually enable the factors influencing dyspnea in a patient to be readily identified.

In analyzing pump function, the ventilation achieved in exercise needs to be related to the impedances of the respiratory system (elastance, resistance, and inertance) and the pressure generated by inspiratory muscles according to the classic expression

$$P\,mus = (E \times V) + (R \times \dot{V}) + (I \times \ddot{V}),$$

in which inertance (I, accelerative impedance) is usually ignored. In terms of the variables measured in exercise

$$P\,mus = (E \times V_T) + (R \times V_T/T_I)$$

where V_T is tidal volume, T_I is inspiratory duration, and V_T/T_I is mean inspiratory flow. An adequate ventilatory response in terms of tidal volume and flow is thus dictated by the balance between the impedances to breathing and the strength of the respiratory muscles. Adaptation to increased impedance may be achieved by a reduction in V_T and increased flow in the case of increased elastance, as seen in pulmonary fibrotic disorders (Burdon et al., 1983), and slower air flow with increase in V_T, in the case of increased resistance, as in obstructive disorders (Jones et al., 1971). However, the effectiveness of these adaptations may be limited by the reductions in muscle strength that accompany muscle shortening and increasing velocity of contraction—the length-tension and force-velocity characteristics. Practically, changes in elastance are assessed by measurement of lung volumes or pressure-volume relationships, and changes in resistance are assessed by measurement of the FEV_1, flow-volume loop, and pressure-flow relationships; the strength of inspiratory muscles is assessed by measurement of the maximal mouth occlusion pressure (MIP).

RESPIRATORY CONTROL. Respiratory control mechanisms contribute to pump function, but abnormalities in control are only rarely encountered in the absence of other respiratory abnormalities. When respiratory function is otherwise normal, the ventilatory response to the increasing carbon dioxide output of exercise provides an assessment of chemoreceptor function. Thus, a reduced ventilatory response to exercise may be found in the alveolar hypoventilation syndrome (Ondine's curse) (Hyland et al., 1978), and a marked increase in the response is seen in some dyspneic patients with normal cardiopulmonary function but very high responsiveness to carbon dioxide.

SKELETAL MUSCLE FUNCTION IN RESPIRATORY DISORDERS. Although for many years, respiratory patients were held to be limited by their reduced capacity to breathe, as reflected in reductions in FEV_1, careful identification of the symptoms limiting maximal exercise revealed that many patients were limited by intolerable muscle effort and an inability to continue pedaling or walking (Killian, 1992). Muscle strength measurements have shown that muscle weakness exerts an effect on maximum exercise capacity that is independent of FEV_1, as expressed in the following equation derived from a study of 784 patients:

$$Wcap = 46 + 3.5(FEV_1 \% \text{ pred}) + 10.3 \text{ (knee extensor strength)}$$

where W is in kpm/min and strength is in kg (Hamilton et al., 1995).

Application of Exercise Testing to Respiratory Disorders

Chronic Airway Obstructive Syndromes

In patients with chronic air flow obstruction (intractable asthma, chronic bronchitis, emphysema),

an exercise test is worth including as part of the clinical evaluation so that individual contributions to disability of a number of mechanisms may be assessed. Limitation is usually related to the increased impedance to breathing (Clark et al., 1969), but this may be compromised by metabolic factors, impaired gas exchange (Jones and Berman, 1984), abnormal respiratory control (Cherniack, 1991), and respiratory muscle weakness.

The demands on the ventilatory pump are often excessive for a number of reasons. Oxygen consumption in patients who are limited by their air flow obstruction is higher than that in healthy subjects studied at comparable exercise intensities (Jones et al., 1971). Because the demands are closely related to carbon dioxide output, any increase in the metabolic respiratory quotient (RQ) tends to reduce $\dot{V}O_2$max; the effect of a carbohydrate load has already been mentioned. Poor ventilation-perfusion ($\dot{V}A/\dot{Q}C$) matching is associated with increases in the VD/VT ratio to 50 per cent or above; although the accompanying increased demands on the ventilatory pump are lessened by a reduction in alveolar ventilation, most patients showing an increase in $PaCO_2$ of at least 5 mm Hg, the total ventilation ($\dot{V}E$) is often increased compared with normal (Jones, 1966). Falls in arterial oxygen saturation, indicating severe gas exchange impairment, are common in emphysema (Fig. 4–1) (Jones, 1966; Keogh et al., 1984) and may contribute a hypoxic stimulus to increase ventilatory drive. Thus, measurement of SaO_2 in exercise may be used to assess the severity of gas exchange impairment owing to loss of alveolar surface area and capillary blood volume and $\dot{V}A/\dot{Q}C$ mismatch. However, falls in SaO_2 seldom contribute directly

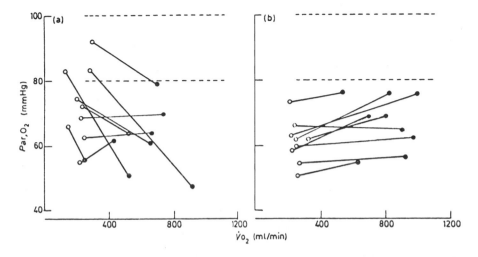

Figure 4–1. Arterial PO_2 in two groups of patients with chronic air flow obstruction—type A (emphysema) *(left)* and type B (chronic bronchitis without significant emphysema) *(right)*. Although resting PO_2 is often lower in type B patients, the fall with exercise is less than in type A. Dotted line indicates normal range of PO_2. (From Jones NL. Pulmonary gas exchange during exercise in patients with chronic airway obstruction. Clin Sci 1966;31:39–50.)

to disability by reducing tissue oxygen delivery; increases in cardiac output and tissue oxygen extraction provide adequate compensation for the hypoxemia, and lactate formation is uncommon (Daly et al., 1967). Furthermore, although oxygen administration completely corrects hypoxemia, the associated increase in $\dot{V}O_2$max is usually due to the accompanying fall in ventilation, allowing a higher power output to be achieved before a ventilatory limit is reached. Because the hypoventilation indicates a rise in $PaCO_2$, regular oxygen administration in exercise requires an objective assessment of its efficacy and risks before its prescription.

CARDIOVASCULAR EFFECTS OF CHRONIC OBSTRUCTIVE PULMONARY DISORDERS. Cardiac output and pulmonary vascular pressures have been studied during exercise on many occasions in the past 30 years (Matthay et al., 1980); generally, a normal cardiac output has been observed (Wade and Bishop, 1962; Jones et al., 1971; Burrows et al., 1972), but pulmonary

artery pressure is elevated (Light et al., 1984), at least in part secondary to hypoxemia. Burrows and colleagues (1972) found that patients with type B syndrome showed a higher cardiac output and more severe pulmonary hypertension than those with the type A syndrome. The importance of the circulation in maintaining oxygen delivery is sometimes seen in very disabled patients whose left ventricular response to exercise is impaired, either as part of the chronic obstructive syndrome or because of coexisting ischemic cardiac disease (Mathur et al., 1985).

PULMONARY MECHANICS. In chronic air flow obstruction, the increase in air flow resistance, particularly in patients with emphysema, is usually far higher in expiration than in inspiration. During exercise, expiratory air flow soon reaches a limiting value, forcing inspiratory flow to increase progressively until it, too, reaches the maximum flow-volume loop (Fig. 4–2); a pattern of breathing results that consists of a relatively well-maintained

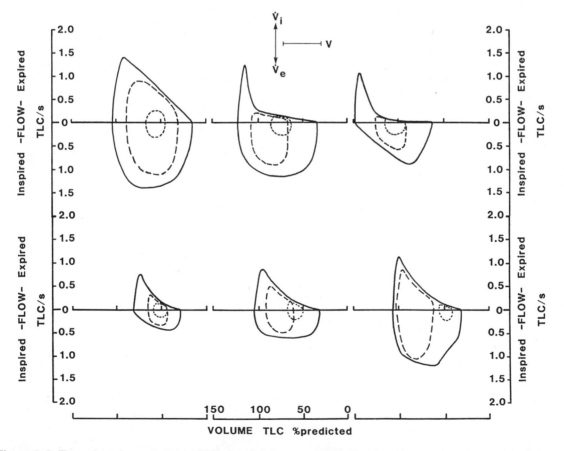

Figure 4–2. Flow-volume loops at rest (solid line) and during exercise (dashed line) in a normal subject *(top left)* and in five patients with air flow limitation. Note that none of the patients reduce end-expiratory lung volume, all are limited by expiratory flow, and there is considerable variation in the extent to which they are able to increase inspiratory flow. TLC = total lung capacity.

tidal volume, a long expiratory time, and a short inspiratory time (T_I), with T_I/T_{tot} often as low as 0.15 (only 15 per cent of the breathing cycle is spent in inspiration). This pattern of breathing throws a heavy load on the respiratory muscles, accounting for the severe dyspnea that most patients experience. Most patients with very reduced flow in the later part of expiration adapt by breathing at an increased lung volume; as long as this does not compromise inspiratory flow as a result of the shortening of the diaphragm, the strategy helps to minimize dyspnea (Noseda et al., 1994). However, this may lead to a high-frequency, low tidal volume pattern of breathing, resulting from the limited capacity to increase end-inspiratory lung volume. Many combinations of tidal volume, frequency, and inspired and expired durations may be encountered in patients with severe air flow limitation; it is usually safe to assume that a particular combination has been adopted unconsciously in an effort to minimize the intensity of dyspnea.

RESPIRATORY MUSCLES. As mentioned above, the muscles of breathing have a daunting task during exercise in patients with severe air flow limitation. They have to generate a high tension, often operate at a shortened length as a result of hyperinflation, and have to contract with a high velocity during inspiration to compensate for a prolonged expiration. These changes might be thought to act as a constant training stimulus for the inspiratory muscles, and for persons who are able to exercise frequently, perhaps they do; however, respiratory muscle weakness is often encountered and is likely to contribute to respiratory failure in some patients (Rochester, 1991). Bye and associates (1985) showed that in severely disabled patients, electromyographic evidence of respiratory muscle fatigue is present in maximal exercise, which may be lessened by oxygen administration. Also, Pardy and colleagues (1981) demonstrated that specific inspiratory muscle training increases endurance and reduces respiratory muscle fatigue in exercise. Thus, exercise tests in chronic air flow obstruction provide clinically valuable information on many facets of structure and function, including mechanical characteristics, respiratory muscles, control of breathing, and gas exchange, as well as being useful in the documentation of responses to treatment, prescription of activity, and occupational assessment and in the making of decisions regarding oxygen therapy.

Cystic Fibrosis

Children with cystic fibrosis exhibit impaired exercise capacity that parallels other clinical indices of severity; responses are similar to those in adults with chronic bronchitis; the major limiting factor is mechanical, but falls in SaO_2 are seen in severely affected children (Godfrey and Mearns, 1971). Patients who survive into adulthood show gas exchange changes that are similar to those of patients with chronic bronchitis. There is a severe ventilation-perfusion mismatch, which improves with exercise; arterial PO_2 remains relatively constant (Dantzker et al., 1982). In addition to pulmonary factors, exercise capacity is limited by reductions in muscle volume and strength; the cardiac output response to exercise is normal (Lands et al., 1992). Respiratory muscle strength is well maintained (Lands et al., 1993).

Pulmonary Fibrotic Conditions

Conditions usually termed *pulmonary fibrosis* or *interstitial lung disease* in North America and *alveolitis* in Europe, characteristically are associated with impaired ventilatory function secondary to an increase in pulmonary elastance, and gas exchange defects, neither of which are closely related to indices of clinical or radiological severity. Because of this, exercise testing may assume even greater importance than in the obstructive syndromes because the measurements may provide the best indication of the structural abnormalities—fibrosis and obliteration of alveolae and vascular bed (Fulmer et al., 1979; Huang et al., 1979). Characteristically, disabled patients are limited by severe dyspnea and show an increased ventilatory response to exercise, low tidal volume and high breathing frequency, decreased arterial oxygen saturation, and evidence of lactate production (Example 6, Chapter 13). Respiratory and skeletal muscle weakness and poor cardiac function may also contribute to the extreme reduction in exercise capacity that is seen in some patients. Increases in exercise capacity achieved by oxygen administration parallel the increase in arterial oxygen saturation (Bye et al., 1981). The exercise abnormalities seen in the different diseases that make up this clinical grouping were recently reviewed (Marciniuk and Gallagher, 1994). The large clinical studies reported from the National Institutes of Health (Keogh et al., 1984) and the Brompton Hospital (Denison et al., 1984) (Fig. 4–3) indicate the value of changes in arterial oxygenation during exercise. Virtually all the patients in these two series who were diagnosed as having interstitial fibrosis (fibrosing alveolitis) showed extremely limited $\dot{V}O_2max$ and falls in PaO_2 with exercise; patients with sarcoidosis showed a more variable response—$\dot{V}O_2max$ was less impaired and many patients did not show a fall in PaO_2. The patterns of exercise response encountered in sarcoidosis were reviewed by Matthews and Hooper (1983), and a study of systemic sclerosis was published by Godfrey and co-workers (1969). The multiple inert gas elimination technique has shown that hypoxemia is

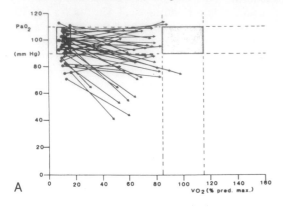

EFFECTS OF EXERCISE ON ARTERIAL PO₂ IN PEOPLE WITH SARCOIDOSIS

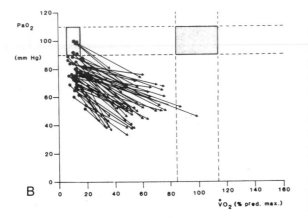

EFFECTS OF EXERCISE ON ARTERIAL PO₂ IN PEOPLE WITH C.F.A

Figure 4–3. Arterial PO₂ at rest and on maximum exercise in patients with sarcoidosis *(A)* and cryptogenic fibrosing alveolitis *(B)*, plotted as a function of predicted maximal VO₂. The slopes of the lines are an indication of the severity of gas exchange impairment, greater in alveolitis than in most of the sarcoid patients. (From Denison D, Al-Hillawi H, Turton C. Lung function in interstitial lung disease. Semin Respir Med 1984;6:40–54.)

due both to ventilation-perfusion mismatch and to a diffusion limitation, with the latter worsening during exercise (Agusti et al., 1991), as the mixed venous oxygen saturation falls (Example 6, Chapter 13). As in chronic air flow obstruction, there appears to be little relationship between hypoxemia and reductions in $\dot{V}O_2$max, but the mechanical effects of fibrosis limit ventilatory capacity (Burdon et al., 1983). However, hypoxemia may be very marked in exercise, and lactate production is not uncommon in this situation; hypoxemia may be associated with pulmonary hypertension and a poor cardiac output response to exercise. The ventilatory response to exercise is often higher than normal owing to a number of factors: increased carbon dioxide output secondary to lactate production, a hypoxic drive to breathing, and increased V_D/V_T

ratio owing to $\dot{V}A/\dot{Q}C$ mismatch. These demands on ventilation are met by a pattern of breathing in which increases in V_T are minimized at the expense of higher air flow, with shorter T_I and increased frequency of breathing (Burdon et al., 1983).

One of the more progressive types of fibrosis is due to asbestosis; because the clinical results of asbestos exposure are varied, exercise testing has been used to assess severity and identify early gas exchange impairment (Picado et al., 1987; Zejda, 1989; Shih et al., 1994). The use of exercise in assessing occupational lung fibrosis is considered below.

As in other respiratory complaints, there are a number of other uses for exercise tests, including assessment of the response to steroid therapy (Jones and Rebuck, 1979).

ASTHMA. In most asthmatic subjects with little current air flow obstruction (FEV₁ > 70 per cent predicted), $\dot{V}O_2$max and other indices of exercise performance are within the normal range, when allowance is made for variations in habitual activity (Bevegård et al., 1976). During exercise, airway obstruction usually improves, but bronchoconstriction often occurs a few minutes after exercise stops (see below). Although few studies have been reported, increasing air flow obstruction is associated with a progressive fall in exercise capacity secondary to the reduction in ventilatory capacity. In some patients with severe obstruction, increases in arterial PCO₂ occur; a defect in respiratory control mechanisms may contribute to this response, which is characteristic of asthmatic subjects who have undergone carotid body removal (Wasserman et al., 1976). Such subjects excluded, gas exchange function is usually well maintained, with little fall in SaO₂ with exercise (Anderson et al., 1972). Apart from documentation of the severity of exercise-induced bronchoconstriction, the main clinical indication for exercise testing in asthma is dyspnea that is out of proportion to the severity of air flow obstruction, in order to detect impairment in cardiopulmonary mechanisms other than simple air flow obstruction.

EXERCISE-INDUCED BRONCHOCONSTRICTION. The identification of a significant increase in airway resistance shortly after heavy exercise has important diagnostic and therapeutic implications (Godfrey, 1975) because it indicates an abnormally high degree of airway reactivity (Anderton et al., 1979). Recent research has identified the important part played by mucosal cooling, which is due to the warming of cool inspired air and the latent heat loss associated with humidification of dry air (McFadden and Ingram, 1979).

Exercise-induced asthma has been extensively studied by R. S. Jones (1966), who devised a "lability index'' calculated on the basis of maximum FEV_1 after administration of a bronchodilator (FEVmax), minimum FEV_1 after exercise (FEVmin), and predicted FEV_1 (FEVpred):

$$\text{Lability index} = \frac{\text{FEVmax} - \text{FEVmin}}{\text{FEVpred}} \times 100$$

Godfrey (1975) has made many contributions in this area that have helped to define the type of exercise that should be used and the responses in normal and asthmatic children. He suggested that the postexercise fall in FEV_1, or PEFR, expressed as a percentage of the resting value, is at least as informative as the lability index. A fall of greater than 10 per cent is considered an abnormal result, obtained in only 5 per cent of nonasthmatic children. A series of studies demonstrated the potency of running compared with other forms of exercise, the relative independence of the percentage fall to the pre-exercise PEFR, and the high (97 per cent) incidence of abnormal responses in asthmatic children and their healthy relatives (32 per cent).

The brilliant series of studies carried out over several years by McFadden and his colleagues (see McFadden, 1984, for a review of their work) demonstrated that the degree of constriction in a given person, whatever the type of exercise, may be explained by the level of ventilation and the humidity and temperature of inspired air. Bronchoconstriction does not occur if air at body temperature and fully saturated with water vapor is breathed, and it may be provoked by hyperventilation of cold dry air at rest. The only exception to these rules is the refractoriness observed with exercise that is repeated after short intervals, and that is thought to be due to the release of inhibitory prostaglandins. There is an obvious need for careful standardization of the conditions under which provocative testing is carried out; indeed, there are arguments for replacing exercise studies for this purpose with hyperventilation of cold air, in which the conditions may be controlled and dose-response curves carried out, relating changes in air flow resistance to respiratory heat loss (O'Byrne et al., 1982).

EVALUATION OF NEUROMUSCULAR FUNCTION

Muscle weakness, fatigue, and pain are frequently difficult to assess clinically; an exercise test may help to establish the severity of these symptoms more or less objectively and may provide indications for further investigation or, alternatively, may provide a basis for reassurance. Also, because exercise is not harmful and may benefit many muscle disorders (Vignos and Watkins, 1966), it is likely to be used as part of a therapeutic regimen and thus requires accurate prescription.

Exercise testing might appear an appropriate tool for assessing a variety of neuromuscular disorders, but owing to the variability in severity between muscle groups, the common forms of testing are usually difficult to apply. More appropriate are methods for measuring muscle power and assessing the fatigue characteristics of muscles under voluntary contraction and neural stimulation; this topic has been reviewed by Edwards (1979). Analysis of movement patterns and measurement of the strength of different muscle groups are also important (Siegel, 1977).

During exercise on a cycle ergometer, a healthy subject may be able to generate as much as 80 per cent of $\dot{V}O_2$max with only one leg; although an untrained subject achieves much less than this, it does imply that a mild degree of muscle weakness may not significantly reduce the capacity to perform the usual progressive incremental exercise test, and that measurements of muscle strength in neuromuscular disorders are usually impaired to a greater relative degree than $\dot{V}O_2$max. However, exercise testing remains a useful technique for assessing impairment related to the normal energy demands of daily living and for following progression of the disorder. In addition, when reduction in exercise capacity associated with a high rating of perceived exertion is unaccompanied by indications of cardiorespiratory impairment, further muscle-directed investigation is warranted. In this situation, we have found maximal isokinetic dynamic ergometry to be helpful; maximal effort is exerted on the pedals of an ergometer at a constant velocity of pedaling for 30 seconds, and the torque exerted is measured by strain gauges (McComas et al., 1986). Maximal power and the fatigue that develops during the test may thus be precisely quantified.

In established local neurological defects, exercise capacity may be difficult to study but may be important in identifying the extent of adaptation that has taken place in unaffected muscles and other systems. Studies of paraplegic athletes with lesions at various levels of the spinal cord have demonstrated the remarkable degree of adaptation that may be achieved and thus these studies may be used as targets in the rehabilitation of spinal cord–injured patients (Wicks et al., 1977). Measurements in patients with hemiplegia may be used for similar reasons and sometimes reveal a defect in unaffected muscles, secondary to inactivity, that may lead to a change in therapy.

In general, two groups of disorders may be recognized in the population of patients referred for exercise testing in which a generalized neuromuscular disorder is suspected. First are syndromes of large muscle group weakness owing to motor unit neuropathy, myasthenia, and muscle degenerative disorders; exercise capacity is reduced, the sense of muscle effort is increased, but cardiorespiratory responses are usually appropriate to the exercise intensity in the absence of coexisting disorders of cardiac or respiratory muscle. The second group consists of patients who have severe exercise intolerance, usually with muscle pain, and in whom weakness is less prominent but fatigue develops rapidly; these features are found in metabolic myopathies, in which depletion of high-energy phosphates or marked falls in muscle pH occur. Interpretation of the exercise test results in such patients may prove difficult because high heart rates and ventilation may mimic cardiac or respiratory disorders (Haller et al., 1983). Also, overlap occurs between different mechanisms, contributing to poor exercise capacity, whatever the initiating cause. For example, a primary neuropathy may be accompanied by reduced acetylcholine release at the motor end-plate and by motor fiber degeneration with loss of contractile protein and impaired activation; inactivity also leads to reductions in the activity of rate-limiting enzymes.

A number of conditions have been studied during exercise to provide a basis for the use of testing in their clinical assessment, and a scheme of diagnostic testing was presented by Mills and Edwards (1983). As with other clinical disorders, measurement of $\dot{V}O_2max$ and the cardiorespiratory responses to exercise are important features of the test, but if a muscle disorder is suspected, it may be helpful to obtain blood samples at rest and at maximal exercise for analysis of metabolites (lactate, glucose, glycerol, and free fatty acids), acid-base status, and enzymes (creatine kinase [CK] isoenzymes).

Muscular Dystrophy

Reductions in $\dot{V}O_2max$ parallel other indices of clinical severity and may vary from the normal range to less than 30 per cent predicted (Sokolov et al., 1977; Carroll et al., 1979). The reduction in capacity is accompanied by a high sense of effort, but if a submaximal power is sustained, fatigue is not prominent. Heart rate, cardiac output, and ventilation are usually normal (Haller and Lewis, 1984), and levels of lactate and other metabolites are not raised; CK is usually markedly elevated. Isokinetic ergometry can precisely quantify the reduction in peak power, but usually fatigue (reduction in power as the test progresses) is not seen. In keeping with the main location of muscle degeneration, $\dot{V}O_2max$ is more impaired in Duchenne's dystrophy than in the facioscapulohumeral type. Patterns of response that are similar to those of muscular dystrophy are also found in conditions of widespread disorders of the spinal cord and motor nerves. Weakness is associated with poor exercise capacity, but other responses are normal, and CK

level is not raised. Involvement of the sympathetic nerves is identified by subnormal blood pressure increases, and respiratory muscle weakness may lead to prominent dyspnea and a ventilatory limitation.

Inflammatory Disorders of Muscle

Myositis may occur alone or as part of a collagen vascular disorder, leading to severe impairment of exercise capacity, usually with elevated lactate and CK levels; sometimes, a hyperkinetic circulatory response is seen in very disabled patients ($\dot{V}O_2max$ less than 50 per cent predicted) (Haller and Lewis, 1984). The site of the lesion in myositis leads to a pattern of response that overlaps metabolic muscle disorders caused by the reduction in enzyme activity, presumably secondary to inactivity (see below).

Primary Disorders of Muscle Metabolism

I will make a few general points only, in view of the rarity of muscle enzyme defects and the excellent reviews that have been published (Morgan-Hughes, 1982). Most of these conditions are associated with abnormal enzyme activity in many organ systems, and patients who present with primary muscle complaints probably represent the less severe examples of the disorders. Considering only the exercise effects, three groups of disorders may be identified: impaired pyruvate production, impaired pyruvate oxidation, and impaired free fatty acid transport.

Myophosphorylase deficiency (McArdle's syndrome) and phosphofructokinase deficiency (Tarui's syndrome) usually present with severe effort intolerance, muscle pain, and myoglobinuria owing to rhabdomyolysis. Maximum power output is limited and is associated with high heart rates and ventilation, probably owing to reflexes originating in ATP-depleted muscle. Lactate is not produced; thus, the hyperventilation, although superficially suggesting the attainment of an anaerobic threshold, is actually associated with a respiratory alkalosis (Hagberg et al., 1982). If exercise is preceded by a long warm-up, endurance is increased because of mobilization and oxidation of fatty acids (a "second wind" effect) (Pernow et al., 1967).

In contrast to disorders of pyruvate production, conditions of impaired pyruvate oxidation (deficiency of pyruvate dehydrogenase or the cytochrome respiratory chain) are associated with markedly increased lactate production; the associated increase in carbon dioxide output leads to dyspnea as a prominent symptom, and ventilation is grossly increased in exercise, as are heart rate and cardiac output (Linderholm et al., 1969).

In conditions of impaired fatty acid transfer into

the mitochondrium (carnitine and carnitine acetyl transferase deficiencies), $\dot{V}O_2$max is less impaired, and abnormalities are more likely to be seen in endurance exercise performance, especially if exercise is repeated or performed in a fasting state, situations in which there is normally a dependence on fatty acids as substrates for exercise. A high respiratory exchange ratio indicates a dependence on glycogen as the main fuel (Carroll et al., 1978) and is accompanied by elevated plasma free fatty acid concentrations (Layzer et al., 1980); adipose tissue fat is mobilized but cannot be used. As in other metabolic defects, plasma CK levels are usually elevated.

Although exercise testing is helpful in the differential diagnosis of these conditions, muscle biopsy and biochemical determination of enzyme activities are required to make a specific diagnosis (Edwards et al., 1980).

Muscle dysfunction probably plays an important role in the disability of most chronic disorders, and the rapidity of its development means that weakness and fatigue are prominent in the recovery from many acute illnesses. Although this seems self-evident in the case of limb immobilization after injury, measurement of muscle strength and endurance after febrile illnesses (Friman, 1977) and myocardial infarction (Jones and McCartney, 1986), for example, indicate that these effects are probably more common than previously appreciated. Because such effects may be prevented or rapidly reversed by appropriate activity, quantitative assessment may be helpful when the mechanisms underlying disability are uncertain. As in primary muscle disorders, there may be contributions from muscle fiber degeneration and from reductions in muscle enzyme activity, depending on the cause and its duration. These changes are expressed in a reduction in maximum power and $\dot{V}O_2$max, with increase in perceived effort (reduced strength) and in excess lactate production (reduced activity of pyruvate dehydrogenase and oxidative enzymes) (MacDougall et al., 1977; Ward et al., 1986). An increase in ventilation is common, secondary to lactate accumulation, and impaired circulatory responses (high heart rate, low blood pressure, and low cardiac output) may also occur (Friman et al., 1985).

EVALUATION OF METABOLIC AND ENDOCRINE FUNCTION

A variety of endocrine disorders may impair exercise performance—thyrotoxicosis (Massey et al., 1967), hypothyroidism (Burack et al., 1971), and diabetes (Berger et al., 1977)—but exercise tests have a relatively minor role in their assessment. On the other hand, the growth hormone response to exercise has yielded a reliable indication of growth hormone deficiency (Sutton and Lazarus, 1976; Johnsonbaugh et al., 1978). The increases in ovarian hormones and gonadotropins that occur in exercise in healthy subjects (Jurkowski et al., 1978) may also prove helpful in assessing pituitary and ovarian disorders.

EVALUATION OF BLOOD DISORDERS

The importance of oxygen delivery to muscle has stimulated several studies of the effects of changes in circulating hemoglobin on $\dot{V}O_2$max that help to define the contributions of anemia and polycythemia to disability. Isovolumic reduction in hemoglobin maintained for several days results in a reduction in $\dot{V}O_2$max that is about two thirds of the percentage reduction in hemoglobin (Woodson et al., 1978; Woodson, 1984). At any given exercise level, cardiac output is higher in the anemic state, but this adaptation is relatively less effective with increasing anemia and increasing time. Similarly, increases in hemoglobin are associated with increases in $\dot{V}O_2$max (Buick et al., 1980). What relevance these studies in healthy humans have to the clinical conditions is not easy to decide; the changes in hemoglobin may be much greater, are maintained for longer, and are often associated with other pathology that may impair exercise. Furthermore, few studies are available in which patients act as their own controls; the comparability of normal standards may be questionable. G. J. Miller and colleagues (1973) studied patients with sickle cell disease, comparing their exercise results with those of a carefully selected control group; $\dot{V}O_2$max was reduced roughly in parallel with reduction in hemoglobin, but reductions in $\dot{V}O_2$max and increases in heart rate were accounted for in part by reductions in muscle mass. Lactate accumulation in blood occurred at a lower $\dot{V}O_2$ and was associated with increases in ventilation. Similar findings were reported by D. M. Miller and associates (1980), who carried out studies before and after exchange transfusion with hemoglobin A–containing cells. Although transfusion was not accompanied by a change in hemoglobin content, exercise performance increased and lactate production lessened, suggesting that the main effect of the exchange was to reduce blood viscosity and improve tissue oxygen delivery. In polycythemia, the increases in oxygen-carrying capacity are offset by increases in blood viscosity that reduce muscle blood flow; even with normal hemoglobin, blood viscosity may limit muscle blood flow in peripheral vascular disease (Yates et al., 1979).

Abnormalities in the molecular structure of hemoglobin, or in red cell enzymes, may influence the characteristics of the oxyhemoglobin dissociation curve, shifting it to the right (high P50) or left (low P50). Oski and co-workers (1971) contrasted a patient with red cell hexokinase deficiency (P50 of 19 mm Hg) with one having pyruvate kinase deficiency (P50 of 38 mm Hg) to show that leftward shifts are associated with impaired offloading of oxygen in the tissues, poor exercise tolerance, and excessive lactate production. In sickle cell disease, the rightward-shifted dissociation curve of hemoglobin S has been thought to play an adaptive role in compensation for anemia but as replacement with normal cells is associated with improved $\dot{V}O_2$max (Miller et al., 1980), this role cannot be important. Miller and associates make the point that many factors contribute to disability in anemia and suggest that measurement of $\dot{V}O_2$max may provide a means for assessing treatment in complex disorders. Also, the experimental studies on the effects of low hemoglobin may allow its contribution to exercise impairment to be assessed in a patient with a primary cardiac or pulmonary disorder who is also anemic.

A number of studies have used exercise to follow erythropoietin treatment of patients with renal failure and anemia (Robertson et al., 1990; McMahon et al., 1992).

One factor frequently encountered in patients referred for exercise testing is an elevated blood carboxyhemoglobin level, which is often increased in smokers, sometimes by as much as 15 per cent. Studies of carbon monoxide inhalation have shown that $\dot{V}O_2$max and the anaerobic threshold are decreased roughly in parallel with the increase in carboxyhemoglobin (Koike and Wasserman, 1992).

EVALUATION OF CHRONIC FATIGUE SYNDROMES

Syndromes consisting of severe effort intolerance without clinical evidence of a specific cause have been recognized for many years (e.g., effort syndrome, soldier's heart, neurocirculatory or vasoregulatory asthenia, postviral syndrome, and benign myalgic encephalomyelitis). The severe handicap, frequent disability, absence of clinical findings, and attitude of frustration with the many physicians that most sufferers have gone to for help have led to a feeling that these conditions straddle the boundary between medicine and psychiatry. Although in a general sense, this is as true as in any chronic disabling disorder, it seems likely that the impairment in physiological function comes first and that the psychological reactions come later and tend to contribute to limitation and its chronicity. The fact that the causative agent or mechanisms have not been isolated should not prevent us from assessing the severity of effort intolerance, identifying the factors contributing to symptoms, and managing the condition logically. Thus, even though criteria have

been proposed for the diagnosis of the chronic fatigue syndrome (e.g., Lloyd et al., 1991), postviral syndrome, and postpoliomyelitis syndrome, the mechanisms remain controversial, and assessment of the severity of the disorders is based on symptom information.

This is a condition characterized by severe handicap, with variable impairment and disability. Because symptoms are prominent and experienced during exercise, a progressive exercise test with measurement of symptom intensity is of great value, not the least because one may use the results to demonstrate to the patient what is wrong and what may be done about it. This carries many benefits, particularly for patients who have been told "it's all in your head." The results also allow a precise prescription of exercise that can be maintained, rather than a recommendation that the patient exercise but not "overdo it."

An exercise test (Example 8, Chapter 13) usually shows one or all of a number of abnormalities, of which an increase in muscle effort is the most consistent and dramatic; the intensity of this sensation at moderate exercise intensities may be as much as four times that expected. Factors contributing to increased effort may include muscle weakness, evidence of impaired blood flow distribution (high heart rate and cardiac output and less than expected blood pressure increase), and lactate production. The increase in lactate concentration suggests that the activity of oxidative muscle enzyme systems, such as pyruvate dehydrogenase, is poorly activated. Conversely, sometimes a low power is unaccompanied by lactate increases, which may be explained by impaired glycolysis or low muscle glycogen stores. Maximum power output is seldom very low and is often in the low expected range (80–90 per cent predicted), but when accompanied by increased effort, these findings suggest that motor command has had to be increased to achieve it. Extensive research by Gandevia and his colleagues (1963) showed that patients do achieve full activation of muscle, indicating that poor motivation and muscle contractile failure are not important contributing factors to the increased effort. When exercise capacity and the associated effort are related to patients' energy demands in their daily lives, it is often found that their job demands exceed a level that can be maintained with any comfort. Dyspnea is often prominent, most commonly related to an increase in carbon dioxide output and ventilation secondary to lactate production, but sometimes associated with respiratory muscle weakness and an inefficient pattern of breathing. Associated respiratory problems are commonly found, including small lungs due to pectus excavatum or infantile pneumonia, exercise-induced asthma, laryngeal dysfunction, and hyperventilation syndrome. Rarely, an exercise test is followed the next day by muscle pain, prostration, and feverishness, but examination has not provided any clues as to the cause of these symptoms, sometimes ascribed to metabolic changes in muscle, such as glycogen or phosphocreatine depletion, or to associated ionic changes, such as potassium loss and low pH. Many of the mechanisms suggested above have not yet been demonstrated, at least partly because of the difficulties in performing invasive studies such as muscle biopsies in group of patients who are experiencing distressing symptoms. Exercise prescription, based on the results of an exercise study, is an important treatment modality (Levander-Lindgren and Ek, 1962).

EVALUATION OF OCCUPATIONAL HEALTH

The assessment of disability related to industrial compensation and the ability of a worker to carry on in his or her job may be major applications for exercise testing. Usually, a patient is referred because of symptoms experienced during work or because of an abnormality found in routine examination, as on a chest radiograph. Often, impairment of pulmonary function has been found, and the clinical question to be answered is whether the impairment is sufficient to prevent the worker from comfortably meeting the physical demands of the job. Impairment of function revealed by tests at rest can identify only those patients with the two extremes of disability—workers who must be disabled because of severe impairment and those unlikely to be disabled because impairment is slight or nonexistent. In most cases, it is impossible to use resting measurements with any degree of confidence, and it is in these cases that exercise assessment helps. Although disability is often used to describe reduced capacity to meet the demands of everyday life and occupation, there are arguments for using the term to define a reduction in exercise capacity. This allows disability to be more or less precisely quantified. A variety of disability gradings have been used in the past, such as the grading put forward by Gaensler and Wright (1966) for diffuse pulmonary disease, recently re-examined by Epler and colleagues (1980). One approach (Ostiguy, 1979) includes exercise test responses (Table 4–1). Having defined *impairment* as the reduction in organ function and *disability* as the reduction in exercise capacity, a third criterion may be recognized, that of *handicap,* which expresses the difficulty experienced in following a given way of life or occupation. Thus, in general, although handicap is related to impairment and disability, there is considerable room for variation. The variation may be accounted for by variations in job requirements, occupational skills, personality, and many other factors.

In the assessment of the suitability for employment in an occupation, a number of approaches are available. In the case of a patient who has recovered from a myocardial infarction, an initial simple approach is to perform a progressive symptom-limited exercise test and examine the results in relation to the known average energy costs of the job (Fig.

Table 4–1. CLASSIFICATION OF IMPAIRMENT

Class	Spirometry*	CO Uptake*	Exercise	Resting Blood Gases
Class I (non)	FEV$_1$ and VC both within $\pm 20\%$ predicted	DLCO within $\pm 25\%$ predicted	$\dot{V}O_2$max > 25 mL/kg/min (Wmax 75% predicted)	Normal Paco$_2$ and A-aPo$_2$ difference
Class II (mild)	FEV$_1$ or VC < 80% predicted	DLCO < 75% predicted	$\dot{V}O_2$max < 25 mL/kg/min (Wmax 50–75% predicted)	Normal Paco$_2$ Pao$_2$ > 70 mm Hg
Class III (moderate)	FEV$_1$ or VC 40–60% predicted	DLCO 50–75% predicted	$\dot{V}O_2$max < 15 mL/kg/min (Wmax 50% predicted)	Normal Paco$_2$ Pao$_2$ > 60 mm Hg
Class IV (severe)	FEV$_1$ or VC < 40% predicted	DLCO < 50% predicted	$\dot{V}O_2$max < 7 mL/kg/min (Wmax 25% predicted)	Normal Paco$_2$ Pao$_2$ < 60 mm Hg
Class V (very severe)	FEV$_1$ or VC < 40% predicted	DLCO < 50% predicted	$\dot{V}O_2$max < 7 mL/kg/min (Wmax 25% predicted)	Paco$_2$ > 45 mm Hg and/or Pao$_2$ < 50 mm Hg

*Predicted values on basis of age, sex, and size: spirometric defect may be obstructive (low FEV/VC) or nonobstructive (low VC with normal or high FEV/VC).

Modified from Ostiguy GL. Summary of the task force report on occupational respiratory disease (pneumoconiosis). Can Med Assoc J 1979;121:414–421. By permission of the publisher.

4–4); these should not exceed 50 per cent of the maximal power in the test and should be below the power that would elicit electrocardiographic changes and heart rates of more than 70 per cent of the measured maximal heart rate. In some patients, it may be important to monitor heart rate during a working day and compare it with the heart rate measured in the exercise test, to estimate the cardiac strain of the occupation. In the case of a subject complaining of dyspnea caused by chronic airway obstruction, the finding of ventilation rates at maximal exercise that equal the maximal voluntary ventilation constitutes important evidence that pulmonary impairment limits exercise. If this limitation occurs at an exercise level encountered during work, even if only for brief periods, then evidence for severe disability is strengthened.

As mentioned previously, the energy costs of a given occupation are not easy to predict, and there is a large variation among persons that leads to a lack of precision in the application of results in the laboratory to everyday situations. Within these limitations, we may use published values for energy demands (Passmore and Durnin, 1955) in the interpretation of exercise tests, realizing that in a small number of cases, observations made during work may be required to supplement the laboratory information (see Fig. 4–4).

THE PRESCRIPTION OF EXERCISE

Exercise has become a popular component of many rehabilitation programs, particularly in coronary artery disease. An adequate prescription of exercise in any patient who has exercise-related symptoms or in whom exercise may be hazardous requires information obtained in a progressive maximal exercise test.

In addition to choosing suitable intensities of training activities (Fig. 4–5) and ensuring that potentially dangerous complications do not occur, the test results are used to identify a training heart rate that may be monitored by the patient (Oldridge et al., 1978). Guidelines for the use of exercise tests in prescribing activity for cardiac and respiratory patients have been published (American College of Sports Medicine, 1986).

In recent years, a limited exercise study has been advocated before a patient recovering from myocardial infarction is discharged from hospital. Exercise-related arrhythmias and myocardial dysfunction may be identified by the study, and precise advice may be given to the patient with regard to activities that may be safely undertaken. The results also may predict outcome over the next year (Théroux et al., 1979).

USE OF EXERCISE TESTING IN PREOPERATIVE EVALUATION

It seems intuitively obvious that there will be a relationship between exercise capacity and the ability to withstand the stress of major operations. The increasing use of major surgical procedures, partic-

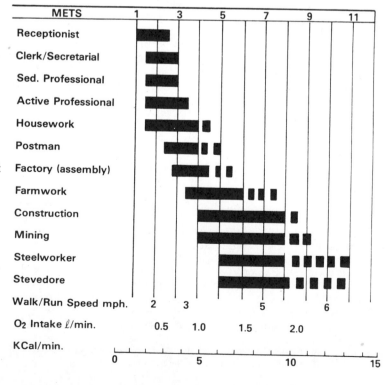

Figure 4–4. Energy costs of various occupations, expressed as mets (1 met = 3.5 mL O_2/kg). The solid bars represent average energy costs; short-term demands are represented by the broken bars. Sed. = sedentary.

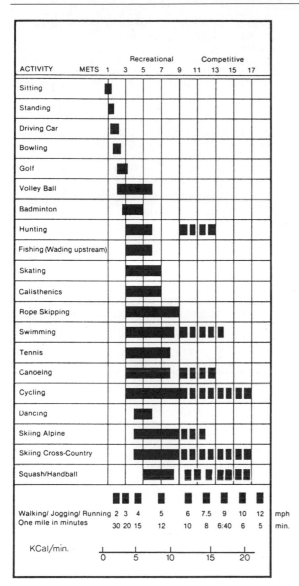

Figure 4–5. Energy costs of various recreational and training activities.

probably to reveal other contributors to disability, in addition to the condition being approached surgically; for example, the identification of muscle weakness and its improvement therapeutically improves outcome in candidates being assessed for transplantation (Howard et al., 1994).

SUMMARY

This chapter has reviewed some of the clinical situations in which an exercise test assessment of cardiac and respiratory reserve may influence patient management. In recent years, methods have been made precise and reference standards have been developed to make exercise testing widely applicable to many clinical conditions. If the techniques and measurements are kept simple and noninvasive, the range of clinical usefulness will inevitably widen. As with any other clinical investigation, the clinical value in terms of cost versus benefit must be kept in mind, but I would suggest that if the staged approach to exercise testing is followed, the cost side of this equation may be kept acceptably small.

REFERENCES

Agusti AGN, Roca J, Gea J, et al. Mechanisms of gas-exchange impairment in idiopathic pulmonary fibrosis. Am Rev Respir Dis 1991;143:219–225.

American College of Sports Medicine. Guidelines for Graded Exercise Testing and Exercise Prescription. Philadelphia: Lea & Febiger, 1986.

Anderson SD, Silverman M, Walker SR. Metabolic and ventilatory changes in asthmatic patients during and after exercise. Thorax 1972;27:718–725.

Anderton RC, Cuff MT, Frith PA, et al. Bronchial responsiveness to inhaled histamine and exercise. J Allergy Clin Immunol 1979;63:315–320.

Areskog NH. Exercise testing in the evaluation of patients with valvular aortic stenosis. Clin Physiol 1984;4:201–208.

Armstrong BW, Workman JN, Hurt HH, et al. Clinico-physiologic evaluation of physical working capacity in persons with pulmonary disease. Am Rev Respir Dis 1966;93:90–99, 223–233.

Arnolda L, Conway M, Doleck M, et al. Skeletal muscle metabolism in heart failure; a ^{31}P nuclear magnetic resonance spectroscopy study of leg muscle. Clin Sci 1990;79:583–589.

Aronow WS, Cassidy J. Five year follow-up of double Master's test, maximal treadmill stress test and resting and post exercise apex cardiogram in asymptomatic persons. Circulation 1975;52:616–618.

Aronow WS, Harris CN. Treadmill exercise test in aortic stenosis and mitral stenosis. Chest 1975;68:507–509.

Auchincloss JH Jr, Gilbert R, Bowman JL. Response of oxygen uptake to exercise in coronary artery disease. Chest 1974;65:500–506.

Barlow CW, Qayyum MS, Davey PP, et al. Effect of physical-training on exercise-induced hyperkalemia in chronic heart-failure: Relation with ventilation and catecholamines. Circulation 1994;89:1144–1152.

Bates DV, Gee JBL, Bentivoglio LG, et al. Diffusion as a limiting factor in oxygen transport across the lung. Proc Int

ularly on the heart and lungs, has led to numerous studies on the use of preoperative exercise testing to predict outcome and the incidence of complications after surgery. Thoracic surgery and lung resection have been most often studied, and in general the intuition has been supported (Olsen, 1989; Gilbreth and Weisman, 1994), with measurements of $\dot{V}o_2max$ predicting morbidity and mortality after lung resection (Bolliger et al., 1995). The capacity to increase ventilation normally during exercise, together with clinical and historical information, helps to predict the incidence of respiratory complications (Dales et al., 1993). The same conclusion applies to heart-lung transplantation (Howard et al., 1994). The most valuable use of exercise testing is

Symp Cardiovasc Respir Effects Hypoxia. Basel/New York: Karger; 1966.

Bendien C, Bossina KK, Buurma AE, et al. Hemodynamic effects of dynamic exercise in children and adolescents with moderate-to-small ventricular septal defects. Circulation 1984;70:929–934.

Berger M, Berchtold P, Cuppers HJ, et al. Metabolic and hormonal effects of muscular exercise in juvenile type diabetics. Diabetologia 1977;13:355–365.

Bergman AB, Stamm SJ. The morbidity of cardiac non-disease in school children. N Engl J Med 1967;276:1008–1013.

Bevegård S, Eriksson BO, Graff-Lonnevig V, et al. Respiratory function, cardiovascular dimensions and work capacity in boys with bronchial asthma. Acta Paediatr 1976;65:289–296.

Bishop JM, Wade OL. Relationships between cardiac output and rhythm, pulmonary vascular pressures and disability in mitral stenosis. Clin Sci 1963;24:391–404.

Blackmon JR, Rowell LB, Kennedy JW, et al. Physiological significance of maximal oxygen intake in "pure" mitral stenosis. Circulation 1967;36:497–510.

Bobbio M, Detrano R, Schmid JJ, et al. Exercise-induced ST depression and ST/heart rate index to predict triple-vessel or left main coronary disease: A multicenter analysis. J Am Coll Cardiol 1992;19:11–18.

Bolliger CT, Jordan P, Soler M, et al. Exercise capacity as a predictor of postoperative complications in lung resection candidates. Am J Respir Crit Care Med 1995;151:1472–1480.

Borg GAV. Psychophysical bases of perceived exertion. Med Sci Sports Exerc 1982;14:377–381.

Borg G, Linderholm H. Exercise performance and perceived exertion in patients with coronary insufficiency, arterial hypertension and vasoregulatory asthenia. Acta Med Scand 1970;187:17–26.

Brown SE, Nagendran RC, McHugh JW, et al. Effects of a large carbohydrate load on walking performance in chronic air-flow obstruction. Am Rev Respir Dis 1985a;132:960–962.

Brown SE, Weiner S, Brown RA. Exercise performance following a carbohydrate load in chronic airflow obstruction. J Appl Physiol 1985b;58:1340–1346.

Bruce RA. Exercise testing for evaluation of ventricular function. N Engl J Med 1977;296:671–675.

Bruce RA, Derouen T, Peterson DR, et al. Noninvasive predictors of sudden cardiac death in men with coronary heart disease. Am J Cardiol 1977;39:833–840.

Bruce RA, Fisher LD, Cooper MN, et al. Separation of effects of cardiovascular disease and age on ventricular function with maximal exercise. Am J Cardiol 1974;34:757–769.

Buick FJ, Gledhill N, Froese AB, et al. Effect of induced erythrocythemia on aerobic work capacity. J Appl Physiol 1980;48:436–442.

Burack R, Edwards RHT, Green M, et al. The response to exercise before and after thyroxine treatment of myxedema. J Pharmacol Exp Ther 1971;176:212–219.

Burdon JGW, Killian KJ, Jones NL. The pattern of breathing during exercise in patients with interstitial lung disease. Thorax 1983;38:778–784.

Burns BH, Howell JBL. Disproportionately severe breathlessness in chronic bronchitis. Q J Med 1969;38:277–294.

Burrows B, Kettel LJ, Niden AH. Patterns of cardiovascular dysfunction in chronic obstructive lung disease. N Engl J Med 1972;286:912–918.

Bye PT, Anderson SD, Woolcock AJ, et al. Bicycle exercise performance of patients with interstitial lung disease breathing air and oxygen. Am Rev Respir Dis 1981;123:1005–1012.

Bye PT, Esau SA, Levy RD, et al. Ventilatory function during exercise in air and oxygen in patients with chronic air-flow limitation. Am Rev Respir Dis 1985;132:236–240.

Caiozzo VJ, Davis JA, Ellis JF, et al. A comparison of gas exchange indices used to detect the anaerobic threshold. J Appl Physiol 1982;53:1184–1189.

Carliner NH, Fisher ML, Pltnick GD, et al. Routine pre-operative exercise testing in patients undergoing major non-cardiac surgery. Am J Cardiol 1985;56:51–58.

Carroll JE, Brooke MH, DeVivo DC, et al. Biochemical and physiological consequences of carnitine palmityltransferase deficiency. Muscle Nerve 1978;1:103–110.

Carroll JE, Hagberg JM, Brooke MH, et al. Bicycle ergometry and gas exchange measurements in neuromuscular diseases. Arch Neurol 1979;36:457–461.

Chaitman BR, Bourassa MG, Davis K, et al. Angiographic prevalence of high-risk coronary artery disease in patient subsets (CASS). Circulation 1981;64:360–367.

Cherniack NS. Control of breathing in COPD. In: Cherniack NS, editor. Chronic Obstructive Pulmonary Disease. Philadelphia: WB Saunders Co.; 1991, pp. 117–126.

Clark TJH, Freedman S, Campbell EJM, et al. The ventilatory capacity of patients with chronic airway obstruction. Clin Sci 1969;36:307–316.

Crawford M, O'Rourke RA, Ramakrishna N, et al. Comparative effectiveness of exercise testing and continuous monitoring for detecting arrhythmias in patients with previous myocardial infarction. Circulation 1974;50:301–305.

Cross AM, Higginbotham MB. Oxygen deficit during exercise testing in heart-failure: Relation to submaximal exercise tolerance. Chest 1995;107:904–908.

Cumming GR. Maximal exercise capacity of children with heart defects. Am J Cardiol 1978;42:613–619.

Cumming GR, Samm J, Borysyk L, et al. Electrocardiographic changes during exercises in asymptomatic men: 3 year follow-up. Can Med Assoc J 1975;112:578–581.

Dagenais GR, Rouleau JR, Hochart P, et al. Survival with painless strongly positive exercise electrocardiogram. Am J Cardiol 1988;62:892–895.

Dales RE, Dionne G, Leech JA, Schweitzer I. Preoperative prediction of pulmonary complications following thoracic surgery. Chest 1993;104:155–159.

Daly JJ, Duff RS, Jackson E, et al. Effect of exercise on arterial lactate, pyruvate and excess lactate in chronic bronchitis. Br J Dis Chest 1967;61:193–197.

Dantzker DR, Patten GA, Bower JS. Gas exchange at rest and during exercise in adults with cystic fibrosis. Am Rev Respir Dis 1982;125:400–405.

Davies H, Gazetopoulos N. Haemodynamic changes on exercise in patients with left-to-right shunts. Br Heart J 1966;28:579–589.

DeBusk RF, Kraemer HC, Nash E. Stepwise risk stratification soon after acute myocardial infarction. Am J Cardiol 1983;52:1161–1166.

Deckers JW, Fioretti P, Brower RW, et al. Prediction of 1-year outcome after complicated and uncomplicated myocardial infarction: Bayesian analysis of predischarge exercise test results in 300 patients. Am Heart J 1987;113:90–95.

Denison D, Al-Hillawi H, Turton C. Lung function in interstitial lung disease. Semin Respir Med 1984;6:40–54.

Devereux RB. Mitral valve prolapse. Am J Med 1979;67:729–731.

Donald KW, Bishop JM, Wade OL. A study of minute to minute changes of arteriovenous oxygen difference, oxygen uptake and cardiac output, and rate of achievement of a steady state during exercise in rheumatic heart disease. J Clin Invest 1954;33:1146–1167.

Dubach P, Froelicher V, Klien J, Detrano R. Use of the exercise test to predict prognosis after coronary artery bypass grafting. Am J Cardiol 1989;63:530–533.

Dubach P, Froelicher V, Klien J, et al. Exercise-induced hypotension in a male population: Criteria, causes and prognosis. Circulation 1988;78:1380–1387.

Edwards RHT. Physiological and metabolic studies of the contractile machinery of human muscle and disease. Phys Med Biol 1979;24:237–249.

Edwards RHT. Weakness and fatigue of skeletal muscles. In:

Sarner M, editor. Advanced Medicine. London: Pitman Medical; 1982;18:100–119.

Edwards RHT, Kristinsson A, Warrell DA, et al. Effects of propranolol on response to exercise in hypertrophic obstructive cardiomyopathy. Br Heart J 1970;32:219–225.

Edwards RHT, Young A, Wiles M. Needle biopsy of skeletal muscle in the diagnosis of myopathy and the clinical study of muscle function and repair. N Engl J Med 1980;302:261–271.

Ekblom B, Goldbarg AN. The influence of physical training and other factors on subjective rating of perceived exertion. Acta Physiol Scand 1971;83:399–406.

Ellestad MH, Wan MKC. Predictive implications of stress testing. Circulation 1975;51:363–369.

Epler GR, Saber FA, Gaensler EA. Determination of severe impairment (disability) in interstitial lung disease. Am Rev Respir Dis 1980;121:647–660.

Epstein SE, Beiser GD, Goldstein RE, et al. Hemodynamic abnormalities in response to mild and intense upright exercise following operative correction of an atrial septal defect or tetralogy of Fallot. Circulation 1973;47:1065–1075.

Evans SA, Watson L, Cowley AJ, et al. Static lung compliance in chronic heart-failure: Relation with dyspnea and exercise capacity. Thorax 1995;50:245–248.

Fixler DE, Laird WP, Dana K. Usefulness of exercise stress testing for prediction of blood pressure trends. Pediatrics 1985;75:1071–1075.

Fletcher GF, Balady G, Froelicher V, et al. Exercise standards: A statement for healthcare professionals from the American Heart Association. Circulation 1995;91:580–615.

Franciosa JA, Leddy CL, Wilen M, Schwartz DE. Relation between hemodynamic and ventilatory responses in determining exercise capacity in severe congestive heart failure. Am J Cardiol 1984;53:127–134.

Franciosa JA, Park M, Levine TB. Lack of correlation between exercise capacity and indices of resting left ventricular performance in heart failure. Am J Cardiol 1981;47:33–39.

Franz IW. Ergometry in the assessment of arterial hypertension. Cardiology 1985;72:147–159.

Friman G. Effects of acute infectious diseases on isometric muscle strength. Scand J Clin Lab Invest 1977;37:303–308.

Friman G, Wright JE, Ilback NG, et al. Does fever or myalgia indicate reduced physical performance capacity in viral infections? Acta Med Scand 1985;217:353–361.

Froelicher VF, Yanowitz FG, Thompson AJ, et al. The correlation of coronary angiography and the electrocardiographic response to maximal treadmill testing in 76 asymptomatic men. Circulation 1973;48:597–604.

Fulmer JD, Roberts WC, von Gal ER, et al. Morphologic-physiologic correlates of the severity of fibrosis and degree of cellularity in idiopathic pulmonary fibrosis. J Clin Invest 1979;63:665–676.

Gaensler EA, Wright GW. Evaluation of respiratory impairment. Arch Environ Health 1966;12:146–189.

Gandevia B. Ventilatory response to exercise and the results of a standardized exercise test in chronic obstructive lung disease. Am Rev Respir Dis 1963;88:66, 406–408.

Gandevia SC, McCloskey DI. Changes in motor commands, as shown by changes in perceived heaviness, during partial curarization and peripheral anesthesia in man. J Physiol 1977;272:673–689.

Garg A, Saxena U. Effects of lifting frequency and technique on physical fatigue with special reference to psychophysical methodology and metabolic rate. Am Ind Hyg Assoc J 1979;40:894–903.

Gazetopoulos N, Davies H, Oliver C, et al. Ventilation and haemodynamics in heart disease. Br Heart J 1966;28:1–15.

Gazetopoulos N, Salonikides N, Davies H. Cardiopulmonary function in patients with pulmonary hypertension. Br Heart J 1974;36:19–28.

Gibson RS, Watson DD, Craddock GB, et al. Prediction of cardiac events after uncomplicated myocardial infarction: A prospective study comparing predischarge exercise thallium-201 scintigraphy and coronary angiography. Circulation 1983;68:321–336.

Gilbreth EM, Weisman IM. Role of exercise stress-testing in preoperative evaluation of patients for lung resection. Clin Chest Med 1994;15:389–403.

Godfrey S. Exercise-induced asthma: Clinical, physiological, and therapeutic implications. J Allergy Clin Immunol 1975;56:1–17.

Godfrey S. Physiological response to exercise in children with lung or heart disease. Arch Dis Child 1970;45:534–538.

Godfrey S, Bluestone R, Higgs BE. Lung function and the response to exercise in systemic sclerosis. Thorax 1969;24:427–434.

Godfrey S, Mearns M. Pulmonary function and response to exercise in cystic fibrosis. Arch Dis Child 1971;46:144–151.

Hagberg JM, Coyle EF, Carroll JE, et al. Exercise hyperventilation in patients with McArdle's disease. J Appl Physiol 1982;52:991–994.

Haller RG, Lewis SF. Pathophysiology of exercise performance in muscle disease. Med Sci Sports Exerc 1984;16:456–459.

Haller RG, Lewis SF, Cook JD, et al. Hyperkinetic circulation during exercise in neuromuscular disease. Neurology 1983;33:1283–1287.

Hamilton AL, Killian KJ, Summers E, Jones NL. Muscle strength, symptom intensity, and exercise capacity in patients with cardiorespiratory disorders. Am J Respir Crit Care Med 1995;152:2021–2031.

Hammond MD, Bauer KA, Sharp JT, Rocha RD. Respiratory muscle strength in congestive heart failure. Chest 1990;98:1091–1094.

Harrison TR, Pilcher C. Studies in congestive heart failure: The respiratory exchange during and after exercise. J Clin Invest 1930;8:291–315.

Hollenberg M, Budge WR, Wisnecki JA, et al. Treadmill score quantifies electrocardiographic response to exercise and improves test accuracy and reproducibility. Circulation 1980;61:276–285.

Hollenberg M, Wisnecki JA, Gertz EW, et al. Computer-derived treadmill exercise score quantifies the degree of revascularization and improved exercise performance after coronary artery bypass surgery. Am Heart J 1983;106:1096–1104.

Hollenberg M, Zoltick JM, Go M, et al. Comparison of a quantitative treadmill exercise score with standard electrocardiographic criteria in screening asymptomatic young men for coronary artery disease. N Engl J Med 1985;313:600–606.

Holm S, Bylund-Fellenius A-C. Continuous monitoring of oxygen tension in human gastrocnemius muscle during exercise. Clin Physiol 1981;1:541–552.

Holmgren A, Jonsson B, Linderholm H, et al. Physical working capacity in cases of mitral valvular disease in relation to heart volume, total amount of hemoglobin and stroke volume. Acta Med Scand 1958;162:99–122.

Holmgren A, Strom G. Blood lactate concentration in relation to absolute and relative work load in normal men, and in mitral stenosis, atrial septal defect and vasoregulatory asthenia. Acta Med Scand 1959;163:185–193.

Hossack KF, Neilson GH. Exercise testing in congenital aortic stenosis. Aust N Z J Med 1979;9:169–173.

Howard DK, Iademarco EJ, Trulock EP. The role of cardiopulmonary exercise testing in lung and heart-lung transplantation. Clin Chest Med 1994;15:405–420.

Huang CT, Heurich AE, Rosen Y, et al. Pulmonary sarcoidosis. Respiration 1979;37:337–345.

Hung J, Chaitman BR, Lam J, et al. A logistic regression analysis of multiple noninvasive tests for the prediction of the presence and extent of coronary artery disease in men. Am Heart J 1985;110:460–468.

Hyland RH, Jones NL, Powles ACP, et al. Primary alveolar hypoventilation treated with nocturnal electrophrenic respiration. Am Rev Respir Dis 1978;117:165–172.

Ikkos D, Jonsson B, Linderholm H. Effect of exercise in pulmonary stenosis with intact ventricular septum. Br Heart J 1966;28:316–330.

Janicki JS, Weber KT, Likoff MJ, et al. Exercise testing to evaluate patients with pulmonary vascular disease. Am Rev Respir Dis 1984;129:S93–S95.

Johnson RL, Taylor HF, Degraff AC. Functional significance of a low pulmonary diffusing capacity for carbon monoxide. J Clin Invest 1965;44:789–800.

Johnsonbaugh RE, Bybee DE, Georges LP. Exercise tolerance test. Single-sample screening technique to rule out growth-hormone deficiency. JAMA 1978;240:664–666.

Jones GL, Killian KJ, Summers E, Jones NL. Inspiratory muscle forces and endurance in maximal resistive loading. J Appl Physiol 1985;58:1608–1615.

Jones NL. Exercise testing in pulmonary evaluation: Clinical application. N Engl J Med 1975a;293:647–649.

Jones NL. Exercise testing in pulmonary evaluation: Rationale, methods and the normal respiratory response to exercise. N Engl J Med 1975b;293:541–544.

Jones NL. Pulmonary gas exchange during exercise in patients with chronic airway obstruction. Clin Sci 1966;31:39–50.

Jones NL. Use of exercise in testing respiratory control mechanisms. Chest 1976;70:171–173.

Jones NL, Berman LB. Gas exchange in chronic air-flow obstruction. Am Rev Respir Dis 1984;129:S81–S83.

Jones NL, Ehrsam R. The anerobic threshold. Exerc Sport Sci Rev 1982;10:49–83.

Jones NL, Goodwin JF. Respiratory function in pulmonary thromboembolic disorders. BMJ 1965;1:1089–1093.

Jones NL, Jones G, Edwards RHT. Exercise tolerance in chronic airway obstruction. Am Rev Respir Dis 1971;103:477–491.

Jones NL, McCartney N. Influence of muscle power on aerobic performance and the effects of training. Acta Med Scand Suppl 1986;711:115–122.

Jones NL, Rebuck AS. Tidal volume during exercise in patients with diffuse fibrosing alveolitis. Bull Eur Physiopathol Respir 1979;15:321–327.

Jones RH, McEwan P, Newman GE, et al. Accuracy of diagnosis of coronary artery disease by radionuclide measurement of left ventricular function during rest and exercise. Circulation 1981;64:585–601.

Jones RS. Assessment of respiratory function in the asthmatic child. BMJ 1966;2:972–976.

Jurkowski JE, Jones NL, Walker WC, et al. Ovarian hormonal responses to exercise. J Appl Physiol 1978;44:109–114.

Keogh BA, Lakatos E, Price D, et al. Importance of the lower respiratory tract in oxygen transfer. Am Rev Respir Dis 1984;129:S76–S80.

Killian KJ. The objective measurement of breathlessness. Chest 1985;88:84S–90S.

Killian KJ, Symptoms limiting exercise. In: Jones NL, Killian KJ, editors. Breathlessness. The Campbell Symposium. Burlington, Canada: Boehringer-Ingelheim; 1992, pp. 132–142.

Killian KJ, Jones NL. The use of exercise testing and other methods in the investigation of dyspnea. Clin Chest Med 1984;5:99–108.

Koike A, Wasserman K. Effect of acute reduction in oxygen transport on parameters of aerobic function during exercise. Ann Acad Med Singapore 1992;21:14–22.

Kveselis DA, Rocchini AP, Roaenthal A, et al. Hemodynamic determinants of exercise-induced ST-segment depression in children with valvular aortic stenosis. Am J Cardiol 1985;55:1133–1139.

Laarman G, Luijten HE, van Zeyl LG, et al. Assessment of silent restenosis and long-term follow-up after successful angioplasty in single vessel coronary artery disease: The value of quantitative exercise electrocardiography and quantitative coronary angiography. J Am Coll Cardiol 1990;16:578–585.

Lands LC, Heigenhauser GJF, Jones NL. Analysis of factors limiting maximal exercise performance in cystic fibrosis. Clin Sci 1992;83:391–397.

Lands LC, Heigenhauser GJF, Jones NL. Respiratory and peripheral muscle function in cystic fibrosis. Am Rev Respir Dis 1993;147:865–869.

Lapin ES, Murray JA, Bruce RA, et al. Changes in maximal exercise performance in the evaluation of saphenous vein bypass surgery. Circulation 1973;47:1164–1173.

Lassen NA, Kampp M. Calf muscle blood flow during walking studied by the Xe[133] method in normals and in patients with intermittent claudication. Scand J Clin Lab Invest 1965;17:447–453.

Layzer RB, Havel RJ, McIlroy MB. Partial deficiency of carnitine palmityltransferase: Physiologic and biochemical consequences. Neurology 1980;30:627–633.

Leblanc P, Bowie DM, Summers E, et al. Breathlessness and exercise in patients with respiratory disease. Am Rev Respir Dis 1986;133:21–25.

Leblanc P, Summers E, Inman MD, et al. Inspiratory muscles during exercise: A problem of supply and demand. J Appl Physiol 1988;64:2482–2489.

Lee SJK, Jonsson B, Bevegård S, et al. Hemodynamic changes at rest and during exercise in patients with aortic stenosis of varying severity. Am Heart J 1970;79:318–331.

Levander-Lindgren MAJ, Ek S. Studies in neurocirculatory asthenia (Da Costa's syndrome). Acta Med Scand 1962; 172:678–683.

Levy S, Broustet JP, Clementy J, et al. Syndrome de Wolff-Parkinson-White. Arch Mal Coeur 1979;72:634–640.

Light RW, Mintz HM, Linden GS, et al. Hemodynamics of patients with severe chronic obstructive pulmonary disease during progressive upright exercise. Am Rev Respir Dis 1984;130:391–395.

Linderholm H, Muller R, Ringqvist T, et al. Hereditary abnormal muscle metabolism with hyperkinetic circulation during exercise. Acta Med Scand 1969;185:153–166.

Linderholm H, Osterman G, Teien D. Detection of coronary artery disease by means of exercise ECG in patients with aortic stenosis. Acta Med Scand 1985;218:181–188.

Lipkin DP, Perrins J, Poole-Wilson PA. Respiratory gas exchange in the assessment of patients with impaired ventricular function. Br Heart J 1985;54:321–328.

Lloyd AR, Gandevia SC, Hales JP. Muscle performance, voluntary activation, twitch properties and perceived effort in normal subjects and patients with the chronic fatigue syndrome. Brain 1991;114:85–98.

MacDougall JD, Ward GR, Sale DG, et al. Biochemical adaptation of human skeletal muscle to heavy resistance training and immobilization. J Appl Physiol 1977;43:700–703.

Magnusson G, Isberg B, Karlberg KE, Sylven C. Skeletal-muscle strength and endurance in chronic congestive heart failure secondary to idiopathic dilated cardiomyopathy. Am J Cardiol 1994;73:307–309.

Mancini DM. Pulmonary factors limiting exercise capacity in patients with heart failure. Prog Cardiovasc Dis 1995;37:347–370.

Mancini DM, Henson D, Lamanca J, et al. Benefit of selective respiratory muscle training on exercise capacity in patients with chronic congestive heart failure. Circulation 1995; 91:320–329.

Mancini DM, Henson D, Lamanca J, Levine S. Evidence of reduced respiratory muscle endurance in patients with heart failure. J Am Coll Cardiol 1994a;24:972–981.

Mancini DM, Wilson JR, Bolinger L, et al. In-vivo magnetic resonance spectroscopy measurement of deoxymyoglobin during exercise in patients with heart failure: Demonstration of abnormal muscle metabolism despite adequate oxygenation. Circulation 1994b;90:500–508.

Marciniuk DD, Gallagher CG. Clinical exercise testing in interstitial lung disease. Clin Chest Med 1994;15:287–303.

Mark DB, Shaw L, Harrell FE, et al. Prognostic value of a

treadmill exercise score in outpatients with suspected coronary artery disease. N Engl J Med 1991;325:849–853.

Massey G, Becklake MR, McKenzie JM, et al. Circulatory and ventilatory response to exercise in thyrotoxicosis. N Engl J Med 1967;276:1104–1112.

Mathur PN, Powles AC, Pugsley SO, et al. Effect of long-term administration of digoxin on exercise performance in chronic airflow obstruction. Eur J Respir Dis 1985;66:273–283.

Matsumara N, Nishijima H, Kojima S, et al. Determination of anaerobic threshold for assessment of functional state in patients with chronic heart failure. Circulation 1983;68:360–370.

Matthay RA, Berger HJ, Davies RA, et al. Right ventricular exercise performance in chronic obstructive pulmonary disease: Radionuclide assessment. Ann Intern Med 1980;93:234–239.

Matthews JI, Hooper RG. Exercise testing in pulmonary sarcoidosis. Chest 1983;83:75–81.

McComas AJ, Belanger AY, Garner S, McCartney N. Muscle performance in neuromuscular disorders. In: Jones NL, McCartney N, McComas AJ, editors. Human Muscle Power. Champaign, IL: Human Kinetics Publishers; 1986, pp. 309–321.

McFadden ER. Exercise performance in the asthmatic. Am Rev Respir Dis 1984;129:S84–S87.

McFadden ER Jr, Ingram RH Jr: Exercise-induced asthma. N Engl J Med 1979;301:763–769.

McKelvie RS, Teo KK, McCartney N, et al. Effects of exercise training in patients with congestive heart failure: A critical review. J Am Coll Cardiol 1995;25:789–796.

McMahon LP, Johns JA, McKenzie A, et al. Haemodynamic changes and physical performance at comparative levels of haemoglobin after long-term treatment with recombinant erythropoietin. Nephrol Dial Transplant 1992;7:1199–1206.

McNeer JF, Margolis JR, Lee KL, et al. The role of the exercise test in the evaluation of patients for ischemic heart disease. Circulation 1978;57:64–70.

McParland C, Krishnan B, Wang Y, Gallagher CG. Inspiratory muscle weakness and dyspnea in chronic heart failure. Am Rev Respir Dis 1992;146:467–472.

Means JH. Dyspnea. Medicine (Baltimore) 1924;3:309–416.

Miller DM, Winslow RM, Klein HG, et al. Improved exercise performance after exchange transfusion in subjects with sickle cell anemia. Blood 1980;56:1127–1131.

Miller GJ, Sergeant GR, Sivapragasam S, et al. Cardio-pulmonary responses and gas exchange during exercise in adults with homozygous sickle-cell disease (sickle-cell anaemia). Clin Sci 1973;44:113–128.

Mills KR, Edwards RHT. Investigative strategies for muscle pain. J Neuro Sci 1983;58:73–88.

Minotti JR, Christoff I, Massie BM. Skeletal muscle function, morphology and metabolism in patients with chronic heart failure. Chest 1992;101:333S–339S.

Minotti JR, Pillay P, Chang L. Impaired skeletal muscle function in patients with congestive heart failure: Relationship to systemic exercise performance. J Clin Invest 1991;88:2077.

Misra M, Thakur R, Bhandari K, Puri VK. Value of the treadmill exercise test in asymptomatic and minimally symptomatic patients with chronic severe aortic regurgitation. Int J Cardiol 1987;15:309–316.

Miyagi K, Asanoi H, Ishizaka S, et al. Importance of total leg muscle mass for exercise intolerance in chronic heart failure. Jpn Heart J 1994;35:15–26.

Moller JA, Satyanarayana R, Lucas RV Jr. Exercise hemodynamics of pulmonary valvular stenosis. Study of 64 children. Circulation 1972;46:1018–1026.

Morgan-Hughes JA. Disorders of mitochondrial metabolism. In: Sarner M, editor. Advanced Medicine 18. London: Pitman Medical Publishing Co.; 1982.

Multiple Risk Factor Intervention Trial Research Group: Exercise electrocardiogram and coronary heart disease mortality in the multiple risk factor intervention trial. Am J Cardiol 1985;55:16–24.

Nakamura M, Chiba M, Ueshima K, et al. Impaired cholinergic peripheral vasodilation and its relationship to hyperemic calf blood-flow response and exercise intolerance in patients with chronic heart failure. Int J Cardiol 1995;48:139–146.

Newman GE, Rerych SK, Upton MT, et al. Comparison of electrocardiographic and left ventricular functional changes during exercise. Circulation 1980;62:1204–1211.

Noseda A, Carpiaux JP, Schmerber J, et al. Dyspnea and flow-volume curve during exercise in COPD patients. Eur Respir J 1994;7:279–285.

O'Byrne P, Ryan G, Morris M, et al. Asthma induced by cold air and its relation to nonspecific bronchial responsiveness to methacholine. Am Rev Respir Dis 1982;125:281–285.

Okin PM, Kligfield P, Amiesen O, et al. Improved accuracy of the exercise electrocardiogram. Identification of three-vessel coronary disease in stable angina pectoris by analysis of peak rate-related changes in ST segments. Am J Cardiol 1985;55:271–276.

Oldridge NB, Wicks JR, McIntosh J. Exercise in coronary rehabilitation: Principles of testing (Part I). Prescription and Program Design (Part II). Physiotherapy (Canada) 1978;30:1–11.

Olsen GN. The evolving role of exercise testing prior to lung resection. Chest 1989;95:218–225.

Oski FA, Marshall BE, Cohen PJ, et al. Exercise with anemia. The role of the left-shifted or right-shifted oxygen-hemoglobin equilibrium curve. Ann Intern Med 1971;74:44–46.

Ostiguy GL. Summary of task force report on occupational respiratory disease (pneumoconiosis). Can Med Assoc J 1979;121:414–421.

Otis AB. The work of breathing. Physiol Rev 1954;34:449–458.

Otterstad JE, Simonsen S, Erikssen J. Hemodynamic findings at rest and during mild supine exercise in adults with isolated uncomplicated ventricular septal defects. Circulation 1985;71:650–662.

Pardy RL, Rivington RN, Despas PJ, et al. The effects of inspiratory muscle training on exercise performance in chronic airflow limitation. Am Rev Respir Dis 1981;123:426–433.

Passmore R, Durnin JVGA. Human energy expenditure. Physiol Rev 1955;35:801–840.

Pernow B, Havel RJ, Jennings DB. The second wind phenomenon in McArdle's syndrome. Acta Med Scand 1967;472(Suppl):294–307.

Picado C, Laporta D, Grassino A, et al. Mechanisms affecting exercise performance in subjects with asbestos related pleural fibrosis. Lung 1987;165:45–57.

Powles ACP, Sutton JR, Wicks JR, et al. Reduced heart rate response to exercise in ischemic heart disease: the fallacy of the target heart rate in exercise testing. Med Sci Sports Exerc 1979;11:227–233.

Puri S, Baker BL, Dutka DP, et al. Reduced alveolar-capillary membrane diffusing capacity in chronic heart failure: Its pathophysiological relevance and relationship to exercise performance. Circulation 1995;91:2769–2774.

Radice M, Alli C, Avanzini F, et al. Role of blood pressure response to provocative tests in the prediction of hypertension in adolescents. Eur Heart J 1985;6:490–496.

Reed JW, Ablett M, Cotes JE. Ventilatory responses to exercise and to carbon dioxide in mitral stenosis before and after valvulotomy: Causes of tachypnoea. Clin Sci Molec Med 1978;54:9–16.

Rhodes KM, Evemy K, Nariman S, et al. Effects of mitral valve surgery on static lung function and exercise performance. Thorax 1985;40:107–112.

Rigg JRA, Jones NL. Clinical assessment of respiratory function. Br J Anesthesiol 1978;50:3–13.

Robertson HT, Haley NR, Guthrie M, et al. Recombinant erythropoietin improves exercise capacity in anemic hemodialysis patients. Am J Kidney Dis 1990;15:325–332.

Rochester DF. Effects of COPD on the respiratory muscles. In:

Cherniack NS, editor. Chronic Obstructive Pulmonary Disease. Philadelphia: WB Saunders Co.; 1991, pp. 134–157.

Ryan M, Lown B, Horn H. Comparison of ventricular ectopic activity during 24-hour monitoring and exercise testing in patients with coronary heart disease. N Engl J Med 1975;292:224–229.

Saltin B, Blomquist B, Mitchell JH, et al. Response to exercise after bed rest and training. Circulation 1968;38(Suppl 17):1–78.

Sannerstedt R. Hemodynamic response to exercise in patients with arterial hypertension. Acta Med Scand 1966;180(Suppl 458):699–706.

Segel N, Hudson WA, Harris P, et al. Circulatory effects of electrically induced changes in ventricular rate at rest and during exercise in complete heart block. J Clin Invest 1964;43:1541, 1550.

Sheffield LT. Editorial: Another perfect treadmill test? N Engl J Med 1985;313:633–635.

Shen WF, Roubin GS, Choong CY-P, et al. Evaluation of relationship between myocardial contractile state and left ventricular function in patients with aortic regurgitation. Circulation 1985;71:31–38.

Shih J-F, Wilson JS, Broderick A, et al. Asbestos-induced pleural fibrosis and impaired exercise physiology. Chest 1994;105:1370–1376.

Siegel IM. The Clinical Management of Muscle Disease: A Practical Manual of Diagnosis and Treatment. London: Heinemann Medical; 1977.

Sietsema KE, Bendov I, Zhang YY, et al. Dynamics of oxygen-uptake for submaximal exercise and recovery in patients with chronic heart-failure. Chest 1994;105:1693–1700.

Silke B, Verma SP, Nelson GIC, et al. The effects on left ventricular performance of verapamil and metoprolol singly and together in exercise-induced angina pectoris. Am Heart J 1985;109:1286–1293.

Smith EE, Guyton AC, Manning RD, et al. Integrated mechanisms of cardiovascular response and control during exercise in the normal human. In: Sonnenblick EH, Lesch M, editors. Exercise and Heart Disease. New York: Grune & Stratton; 1976.

Smith TP, Kinasewitz GT, Tucker WY, et al. Exercise capacity as a predictor of post-thoracotomy morbidity. Am Rev Respir Dis 1984;129:730–734.

Sokolov R, Irwin B, Dressendorfer R, et al. Exercise performance in 6- to 11-year-old boys with Duchenne muscular dystrophy. Arch Phys Med Rehabil 1977;58:195–201.

Stevens SS. Issues in psychophysical measurement. Psychol Rev 1971;78:426–450.

Stratton JR, Dunn JF, Adamopoulos S, et al. Training partially reverses skeletal-muscle metabolic abnormalities during exercise in heart failure. J Appl Physiol 1994;76:1575–1582.

Sue DY, Wasserman K, Moricca RB, et al. Metabolic acidosis during exercise in patients with chronic obstructive pulmonary disease. Chest 1988;94:931–938.

Sugushita Y, Matsuda M, Ito I, et al. Evaluation of left ventricular reserve in left ventricular diseases: Non-invasive analysis of its determinants by dynamic exercise echocardiography. Acta Cardiol 1983;38:103.

Sullivan M, Atwood JE, Myers J, et al. Increased exercise capacity after digoxin administration in patients with heart failure. J Am Coll Cardiol 1989;13:1138–1143.

Sullivan MJ, Green HJ, Cobb FR. Skeletal muscle biochemistry and histology in ambulatory patients with long-term heart failure. Circulation 1990;81:518–527.

Sullivan MJ, Higginbotham MB, Cobb FR. Increased exercise ventilation in patients with chronic heart failure: Intact ventilatory control despite hemodynamic and pulmonary abnormalities. Circulation 1988;77:552–559.

Sutton J, Lazarus L. Growth hormone in exercise: Comparison of physiological and pharmacological stimuli. J Appl Physiol 1976;41:523–527.

Swedberg K. Exercise testing in heart failure: A critical review. Drugs 1994;47(Suppl 4):14–24.

Sylven C, Borg G, Holmgren A, Astrom H. Psychophysical power functions of exercise limiting symptoms in coronary heart disease. Med Sci Sports Exerc 1991;23:1050–1054.

Théroux P, Waters DD, Halphen C, et al. Prognostic value of exercise testing soon after myocardial infarction. N Engl J Med 1979;301:341–345.

Thomson PD, Kelemen MH. Hypotension accompanying the onset of exertional angina. Circulation 1975;52:28–32.

Thulesius O. Pathophysiological classification and diagnosis of orthostatic hypotension. Cardiology 1976;61(Suppl 1):180–190.

Tjahja IE, Reddy HK, Janicki JS, Weber KT. Evolving role of cardiopulmonary exercise testing in cardiovascular disease. Clin Chest Med 1994;15:271–285.

Vacek JL, Valentin-Stone P, Wolfe M, Davis WR. The value of standardized exercise testing in the noninvasive evaluation of mitral stenosis. Am J Med Sci 1986;292:335–343.

Vignos PJ, Watkins MP. The effect of exercise in muscular dystrophy. JAMA 1966;197:843–848.

Wade OL, Bishop JM. Cardiac output and regional blood flow. Oxford: Blackwell Scientific Publications; 1962.

Ward GR, MacDougall JD, Sutton JR, et al. Activation of human muscle pyruvate dehydrogenase with activity and immobilization. Clin Sci 1986;70:207–210.

Wasserman K, Sue D. Impact of integrative cardiopulmonary exercise testing on clinical decision making. Chest 1991;99:981–992.

Wasserman K, Whipp BJ, Koyal SN, Cleary MG. Effect of carotid body resection on ventilatory and acid-base control during exercise. J Appl Physiol 1976;39:354–358.

Weber KT, Janicki JS. Cardiopulmonary exercise testing for evaluation of chronic cardiac failure. Am J Cardiol 1985;55:22A–31A.

Weber KT, Janicki JS, Fishman AP. Respiratory gas exchange during exercise in the noninvasive evaluation of the severity of chronic cardiac failure. In: Braunwald E, Mock MB, Watson JT, editors. Congestive Heart Failure. New York: Grune & Stratton;. 1982b, pp. 221–235.

Weber KT, Janicki JS, McElroy PA. Cardio-pulmonary exercise testing in the evaluation of mitral and aortic valve incompetence. Herz 1986;11:88–96.

Weber KT, Janicki JS, McElroy PA, Reddy HK. Concepts and applications of cardiopulmonary exercise testing. Chest 1988;93:843–847.

Weber KT, Kinasewitz GT, Janicki JS, et al. Oxygen utilization and ventilation during exercise in patients with chronic cardiac failure. Circulation 1982a;65:1213–1223.

Weber KT, Wilson JR, Janicki JS, Likoff MJ. Exercise testing in the evaluation of the patient with chronic cardiac failure. Am Rev Respir Dis 1984;129:S60–S62.

Weiner DA. Prognostic value of exercise testing early after myocardial infarction. J Cardiac Rehabil 1982;2:562–568.

Weiner DA, McCabe CH, Ryan TJ. Identification of patients with left main and three vessel disease with clinical and exercise test variables. Am J Cardiol 1980;46:21.

Weiner DA, McCabe CH, Ryan TJ. Prognostic assessment of patients with coronary artery disease by exercise testing. Am Heart J 1983;105:749–755.

Werko L. Mitral Valvular Disease: Hemodynamic Studies of the Consequences for the Circulation. Stockholm: Almqvist & Wiksell; 1964.

Wicks JR, Lymburner K, Dinsdale SM, et al. The use of multistage exercise testing with wheelchair ergometry and arm cranking in subjects with spinal cord lesions. Paraplegia 1977;15:252–261.

Wilhelmsen L, Selander S, Soderholm B, et al. Recurrent pulmonary embolism. Medicine 1963;42(5):335–355.

Wilson JR. Exercise intolerance in heart failure: Importance of skeletal muscle. Circulation 1995;91:559–561.

Wilson JR, Fink LI, Ferraro N, et al. Use of maximal bicycle performance in patients with congestive heart failure secondary to coronary artery disease or to idiopathic dilated cardiomyopathy. Am J Cardiol 1986;15:601–606.

Wilson JR, Mancini DM, McCully K, et al. Noninvasive detection of skeletal muscle underperfusion with near-infrared spectroscopy in patients with heart failure. Circulation 1989; 80:1668–1674.

Woodson RD. Hemoglobin concentration and exercise capacity. Am Rev Respir Dis 1984;129:S72–S75.

Woodson RD, Wills RE, Lenfant C. Effect of acute and established anemia on O_2 transport at rest, submaximal and maximal work. J Appl Physiol 1978;44:36–43.

Yamabe H, Itoh K, Yasaka Y, et al. Lactate threshold is not an onset of insufficient oxygen supply to the working muscle in patients with chronic heart failure. Clin Cardiol 1994;17:391–394.

Yates CJP, Andrews V, Berent A, et al. Increase in leg blood-flow by normovolaemic haemodilution in intermittent claudication. Lancet 1979;2:941–943.

Zejda J. Diagnostic value of exercise testing in asbestosis. Am J Ind Med 1989;16:305–319.

Zimmerman P, Heigenhauser GJF, McCartney N, et al. Impaired cardiovascular "acceleration" at the onset of exercise in patients with coronary artery disease. J Appl Physiol 1982;52:71–78.

5

Approaches to Clinical Exercise Testing

Clinical exercise testing is plagued by a lack of standardization. Unlike many procedures in clinical physiology, there is a lack of agreement as to how an exercise test should be carried out, what measurements should be made, how to interpret the results, and what clinical use can be made of them. However, recently published guidelines will help to develop a more consistent approach to these problems (Fletcher et al., 1995). In this chapter, we review some of the considerations involved in the choice of exercise tests suitable for routine clinical use. These considerations have led us to advocate a series of procedures, which we have termed stages 1 to 4. The stage 1 test may be used in all the usual clinical situations; it is acceptable to most patients and is of short duration. It consists of a progressive incremental power test on a cycle ergometer or treadmill to a symptom-limited or sign-limited maximum and in which noninvasive measurements are made. Stage 2 is a noninvasive test carried out in a steady state to examine interrelationships among metabolism, cardiac output, and pulmonary gas exchange. The stage 3 procedure uses arterial or capillary blood sampling to measure cardiac output and pulmonary gas exchange, and stage 4 adds right-sided heart catheterization for measurement of pulmonary hemodynamics. Thus, stage 1 is used in all cases, and the more complex stages (2 through 4) are reserved for the solution of complex problems. Our adoption of this system was partly for practical reasons and partly for reasons of patient acceptance and clinical usefulness. We would be unable to offer a "routine" laboratory service for exercise testing if the routine technique were lengthy and costly in terms of personnel. Furthermore, most clinical problems that are helped through an exercise test do not require a complex procedure. Improvements in the technology of exercise testing measurements have blurred some of these distinctions for many reasons. First, because many of the measurements were complex, necessitating gas collection and chemical analysis of gas concentrations, we initially proposed an extremely simple protocol and resorted to more complex measurements only if indicated from the initial results. It is now possible to obtain reliable measurements more or less automatically and even on a breath-by-breath basis if required. Second, some of the measurements were considered to require a steady state and could not be made reliably in a progressive incremental exercise study; these variables included cardiac output and pulmonary gas exchange (V_D/V_T and A-a P_{O_2} difference). Our later experience suggested that as long as some precautions were observed, such measurements were feasible (McKelvie et al., 1987). Third, arterial puncture was associated with anxiety in both patients and observers that could interfere with the quality of other features of the test and was thus reserved for specific indications. However, capillary blood sampling may safely be used instead, and for screening purposes, oximetry is effective in identifying significant changes in arterial oxygen saturation with exercise. However, there are drawbacks to making a routine test too complex and too expensive, and such decisions should be made in the context of the clinical problems that are usually referred to the laboratory. Our approach is described in this chapter and is elucidated in the examples provided later in this book.

The study of exercise physiology from its beginnings in the early years of this century has used a variety of exercise situations—walking and running ("free range"), steps, uphill treadmill walking and running, and cycle ergometry. Although all modes continue to be used clinically, the treadmill and cycle are most commonly used now.

In the early days of clinical exercise testing, measurements were made at rest and at exercise; there was often no indication of the power, either in absolute terms or relative to the patient's maximum. Later, it became clear that precision was important, and interpretation was helped by knowledge of the power or oxygen uptake at which measurements were made and the power or oxygen uptake relative to a measured or predicted maximum power, or $\dot{V}_{O_2}max$.

Many protocols—combinations of intensity and duration—have been advocated for exercise testing. We review some of the more popular to give the reader an idea of the large variation among the methods in current use. A more detailed comparison and review is given by Arstila (1972).

PROTOCOLS

THE MASTER STEP TEST. A simple stepping test of cardiac function was proposed by Selig (1905) at the turn of the century, and Master and Oppenheimer (1929) developed a more standardized step test that became widely used in North America. With later modifications (Master and Rosenfeld, 1967), it is still used sometimes in exercise electrocardiographic screening (Fig. 5–1) (Stuart and Ellestad, 1980). However, the trend in recent years has been toward treadmill and cycle testing because these methods allow more precisely graded increments of exercise to be used.

Step tests have the advantage of simplicity, which makes them suitable for office testing and field studies. A number of protocols have been proposed in which changes in work rate may be made by altering the step height and the frequency of stepping (Nagle et al., 1965). Shephard (1966), in reviewing several methods, suggested that the height be kept constant and the rate of stepping gradually be increased; this is the basis of the Canadian Home Fitness Test (Bailey et al., 1976); music of increasing tempo is used to control increases in stepping rate, and the subject is prompted to record pulse rate at intervals. A similar test was described and validated by Siconolfi and colleagues (1985). Gupta and associates (1973) described a progressive step test in which both height and rate are varied. Precise measurement of power is difficult because of uncertainty in the work done in stepping down, and Cumming and Glenn (1977) showed that predictions of maximal oxygen uptake are subject to large errors. On the other hand, Siconolfi and associates (1985) suggested that a valid estimate of $\dot{V}o_2$max is obtained by their technique. Suitable methods for direct measurement of $\dot{V}o_2$max during a step test include a lightweight anemometer (Wright, 1958) and a system for expired gas collection (Gupta et al., 1973).

THE BRUCE PROTOCOL. This protocol is widely used in North America for exercise stress testing for coronary artery disease (Bruce and McDonough, 1969; American College of Sports Medicine, 1986; Fletcher et al., 1995). The test is carried out with a treadmill, and four stages are used to produce a graded increase in power, each stage being maintained for 3 minutes: stage 1, 1.7 mph and 10 per cent grade; stage 2, 2.5 mph and 12 per cent grade; stage 3, 3.4 mph and 14 per cent grade; and stage 4, 4.2 mph and 16 per cent grade. A disadvantage of this approach is the high oxygen cost of the initial stage and of each increment (see Fig. 5–1); smaller increments allow the more disabled patient to adapt gradually to the stress.

THE BALKE PROTOCOL. This protocol is also carried out on a treadmill, but the speed is kept constant, and the grade is increased from an initial zero grade by equal steps of 2.5 per cent every 1 minute or, in disabled patients, every 2 minutes (Nagle et al., 1965). These smaller increments amount to approximately 1 met (metabolic equivalent of resting oxygen intake) each and thus produce a smoother gradation from rest to maximal work; our experience with this procedure had led us to adopt it for routine (stage 1) tests, with the minor modification of an initial minute at 1 mph at zero grade, followed by 2 mph at zero grade before the protocol just outlined is started (see Fig. 5–1). Equivalent work rates and oxygen uptakes may be calculated from the treadmill settings and the patient's weight (Appendix C, Fig. C–2), allowing comparison with results obtained on a cycle ergometer.

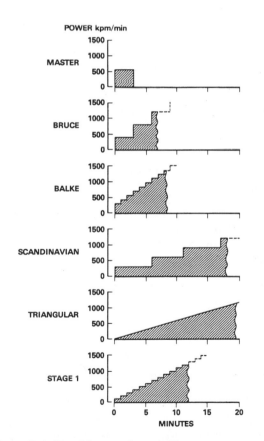

Figure 5–1. Pictorial comparison of different test protocols showing the increase in power (kpm/min) as a function of the duration of the test (minutes). To aid comparison, an 80-kg 40-year-old male is used as the example; the shaded area shows the average duration of the tests for a healthy untrained subject.

Other protocols may be considered to be compromises between the Bruce and the Balke approaches. The reader is referred to the useful review of Sheffield and Roitman (1977) for a critical comparison of a number of these protocols.

THE SCANDINAVIAN PROTOCOL. This protocol uses a cycle ergometer, with increments in power of 50 W (300 kpm/min) for men and 33 W (200 kpm/min) for women, each step being maintained for 4 to 6 minutes (Sjöstrand, 1960; Atterhog et al., 1979) (see Fig. 5–1). As with the Bruce protocol, steps of this size may mean that the patient completes only one or two increments, thus limiting the useful information to be obtained. Our experience with this protocol led us to adopt steps of 16 W (100 kpm/min), each maintained for 1 minute, with measurements being made at the end of each minute (Jones et al., 1967; Spiro et al., 1974). This is part of the stage 1 procedure (see Fig. 5–1). Smaller steps (8 W, 50 kpm/min) may be used for small or very disabled subjects.

THE "TRIANGULAR" PROTOCOL. Developed by Arstila in 1972, this protocol uses an electrically controlled and braked cycle ergometer to increase power continuously at a rate that may be chosen by the observer. This "ramp" test usually causes the oxygen intake to increase (10 W/min) at a slightly slower rate than that of the stage 1 procedure (17 W/min) outlined later in this chapter. Normal reference values for such a test have been provided by Nordenfelt and co-workers (1985).

WALKING TESTS. For some very disabled patients, tests using treadmills and cycles give limited information; often, a test using walking is all that is required to assess exercise tolerance. McGavin and colleagues (1977) used a test in which the distance walked in 12 minutes is measured in order to assess patients with limited respiratory reserve and to measure improvement after rehabilitation exercise training. A similar test for healthy subjects—the 12-minute run test—was popularized by Cooper (1970), who showed reasonable agreement between the 12-minute distance and aerobic capacity ($\dot{V}O_2$max). Guyatt and colleagues (1985) have examined the validity and application of shorter walking tests in the evaluation of severe cardiopulmonary disorders. They found that a 6-minute test was more reproducible and clinically useful than a 2-minute test, that at least two repetitions are required for consistency to be obtained, and that encouragement led to a significant improvement in walking distance. These factors have to be adequately controlled if such a test is to be used to evaluate the efficacy of a therapeutic regimen. Walking tests have been successfully used in the assessment of chronic air flow limitation (Knox et al., 1988; Spence et al., 1993).

Several groups have found the measurement of walking speed at a self-selected pace to be a valid reflection of exercise capacity (Bassey et al., 1976; Cunningham et al., 1982) that is particularly useful in evaluating elderly subjects (Himann et al., 1988) and in following the effects of training (Cunningham et al., 1986).

THE WINGATE TEST. This test was introduced as a simple test of short-term maximal power output (Bar-Or et al., 1980; Dotan and Bar-Or, 1983). Briefly, the braking force of a mechanical cycle ergometer (Monark type) is set by reference to the subject's body size; the subject then pedals at a maximal frequency for 30 to 45 seconds. The frequency is recorded and multiplied by the braking force to obtain power for each pedal stroke, or an average for each 5 seconds of the test. From these measurements, maximum power and index of fatigue resistance may be obtained. The test provides an assessment of muscle performance in dynamic exercise that may be useful in population studies of fitness, particularly in children, in athletes, and in patients with muscle disorders. A disadvantage is that the velocity of muscle contraction varies through the test; also it is difficult to factor in the work performed against the inertia of the flywheel. More precise measurements may be obtained by measuring the force exerted on the pedals of the ergometer using strain gauges; this is, however, more complex technically.

ISOKINETIC CYCLE ERGOMETRY. In the Wingate test, a constant braking force is set on a mechanical ergometer, and pedaling rate is recorded to obtain measurements of power and the total work performed; the velocity of muscle contraction is thus high to begin with and falls progressively as the test proceeds. In view of the important effects of velocity on the forces produced by muscle, Sargeant (1980) proposed an isokinetic procedure in which power and work may be measured at controlled pedal frequencies. This may be achieved by asking the subject to exert maximal effort on the pedals of a cycle ergometer that is connected to a motor that prevents the predetermined speed to be exceeded; the forces exerted are measured by strain gauges bonded to the pedals, allowing power and work to be calculated (McCartney et al., 1983b). Studies with this technique have proved sensitive enough to demonstrate differences between athletes having different muscle fiber properties (McCartney et al., 1983a), the effects of training at different ages, and the effects of neuromuscular disorders; normal values have been published by Makrides and associates (1985).

ASSESSMENT OF EXERCISE DEMANDS IN EVERYDAY LIFE. At their simplest, exercise tests are an extension of the clinical examination in which the patient is observed walking a standard distance or climbing stairs; the observer times the activity, measures the heart rate and breathing frequency, and listens to the heart. However, it is sometimes important to know what happens in daily activity and at work. The most practical methods probably use lightweight portable recording systems to measure heart rate and record the electrocardiogram (Holter, 1961; Weiner and Lourie, 1969). For field studies in industry of the metabolic demands of occupations, measurements of oxygen intake may be made by use of portable apparatus, such as the Kofranyi-Michaelis respirometer (Müller and Franz, 1952) or the Wolff integrating pneumotachograph (IMP) (Wolff, 1958).

MAXIMAL OXYGEN UPTAKE

Classically, the estimation of maximal oxygen intake ($\dot{V}O_2$max) was made by measuring $\dot{V}O_2$ during exercise of short duration at increasing power output; brief collections of expired gas were used, to the point that $\dot{V}O_2$ did not increase in spite of an increase in power (Åstrand and Rodahl, 1970). Later, a similar criterion was applied to a continuous incremental exercise test. Although a plateau of oxygen uptake may sometimes be measured during maximal power in an incremental test, this is not an invariable finding, even in healthy subjects. For this reason, a second criterion, a peak plasma lactate concentration of more than 8 mmol/L, may be used. Alternatively, a "supramaximal" power output that may be maintained for 2 minutes is used to demonstrate that a peak oxygen uptake has been attained.

It is unlikely that the demonstration of a plateau of oxygen uptake is important in clinical evaluation. Because the peak oxygen uptake in an incremental power output test taken to a symptom-limited maximum yields a reasonable estimate of $\dot{V}O_2$max (Froelicher et al., 1974), we have used it as an acceptable alternative. Furthermore, the risk of a supramaximal test is not justified in patients. Some workers in the field of exercise physiology believe in the concept of a "true" $\dot{V}O_2$max, an independent variable representing a point at which oxygen delivery mechanisms have reached their limit. This concept carries the inference that maximal exercise capacity is limited by such factors, which may not be the case. Thus, it seems preferable to consider $\dot{V}O_2$max as merely the $\dot{V}O_2$ observed in a given individual who has reached a power output that cannot be sustained. $\dot{V}O_2$max may then be viewed as a variable that is dependent on many factors, usually acting in a complex and interactive fashion.

Although the extrapolation of $\dot{V}O_2$max from measurements made at submaximal power outputs is reasonable in healthy subjects, it assumes that a limiting factor—usually cardiac frequency—is known for the patient. This assumption is not justified in patients, a further argument for incremental tests that take the subject to a symptom-limited maximum power. There are two main methods for estimating maximal oxygen intake from submaximal cardiac frequency; both require at least two observations, with one reaching a frequency of at least 150 beats per minute (b/min). The line joining the points of f_c and $\dot{V}O_2$ is extrapolated (a) to an f_c of 170 b/min in order to obtain the physical work capacity (the PWC_{170}) of the patient (Wahlund, 1948), or (b) to a maximum f_c predicted from age (Maritz et al., 1961). In clinical situations, there is no point in carrying out these extrapolations. They merely reflect the slope of the f_c:$\dot{V}O_2$ relationship, and unless the subject's own maximal f_c is known, the extrapolation is subject to considerable error, owing to the variation in maximal f_c of $\pm$ 20 b/min in normal populations. Although this variation seems small, the slope of f_c $\dot{V}O_2$ is so shallow that an error of 20 b/min leads to an error in $\dot{V}O_2$max of as much as 20 per cent. An extrapolation procedure has been advocated for patients with respiratory disease in which maximal ventilation is predicted from spirometric measurements (Armstrong et al., 1966). The variation in the ventilatory response to exercise and in the maximal ventilation in these patients militates against such an extrapolation.

The difficulty in deriving a maximal power by extrapolation from submaximal measurements is further argument for extending observations in patients to a symptom-limited or a sign-limited maximum.

MODE OF TESTING

Cycle ergometer or treadmill? Carried on for many years, this contest appears to have been won by the cycle ergometer in Europe (Atterhog et al., 1979) and by the treadmill in North America (Stuart and Ellestad, 1980). The arguments have practical and physiological aspects. It is said in the treadmill's favor that everyone walks but many do not cycle or have not done so for years. However, walking on a moving belt without holding a handrail may be difficult for some patients, particularly if the treadmill speed cannot be sufficiently reduced. Also, breathing through a respiratory mouthpiece on a treadmill requires more cooperation by the patient than is needed on a cycle; measuring blood pressure, sampling blood, and rebreathing are all easier on a cycle. Other practical drawbacks to many treadmills are their cost, size, and weight; some are noisy and some cannot be stopped instantly in case of emergency. The differences in physiological responses to the two forms of exercise are not large. A change in the braking power of a calibrated cycle ergometer leads to a predictable ($\pm$ 10 per cent) increase in oxygen intake, and in a given subject, oxygen intake is reproducible to $\pm$ 5 per cent. With the treadmill, power is calculated from the subject's weight and the treadmill settings; if the speed is kept constant, equal increments in elevation lead to equal increments in oxygen intake ($\pm$ 10 per cent). In some patients with limited exercise tolerance, a learning effect may be seen; small reductions in oxygen intake occur with repeated testing, presumably because of a more efficient stride length and cadence. An advantage of the treadmill is that standard settings for speed and grade may be used for subjects of all sizes; because body weight is a determinant of the power, at a given setting, an approximately equivalent power, expressed as $\dot{V}O_2$/kg, will be used by all subjects.

The best-known difference between the two testing modes lies in the maximal oxygen intake, which in untrained subjects is usually higher on the treadmill than on the cycle ergometer by an average of 7 per cent (Shephard, 1971). The difference is explained by the brunt of the loads being carried by the thigh muscles in cycling, leading to local muscle fatigue, which may be minimized by optimal positioning on the cycle and pedaling at a high frequency. Although maximal oxygen intake is lower, ventilation and blood lactate values tend to be slightly higher in cycling (Shephard, 1966). Because higher power and higher maximal heart rates are found in cardiac patients exercising on a treadmill, many cardiac laboratories prefer this mode for routine testing. However, the differences are small, and a formal comparison of the two modes in patients with coronary artery disease showed identical electrocardiographic changes; although maximal heart rate was slightly lower in cycling, this was offset by a slightly higher arterial pressure, and the rate:pressure product was comparable (Wicks et al., 1978).

Some studies of exercise-induced asthma suggest that treadmill exercise is associated with greater bronchoconstriction (Godfrey, 1975), but others have shown similar degrees of bronchoconstriction with cycle ergometry (Anderton et al., 1979). Probably for this application the mode of testing is less important than control of temperature and humidity of inspired air (McFadden and Ingram, 1979).

Extensive experience with both these modes of exercise testing has led us to prefer the cycle ergometer for most studies, the treadmill being used in some clinical situations—for exercise prescription, particularly in patients tested soon after myocardial infarction; for intermittent claudication; in young children; and in very disabled respiratory patients.

THE APPROACH DESCRIBED IN THIS BOOK

It is apparent from the descriptions in earlier chapters of the physiology and clinical applications of exercise that measurement of all the physiological variables in all the patients who might benefit from exercise studies is an impossible aim. The information required is dictated by the clinical question being asked and is usually obtained through simple measurements made in a progressive incremental exercise test. More complex measurements are reserved for complex problems identified by the simple studies.

Experience and experimentation with a number of approaches led us to develop a series of tests, of which the first may be considered a "basic" or "screening" procedure capable of application to nearly all patients, and the more complex are reserved for those situations in which more detailed information is required. We termed these stages 1 to 4.

The Stage 1 Test

The objective of this simple, economical procedure is to obtain measurements related to metabolic, cardiovascular, and respiratory adjustments as they evolve from the resting state to maximal exercise. *Maximal exercise* is defined as the point at which the patient is unable to continue because of symptoms or because safety limits have been reached. The test is performed on a cycle ergometer or treadmill: the power settings are standardized with the aim of obtaining a total duration for the test of 8 to 20 minutes (Buchfuhrer et al., 1983). The settings are increased by equal amounts at the end of each minute, and measurements are made toward the end of each minute.

The reasons for making measurements are implicit in the previous descriptions of physiological responses and also in the examples presented in later chapters and briefly introduced here:

Power: in a test carried out on a calibrated cycle ergometer, this measurement is the most reliable indicator of relative and absolute exercise capacity, with which other variables may be compared.

Symptom intensity, Borg scale: at one level, recording symptoms provides an indication of the stress or pain being experienced by the patient as the test progresses, and at another, it provides variables that need to be related to physiological changes in systems.

Oxygen intake: reflects the metabolic demands of exercise, and in particular, the cardiac output and pulmonary gas exchange (venous admixture).

Carbon dioxide output: provides an index of the oxidative fuels being used and of lactate entry into blood; it is the parameter used to assess the responses of ventilation and gas exchange (VD/VT ratio).

Heart rate: reflects cardiac output and stroke volume, when related to $\dot{V}O_2$, and chronotropic control mechanisms.

Systemic blood pressure: monitors left ventricular function and assesses neurovascular control.

12-lead electrocardiography: assesses myocardial perfusion and identifies arrhythmias.

Ventilation: assesses pulmonary gas exchange efficiency and respiratory control mechanisms.

Pattern of breathing (VT and f_b): influenced by the responses to pulmonary impedance (elastic and resistive), ventilatory capacity, and respiratory muscle strength.

Arterial O_2 saturation: in relation to $\dot{V}O_2$, assesses pulmonary gas exchange and intracardiac shunts.

Capillary blood is not routinely sampled but can provide information on pulmonary gas exchange, acid-base status, and lactate accumulation.

Of course, other measurements might be added, but they are often difficult to make within the time available.

We are often asked, particularly in relation to cardiac stress testing, to defend the importance of ventilation measurements; we do so mainly on two counts. First, in submaximal exercise, the ventilatory response offers a check on the metabolic (oxygen intake, carbon dioxide output) requirements of the exercise and of the ergometer calibration. Second, if the normal linear increase of ventilation, with increasing power, changes to a disproportionate increase (anaerobic threshold; see Chapter 2), this may be taken as reliable evidence of lactate accumulation in blood.

Stage 2, 3, and 4 Tests

These tests use increasingly complex techniques for measuring variables that require steady state conditions for valid results. They are performed with a cycle ergometer at two or more power outputs, which are always chosen on the basis of results obtained in a stage 1 test. The cycle ergometer is used because the required oxygen intake may be reliably maintained for several minutes in a steady state and because measurements using rebreathing or blood sampling are easier than on a treadmill. The results of a stage 1 test allow the submaximal steady state results to be accurately placed in the subject's own scale of performance.

Measurements of cardiac frequency and mixed expired gas concentrations are used to identify a steady state, which is usually present after 3 to 5 minutes of exercise.

In the stage 2 test, the following measurements are made: cardiac frequency; blood pressure; ventilation, tidal volume, and frequency of breathing; mixed expired gas oxygen and carbon dioxide concentrations; mixed venous PCO_2 (by rebreathing); and end-tidal PCO_2. These measurements are noninvasive, but their application to carbon dioxide transport may be interpreted in terms of alveolar ventilation and arterial PCO_2, gas exchange (dead space–tidal volume ratio), cardiac output and stroke volume, and lactic acid production.

In the stage 3 test, arterial or capillary blood is sampled for measurement of blood gases, pH, and lactate concentration. In conjunction with the stage 2 measurements, calculations are made of alveolar ventilation, pulmonary gas exchange–dead space and venous admixture, and cardiac output. The blood measurements lead to a greater precision than is usually obtained from the noninvasive stage 2 test. Why perform a stage 2 test, in which only estimates and limits may be obtained for several important variables, when blood sampling (stage 3) yields the values with greater precision? The answer lies in the noninvasive nature of the stage 2 test, its simplicity and brevity, and the accuracy of the estimates obtained, which often cannot be significantly improved on by blood measurements.

The stage 4 test is reserved for clinical situations in which central venous blood sampling and hemodynamics are necessary. A Swan-Ganz catheter is "floated" into the pulmonary artery.

Our experience has been that for most (> 90 per cent) patients referred for exercise testing, an adequate assessment is obtained from a stage 1 test. This test has many practical advantages, being technically simple and standardized for routine laboratory application and requiring only a modest outlay in terms of equipment, staff, and time.

Modifications for Some Applications

This series of tests may be applied to nearly all the clinical situations in which an exercise test may be helpful and allows a reasonably flexible approach to be taken in the laboratory. The choice between the procedures is usually dominated by the physiological information needed. However, there are a number of clinical situations in which some modification of the procedures just outlined may be required.

VERY DISABLED SUBJECTS. The first question may be whether any useful information will be gained from subjecting the patient to an exercise test. If the answer is "yes," the choice usually is among a progressive (stage 1) test with small (50 kpm/min) increments of power, an endurance test at a constant low power output (100 or 200 kpm/

min or 1 or 2 mph at zero grade), and a 6-minute walk test (Guyatt et al., 1985).

ARM ERGOMETRY. A progressive exercise test of the stage 1 type may be used with arm cranking in paraplegic subjects (Wicks et al., 1983), in patients who experience symptoms when working with their arms, and in patients with severe vascular disease of the legs. Power increments of 50 kpm/min are usually appropriate, but normal standards for leg exercise do not apply (Reybrouck et al., 1975). The topic was reviewed recently by Celli (1994).

EXERCISE-INDUCED BRONCHOCONSTRIC-TION. A wide range of tests has been used, from "free range" running to the measurement of respiratory heat exchange during cycle ergometry. Godfrey (1975) compared bronchoconstrictor responses to a variety of procedures; for a routine laboratory screening test, he suggested a treadmill test lasting for 8 minutes at power settings, usually 3 mph and 10 per cent incline, associated with a heart rate of 160 to 180 b/min. An equivalent exercise intensity is usually achieved in a stage 1 test on a treadmill or cycle ergometer, and the bronchoconstrictor effect is comparable (Anderton et al., 1979). For this reason, our usual practice is to use a stage 1 test as a screening procedure, going on to histamine or methacholine inhalation challenge to identify lesser degrees of airway reactivity if no bronchoconstriction is found. More critical studies of exercise-induced bronchoconstriction require control of temperature and humidity of inspired air, using a technically demanding system of refrigerated air delivery with heat exchange measurements (McFadden and Ingram, 1979).

AMBULATORY OXYGEN ADMINISTRA-TION. Several portable oxygen systems are available for patients whose activity is limited by arterial oxygen desaturation. Because of the expense and inconvenience involved, objective evidence of improved exercise tolerance in addition to increased oxygen saturation is required before ambulatory oxygen is prescribed. Because most patients with this condition are severely disabled, a useful approach is to use a treadmill setting (usually 2 or 3 mph at zero incline) that the patient cannot tolerate for more than 2 to 4 minutes. Exercise is performed with air or 30 per cent oxygen delivered from a Douglas bag or Tissot spirometer, without the patient knowing whether he or she is receiving air or oxygen. Arterial oxygen saturation is monitored by an ear oximeter. A doubling of the endurance time is taken as evidence of a clinically useful effect of oxygen (Cotes, 1963). The 6-minute walk test may also be used for this purpose.

REFERENCES

American College of Sports Medicine: Guidelines for graded exercise testing and prescription. Philadelphia: Lea & Febiger, 1986.

Anderton RC, Cuff MT, Frith PA, et al. Bronchial responsiveness to inhaled histamine and exercise. J Allergy Clin Immunol 1979;63:315–320.

Armstrong BW, Workman JN, Hurt HH, et al. Clinico-physiologic evaluation of physical working capacity in persons with pulmonary disease. Ann Rev Respir Dis 1966;93:90–99, 223–233.

Arstila M. Pulse-conducted triangular exercise: ECG Test. A feedback system regulating work during exercise. Acta Med Scand 1972;529(Suppl):3–109.

Åstrand PO, Rodahl K. Textbook of Work Physiology. New York: McGraw-Hill; 1970.

Atterhog JH, Jonsson B, Samuelsson R. Exercise testing in Sweden: A survey of procedures. Scand J Clin Lab Invest 1979;39:87–92.

Bailey DA, Shephard RJ, Mirwald RL. Validation of a self-administered home test of cardiorespiratory fitness. Can J Appl Sport Sci 1976;1:67–78.

Bar-Or O, Dotan R, Inbar O, et al. Anaerobic capacity and muscle fiber type distribution in man. Int J Sports Med 1980;1:89–92.

Bassey EJ, Fentem PH, MacDonald IC, Scriven PM. Self-paced walking as a method for exercise testing in elderly and young men. Clin Sci Mol Med 1976;51:609–612.

Borg G. Perceived exertion as an indicator of somatic stress. Scand J Rehabil Med 1970;2:92–98.

Bruce RA, McDonough JR. Stress testing in screening for cardiovascular disease. Bull NY Acad Med 1969;45:1288–1305.

Buchfuhrer MJ, Hansen JE, Robinson TE, et al. Optimizing the exercise protocol for cardiopulmonary assessment. J Appl Physiol 1983;55:1558–1564.

Celli BR. The clinical use of upper extremity exercise. Clin Chest Med 1994;15:339–349.

Cooper KH. New Aerobics. New York: Bantam Books; 1970.

Cotes JE. Continuous versus intermittent administration of oxygen during exercise to patients with chronic lung disease. Lancet 1963;1:1075–1076.

Cumming GR, Glenn J. Evaluation of the Canadian Home Fitness Test in middle-aged men. Can Med Assoc J 1977; 117:346–349.

Cunningham DA, Rechnitzer PA, Donner AP. Exercise training and the speed of self-selected walking pace in men at retirement. Can J Aging 1986;5:19–26.

Cunningham DA, Rechnitzer PA, Pearce ME, Donner AP. Determinants of self-selected walking pace across ages 19 to 66. J Gerontol 1982;37:560–564.

Dotan R, Bar-Or O. Load optimization for the Wingate anaerobic test. Eur J Appl Physiol 1983;51:409–417.

Fletcher GF, Balady G, Froelicher VF, et al. Exercise standards: A statement for health-care professionals from the American Heart Association. Circulation 1995;91:580–615.

Froelicher VF Jr, Brammell H, Davis G, et al. A comparison of three maximal treadmill exercise protocols. J Appl Physiol 1974;36:720–724.

Godfrey S. Exercise-induced asthma: Clinical, physiological, and therapeutic implications. J Allergy Clin Immunol 1975;56:1–17.

Gupta S, Fletcher CM, Edwards RHT. A progressive exercise step test. J Assoc Physicians India 1973;21:555–564.

Guyatt GH, Sullivan MJ, Thompson PJ, et al. The 6-minute walk: A new measure of exercise capacity in patients with chronic heart failure. Can Med Assoc J 1985;132:919–923.

Himann JE, Cunningham DA, Rechnitzer PA, Paterson DH. Age-related changes in speed of walking. Med Sci Sports Exerc 1988;20:161–166.

Holter NL. New method for heart studies. Science 1961; 134:1214–1220.

Jones NL, Campbell EJM, McHardy GJR, et al. The estimation of carbon dioxide pressure of mixed venous blood during exercise. Clin Science 1967;32:311–327.

Knox AJ, Morrison JF, Muers MF. Reproducibility of walking test results in chronic obstructive airways disease. Thorax 1988;43:388–392.

Makrides L, Heigenhauser GJF, McCartney N, Jones NL. Maximal short term exercise capacity in healthy subjects aged 15–70 years. Clin Sci 1985;69:197–205.

Maritz JS, Morrison JF, Peter J, et al. A practical method of estimating an individual's maximum oxygen intake. Ergonomics 1961;4:97–122.

Master AM, Oppenheimer ET. A simple exercise tolerance test for circulatory efficiency with standard tables for normal individuals. Am J Med Sci 1929;177:223–243.

Master AM, Rosenfeld I. Exercise electrocardiography as an estimate of cardiac function. Dis Chest 1967;51:347–382.

McCartney N, Heigenhauser GJF, Jones NL. Power output and fatigue of human muscle in maximal cycling exercise. J Appl Physiol 1983a;55:218–224.

McCartney N, Heigenhauser GJF, Sargeant AJ, Jones NL. A constant velocity cycle ergometer for the study of dynamic muscle function. J Appl Physiol 1983b;55:212–217.

McFadden ER Jr, Ingram RH Jr. Exercise-induced asthma. N Engl J Med 1979;301:763–769.

McGavin CR, Gupta SP, Lloyd EL, et al. Physical rehabilitation for the chronic bronchitic: Results of a controlled trial of exercises in the home. Thorax 1977;32:307–311.

McKelvie RS, Heigenhauser GJF, Jones NL. Measurement of cardiac output by CO_2 rebreathing in unsteady state exercise. Chest 1987;92:777–782.

Müller EA, Franz H. Energieverbrauchsmessungen bei beruflicher Arbeit mit einer verbesserten Respirations-gesuhr. Int Z Angew Physiol 1952;14:499–504.

Nagle FJ, Balke B, Naughton JP. Gradational step tests for assessing work capacity. J Appl Physiol 1965;20:745–748.

Nordenfelt I, Adolfsson L, Nilsson JE, Olsson S. Reference values for exercise tests with continuous increase in load. Clin Physiol 1985;5:161–172.

Reybrouck T, Heigenhauser GF, Faulkner JA. Limitation of maximum oxygen uptake during arm, leg and combined arm-leg ergometry. J Appl Physiol 1975;38:774–779.

Sargeant AJ. Measurement of maximal short-term (anaerobic) power output in man. J Physiol (Lond) 1980;307:12P–13P.

Selig A. Die funktionelle herzdiagnostik Prag. Med Wochenschr 1905;30:418–423.

Sheffield LT, Roitman D. Stress testing methodology. In: Sonnenblick EH, Lesch M, editors. Exercise and Heart Disease. New York: Grune & Stratton; 1977, pp 145–162.

Shephard RJ. The relative merits of the step test, bicycle ergometer and treadmill in the assessment of cardio-respiratory fitness. Int Z Angew Physiol 1966;23:219–230.

Shephard RJ. Standard tests of aerobic power. In: Shephard RJ, editor. Frontiers of Fitness. Springfield, IL: Charles C Thomas Publisher; 1971, pp. 233–264.

Siconolfi SF, Garber CE, Lasater TM, Carleton RA. A simple, valid step test for estimating maximal oxygen uptake in epidemiological studies. Am J Epidemiol 1985;121:382–390.

Sjöstrand T. Functional capacity and exercise tolerance in patients with impaired cardiovascular function. In: Gordon BI, editor. Clinical Cardiopulmonary Physiology. New York: Grune & Stratton; 1960.

Spence DPS, Hay JG, Carter J, et al. Oxygen desaturation and breathlessness during corridor walking in chronic obstructive pulmonary disease. Thorax 1993;48:1145–1150.

Spiro SG, Juniper E, Bowman P, et al. An increasing work rate for assessing the physiological strain of submaximal exercise. Clin Sci 1974;46:191–206.

Stuart RJ Jr, Ellestad MH. National survey of exercise stress testing facilities. Chest 1980;77:94–97.

Wahlund H. Determination of the physical working capacity. Acta Med Scand 1948;215(Suppl):1–78.

Weiner JS, Louric JA. Human Biology: A Guide to Field Methods. Oxford: Blackwell Scientific Publications; 1969.

Wicks JR, Oldridge NB, Cameron BJ, Jones NL. Arm cranking and wheel chair ergometry in elite spinal cord-injured athletes. Med Sci Sports Exerc 1983;15:224–231.

Wicks JR, Sutton JR, Oldridge NB, et al. Comparison of the electrocardiographic changes induced by maximum exercise testing with treadmill and cycle ergometer. Circulation 1978;57:1066–1070.

Wolff HS. The integrating pneumotachograph: A new instrument for the measurement of energy expenditure by indirect calorimetry. Q J Exp Physiol 1958;43:270–283.

Wright BM. A respiratory anemometer. J Physiol (Lond) 1958;127:25P.

6

Conduct of the Stage 1 Test

This chapter describes the general conduct of exercise tests and details the procedure and calculations performed in the stage 1 test that were outlined in Chapter 5.

A number of general points may be made regarding the initial contact with the patient. Often, patients come to the laboratory anxious and ignorant about what is to happen during the test. Because this may influence their ability to cooperate, it is helpful to counteract these problems before they occur by educating referring physicians in test procedures; by giving patients, when an appointment is made, a description of the test and advice about clothing and meals; by employing a pleasant receptionist; by using professionalism and good humor in the laboratory; and by communicating well with the patient during the test. When the patient arrives in the laboratory, the test procedure should be explained in detail, and a consent form should be signed and witnessed. The patient should bring or be given suitable clothing; changing and showering facilities should be satisfactory.

SAFETY

The risks of an exercise test to the patient are very small, provided that simple precautions are observed. Although the danger of myocardial infarction or serious arrhythmia is estimated to be at about 1 in 10,000 submaximal tests (Rochmis and Blackburn, 1971), the incidence increases with maximal tests and rises to about 1 in 2500 in patients who have had a myocardial infarction in the past (Shephard, 1970; Gibbons et al., 1989). The referring physician takes some responsibility for deciding that an exercise test does not carry undue risk, but often he will be unfamiliar with the procedure. A physician experienced in the procedure should review the patient's history and physical findings and supervise the test. Occasionally, it may be necessary to obtain more information from the referring physician before proceeding with the test. In some patients, exercise tolerance is so limited that formal testing leads to little useful information and is too distressing; in this case, it may be advisable to abandon or defer the test. Various aspects related to the conduct of exercise testing,

safety, and personnel training are reviewed in a special report published by the American Heart Association (Fletcher et al., 1995).

A number of absolute or relative contraindications to exercise testing are listed in Table 6–1. The risks in patients showing relative contraindications may outweigh the possible clinical benefit expected from the test but depend also on whether a maximal or submaximal test is planned and on the facilities and personnel available to cope with any emergency that may occur.

In any patient older than 40 years of age, a 12-lead electrocardiogram should precede the test to exclude the possibility of recent ischemic changes and to provide a baseline for any abnormalities that might follow the test.

It is usual to obtain a signature of consent. In North America, there are good legal reasons for doing so, although such consent does not absolve the laboratory from taking adequate precautions. Within the consent form, the test and possible risks are described, and this occasionally leads to a patient's refusal to take the test, a situation that is unavoidable. An example of a consent form is shown in Appendix E.

During the procedure, the observers should be alert to the possibility of untoward effects, and the laboratory must be equipped to handle emergencies. In our laboratory, a physician is within call in all tests performed on patients. The technologists are trained and certified in cardiopulmonary resuscitation, and emergency procedures are established and periodically rehearsed. Some laboratories employ a registered nurse with coronary unit experience instead of a physician, but even then a physician should be available in the department for consultation. During the test, the patient is observed and questioned periodically regarding symptoms. The American Heart Association (1972) has recommended that for any patient known or suspected to have heart disease, a predetermined heart rate should not be exceeded, usually 85 per cent of the predicted maximum heart rate. We have not followed this practice, mainly because of the variability in the heart rate response in patients and because we have not encountered problems with maximal testing.

Table 6–1. CONTRAINDICATIONS TO EXERCISE TESTING

Absolute Contraindications	Acute febrile illness
	Acute electrocardiographic changes of myocardial ischemia
	Uncontrolled heart failure
	Pulmonary edema
	Unstable angina
	Acute myocarditis, pericarditis
	Uncontrolled hypertension (> 250 mm Hg systolic, 120 mm Hg diastolic)
	Uncontrolled asthma
Relative Contraindications	Recent (< 4 weeks previous) myocardial infarction
	Aortic valve disease
	Resting tachycardia (heart rate > 120 b/min)
	Severe electrolyte disturbances
	Thromboembolic disorders
	Resting electrocardiographic abnormalities
	Poorly controlled diabetes
	Epilepsy
	Cerebrovascular disease
	Respiratory failure

All laboratories should establish indications for stopping an exercise test and should ensure that they are known to all those performing the test. The indications we use are listed in Table 6–2.

After completion of the test, the electrocardiogram is observed for at least 15 minutes for postexercise changes. Should the test have been stopped because of any of the indications listed in Table 6–2, the patient rests in the laboratory until symptoms or signs have completely cleared. In this situation, care should also be taken that a member of the laboratory staff is within call while the patient showers and dresses. On rare occasions, admission to hospital for observation may be necessary in a patient showing pulmonary edema, acute electrocardiographic changes that do not resolve, or unstable cardiac rhythm. These complications are uncommon, with an incidence of 3 to 5 per 1000 tests. It is in the best interests of the patient and the laboratory to establish a careful routine to prevent compli-

---

Table 6–2. INDICATIONS FOR STOPPING AN EXERCISE TEST

General Signs and Symptoms	Severe chest pain suggestive of angina
	Severe dyspnea
	Dizziness or faintness
	Marked apprehension, mental confusion, or lack of coordination
	Sudden onset of pallor and sweating
	Onset of cyanosis
Electrocardiographic Signs	Frequent ventricular premature beats, particularly when showing the R on T wave, frequent runs of three or more, and paroxysmal ventricular tachycardia
	Atrial fibrillation when absent at rest
	Second or third degree heart block
	Ischemic changes: marked ST depression, T wave inversion, or the appearance of a Q wave
	Appearance of bundle branch block pattern
Blood Pressure Signs	Any fall in systolic pressure below the resting value
	A fall of more than 20 mm Hg in systolic pressure occurring after the normal exercise rise
	Systolic blood pressure in excess of 300 mm Hg or diastolic pressure in excess of 140 mm Hg

cations insofar as possible, to detect them promptly, and to deal with them adequately. This is not because the true risks are high, but because patients referred for exercise tests inevitably include a number who are liable to coincidental deterioration. The charge of *post hoc ergo propter hoc* is easier to refute if a laboratory discipline has been established.

CONDUCT OF A STAGE 1 TEST

Measurements Made Before the Test

Many important measurements may be made before the exercise test is carried out, partly to ensure safety; partly to assess the severity of neuromuscular, respiratory, and cardiovascular impairment; and partly to aid in the interpretation of results.

HEIGHT AND WEIGHT. Maximum power output and ideal weight are predicted on the basis of age, gender, and height; weight may be considered when it is below the ideal because it indicates a reduction in lean body (and muscle) mass. In overweight subjects, weight is considered in relation to the metabolic cost of everyday activities. In research applications, an estimate of lean body mass may be obtained from anthropometric measurements, including skinfold thickness, or by complex techniques, such as dual-photon absorptiometry and whole-body counting of the naturally occurring isotope ^{40}K, all of which yield comparable estimates (Lands et al., 1993) but are not needed for routine exercise testing.

SPIROMETRY AND FLOW:VOLUME LOOP. Estimates of maximal ventilatory capacity conventionally have been obtained from measurement of the 1-second forced expired volume (FEV_1) by multiplying FEV_1 by 35 or 40 (Freedman, 1970; Dillard et al., 1993). However, because this measurement is obtained from a forced expired maneuver, there is considerable variability in the prediction, at least in part because inspiratory flow is ignored. Thus, measurement of both inspiratory and expiratory flow with a flow-volume loop may be very revealing and improves prediction of maximal ventilatory capacity (Jones and Killian, 1991). The measurements are essential to the assessment of ventilatory capacity and the factors contributing to dyspnea.

DIFFUSING CAPACITY OF THE LUNGS FOR CARBON MONOXIDE (D_{LCO}). Long established as a routine measurement in the assessment of pulmonary gas exchange impairment (Cotes, 1993), the single-breath D_{LCO} also predicts exercise capacity as well as any other single vari-

able, probably because several physiological mechanisms contribute to gas exchange capacity (blood hemoglobin content, lung volume, $\dot{V}A/\dot{Q}C$ distribution, and alveolar-capillary diffusion). Indeed, it has been argued that the association is so close as to make exercise testing unnecessary (Owens et al., 1984). However, even in the largest studies, D_{LCO} explains only about 50 per cent of the variance in the exercise capacity of pulmonary patients (Jones and Killian, 1991). Its measurement is worthwhile in assessing the role of these mechanisms in disability and particularly in assessing the reasons for exercise-induced hypoxemia. We include capillary blood measures of hemoglobin and carboxyhemoglobin because reductions in hemoglobin and increases in carboxyhemoglobin may reduce the measured apparent carbon monoxide uptake; they may also contribute to a reduction in exercise capacity through their effect on oxygen delivery.

MAXIMUM INSPIRATORY PRESSURE (MIP) AND MAXIMUM EXPIRATORY PRESSURE (MEP). These two simple measurements provide an estimate of the static strength of the inspiratory muscles (MIP), mainly the diaphragm, and expiratory muscles (MEP), mainly the abdominal musculature. They reflect the capacity of both respiratory and skeletal muscles and provide insight into the role of muscle weakness in both dyspnea and effort.

STATIC SKELETAL MUSCLE STRENGTH. These simple measures provide information that exceeds the cost and time expended in obtaining them. We prefer measurements of dynamic movement around the knee joint (flexion, extension) and in the arms (pushing, pulling) for assessments of lower and upper limb strength, but static measurements probably provide similar information. Studies in a large population have shown that they contribute importantly to maximum exercise capacity and the sense of effort in incremental exercise tests (see Chapters 3 and 14).

Equipment Required

The following equipment is needed for a stage 1 exercise test (see also Chapter 14):

- Calibrated cycle ergometer or treadmill
- Respiratory valves, tubing, noseclip
- Dry gas meter, Tissot spirometer or flowmeter for recording ventilation
- 12-Lead electrocardiograph
- 3-Channel recorder-electrocardiograph, ventilation, and time
- Sphygmomanometer

- Resuscitation equipment (e.g., defibrillator)
- Oxygen and carbon dioxide analyzers or automated gas analysis system
- Ear oximeter

Procedure

The equipment is set up and checked before the patient arrives to ensure that the procedure runs smoothly. The test is explained to the patient, and the equipment is described in order to reduce possible anxiety. The supervising physician obtains a brief history, concentrating on exercise-related symptoms and any drugs that the patient may be taking. Usually, the standard protocol described here is followed, but if the patient is very disabled, smaller steps in power are used, and a number of other situations may call for minor modification of the test. For example, if the test is being performed in a patient before discharge from hospital after a myocardial infarction, a maximum power (usually 100 W or 600 kpm/min) and a maximum cardiac frequency (usually 130 beats per minute [b/min]) are usually not exceeded. If exercise-induced bronchoconstriction is suspected, spirometry is repeated immediately after maximum exercise and at intervals during recovery. If a treadmill test is being performed, the patient's weight is used for calculating the increments in treadmill elevation. The increments are calculated in order to obtain increases in oxygen uptake of 150 to 200 mL/min; this may be simply performed by use of the graph in Appendix C, Fig. C-2.

The electrocardiograph electrodes are carefully placed and secured. Twelve leads in the conventional positions are usually used (Fletcher et al., 1995). There are many varieties of self-adhesive electrodes, including disposable models, which tend to be expensive. An acceptable compromise is provided by small (1.4-cm-diameter) nondisposable silver–silver chloride electrodes, which are mounted in plastic to leave a space for conducting jelly and are attached to the skin by adhesive disks. The skin is first prepared by acetone and abrasion with a nylon scourer, after shaving, if necessary. Excessive electrode movement during exercise sometimes necessitates the use of a surgical net vest or bra. A sphygmomanometer cuff is placed on the upper arm and taped in position (de Sweit et al., 1989; Hill and Grim, 1991); the site of maximal pulse intensity is identified, and the stethoscope diaphragm is taped into position.

So that valid measurements of symptom intensity are obtained, the intention of the Borg scale (Borg and Noble, 1974) is explained to the patient; the distinction between leg effort, dyspnea, and chest discomfort is made; and the descriptors and their associated numbers are made clear. The last elements are printed on a large card in view of the patient so that they may be readily indicated by pointing.

If a cycle ergometer is being used, the patient is seated on the saddle and adjustments are made to ensure a comfortable cycling position—the knee should be almost fully extended at the bottom of the pedal stroke, the handlebars should be at waist height, and the mouthpiece and respiratory valve assembly are positioned so that the patient is leaning forward and has a comfortable neck position. The patient is then instructed to pedal without any added load in order to obtain the necessary pedalling frequency and to become accustomed to breathing through the valve. At this point, the initial load, usually 16 W (100 kpm/min), is imposed. If a treadmill is being used, one of the observers demonstrates its use, and the patient becomes accustomed to walking at a low treadmill setting of 1 or 1.5 mph on the level. The patient is encouraged to look straight ahead, to develop a long easy stride, and to walk without holding the handrails.

During the test, the recorder is run at a slow speed in order to obtain ventilation and to monitor the electrocardiogram; during the last 15 seconds of each minute, the blood pressure is recorded, and the recorder speed is increased in order to measure cardiac frequency and display the electrocardiogram. Usually, it is not necessary to obtain blood pressure measurement or a 12-lead electrocardiogram at each workload; they may be taken every second or third increase and if chest pain is experienced. At the end of each minute, the power is increased by an equal amount; with a cycle ergometer, this usually amounts to 16 W (100 kpm/min). In a treadmill test, the initial minute is carried out at zero elevation and 1 or 1.5 mph, followed by a second minute at 2 mph and a third minute at 3 mph; after this, the speed is kept constant at 3 mph, but at every minute, the elevation is increased by a predetermined amount (2.5 per cent for a 70-kg man).

At the end of each minute, the patient is asked to rate the severity of perceived leg effort (Borg and Noble, 1974), effort in breathing (dyspnea) (Killian and Jones, 1984), and chest discomfort (Borg et al., 1981). The test is continued until the patient stops because of severe symptoms or the observer ends the procedure according to the guidelines described earlier. Throughout the test, the patient is encouraged to pedal or walk steadily and regularly and is kept reassured and informed regarding progress in the test. If obvious tachypnea is observed, the patient is advised to breathe at a slower rate. There is no doubt that communication increases confidence and helps patients perform their best, but usually there is no point in trying to push patients past the stage of distress.

When the patient stops pedaling or walking, a

12-lead electrocardiogram is immediately recorded. The patient is then told to turn the pedals against minimal load or to walk at a slow rate on the treadmill in order to prevent fainting. After a minute, another electrocardiogram is recorded, and the patient sits on a chair. Information is obtained regarding symptoms that prevented further exercise—severity of chest pain, dyspnea, general fatigue, and leg discomfort or pain. Additional 12-lead electrocardiograms are recorded 3 minutes, 5 minutes, and 10 minutes after exercise. During this time, the physician is able to tell the patient about performance during the test and answer any questions.

Recordings and Calculations

During the test, measurements are recorded by hand, multichannel recorder, or microprocessor/ computer; although modern instruments are very reliable, recording some basic measurements by hand as well as automatically has its advantages, and the ability to record measurements independently of an automated measurement system is essential for quality control. In our laboratory, blood pressure and Borg scale recordings (Borg and Noble, 1974; Borg et al., 1981) are directly noted on a work sheet, together with heart rate and oximeter readings taken from the instruments; the electrocardiogram is obtained in hard copy.

In previous editions of the book, the measurements and calculations were detailed as part of the stage 1 procedure; they are included in Appendix D not only to allow the algorithms used in automated systems to be checked but also to allow periodic quality control checks to be made. Often, malfunction of analyzers or ergometers is difficult to detect, and a routine is required in the laboratory for establishment quality; this topic is discussed in Chapter 10.

Many automated systems provide a report form on which the recordings are entered in a suitable format for sending to referring physicians and for inclusion in a patient's health record. Although such output may be "customized," our own experience has led us to develop our own form by interfacing a computer to the automated system. This report is on a single sheet and is designed to accompany a letter providing the interpretation. It is possible to semiautomate the interpretation letter by an interactive program, but the benefit afforded by this option is only marginal.

The report includes some clinical details, anthropometry, drugs being taken, resting pulmonary function, electrocardiogram, hemoglobin determination, and muscle strength measurements. Exercise

data include a table containing power output, symptom rating, oxygen intake, carbon dioxide output, respiratory exchange ratio, heart rate and blood pressure, ventilation and pattern of breathing, and oxygen saturation. Changes in spirometry after exercise are noted. Symptom ratings, heart rate, and ventilation are recorded on graphs containing the normal responses as well as the patient data. Variables at maximum exercise are expressed as per cent predicted. Together with the electrocardiogram, this report contains all the data needed for the interpretation.

REFERENCES

American Heart Association: Exercise Testing and Training of Apparently Healthy Individuals: A Handbook for Physicians. New York: The American Heart Association, 1972.

Borg G, Holmgren A, Lindblad I. Quantitative evaluation of chest pain. Acta Med Scand Suppl 1981;664:43–45.

Borg G, Noble B. Perceived exertion. Exerc Sport Sci Rev 1974;12:131–153.

Cotes JE. Lung Function. Assessment and Application in Medicine, 5th ed. Oxford: Blackwell Scientific Publications; 1993.

de Sweit M, Dillon MJ, Littler W, et al. Measurement of blood pressure in children: Recommendations of a working party of the British Hypertension Society. BMJ 1989;299:497.

Dillard TA, Hnatiuk OW, McCumber R. Maximum voluntary ventilation: Spirometric determinants in chronic obstructive pulmonary disease patients and normal subjects. Am Rev Respir Dis 1993;147:870–875.

Fletcher GF, Balady G, Froelicher V, et al. Exercise standards: A statement for healthcare professionals from the American Heart Association. Circulation 1995;91:580–615.

Freedman S. Sustained maximum voluntary ventilation. Respir Physiol 1970;8:23–244.

Gibbons L, Blair SN, Kohl HW, Cooper K. The safety of maximal exercise testing. Circulation 1989;80:846–852.

Hill MN, Grim CM. How to take a precise blood pressure. Am J Nursing 1991;91:38–42.

Jones NL, Killian KJ. Limitation of exercise in chronic airway obstruction. In: Cherniack NS, editor. Chronic Obstructive Pulmonary Disease. Philadelphia: WB Saunders Co.; 1991, pp. 196–206.

Killian KJ, Jones NL. The use of exercise testing and other methods in the investigation of dyspnea. Clin Chest Med 1984;5:99–108.

Lands LC, Gordon C, Bar-Or O, et al. Comparison of three techniques for body composition analysis in cystic fibrosis. J Appl Physiol 1993;75:162–166.

McKelvie RS, Heigenhauser GJF, Jones NL. Measurement of cardiac output by CO_2 rebreathing in unsteady state exercise. Chest 1987;92:777–782.

Noble BJ. Clinical applications of perceived exertion. Med Sci Sports Exerc 1982;14:406–411.

Owens GR, Rogers RM, Pennock BE, Lewis D. The diffusing capacity as a predictor of arterial oxygen desaturation during exercise in patients with chronic obstructive pulmonary disease. N Engl J Med 1984;310:1218–1221.

Rochmis P, Blackburn H. Exercise tests. A survey of procedures, safety and litigation experience in approximately 170,000 tests. JAMA 1971;17:1061–1066.

Shephard RJ. For exercise testing: A review of procedures available to the clinician. Bull Physiopathol Respir 1970;6:425–474.

7

The Exercise Electrocardiogram

This chapter provides a brief discussion of the electrocardiographic changes seen in normal subjects during exercise, the electrocardiographic criteria of coronary artery disease, some effects of commonly prescribed drugs, and a listing of the dysrhythmias that may be brought on by exercise. Also included are some observations on the electrocardiogram in athletes, for which I am indebted to the late Dr. John Sutton.

Technical aspects of electrocardiography were mentioned earlier but cannot be overemphasized; electrocardiograms of the highest quality are required for the interpretation of exercise-related changes. Details are provided in a recent statement by the American Heart Association (Fletcher et al., 1995). Good skin preparation, firm electrode attachment, and high-quality electronic equipment usage are all important in obtaining accurate recordings that are free from drift and interference. Computer-aided signal conditioning and averaging have led to increased quality of recordings (Simoons, 1977; Sheffield, 1978). There has been argument regarding the best leads to use during exercise. The easiest method is to place one electrode in the V_4 or V_5 position and an indifferent electrode in an area free of muscle on the sternum or forehead. This electrode placement is excellent for monitoring purposes and identifies 90 per cent of ischemic electrocardiographic changes (McHenry et al., 1972). However, a significantly higher yield is obtained with the standard 12-lead system (Chaitman et al., 1978). Although the use of X, Y, and Z leads introduced by Frank has been recommended for exercise testing, and although computer analysis has been available for many years (Blomqvist,

1965), these methods have not been widely used and probably do not offer any advantages over 12-lead systems (Sheffield and Roitman, 1976).

NORMAL RESPONSE TO EXERCISE

Associated with the increase in cardiac frequency during exercise are a number of minor electrocardiographic changes (Sandberg, 1961). The P wave may increase slightly in amplitude, and the PR interval shortens. The duration of the QRS does not change, but a rate-dependent shift in the axis to the right, of up to 30 degrees, is often seen (Simoons and Hugenholz, 1975). Depression of the J point with upward-sloping ST segment is also rate dependent but may be difficult to distinguish from ST depression associated with coronary artery disease. Usually, in healthy subjects, depression of the ST segment is less than 1 mm and lasts for less than 40 msec (Fig. 7–1); J-point depression of over 1.5 mm is associated with an increased probability of coronary artery disease (Kurita, 1977). The T wave normally does not change in direction, except in some athletes showing T-wave inversion at rest (see below), but the amplitude commonly decreases. The amplitude of the U wave may increase in exercise (Lepeschkin, 1969), and fusion of T, U, and P waves is common at high cardiac frequencies. The fusion of T and P waves may make identification of the isoelectric level difficult (see Fig. 7–1).

CHANGES ASSOCIATED WITH CORONARY ARTERY DISEASE

In spite of a huge amount of research, problems associated with the development of diagnostic crite-

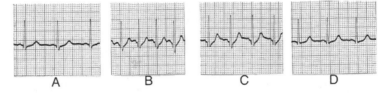

Figure 7–1. Lead V_4 obtained in a 45-year-old female investigated for atypical chest pain. *A*, rest; *B*, exercise, 700 kpm/min; *C*, maximum exercise, 800 kpm/min; *D*, recovery, 5 min. There is fusion of T and P waves, downward-sloping PQ, and J-point depression, interpreted as normal. Thallium scintigram was normal.

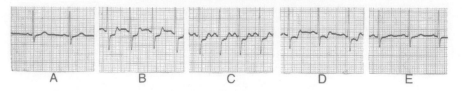

Figure 7–2. Lead V_5 in a 40-year-old male complaining of angina. *A,* rest; *B,* 900 kpm/min; *C,* maximum exercise, 1100 kpm/min; *D,* recovery, 1 min; *E,* recovery, 10 min. During exercise, 2-mm ST depression and chest pain developed; both resolved rapidly in recovery. Coronary artery narrowing was confirmed by angiography.

ria for coronary artery disease continue to exist. Many studies have reported the relationship of angiographic abnormalities to the exercise electrocardiogram, but a number of questions remain unanswered; ST segment depression has been well studied, but other associated changes are less well established, leaving room for uncertainty in the interpretation of some tests. This is why interpretation always should be made in relationship to clinical features, the occurrence of symptoms, and any associated features during exercise, such as in cardiac frequency or blood pressure, overall exercise capacity, and development or abolition of any arrhythmias.

ST SEGMENT DEPRESSION. There is agreement that the presence of horizontal or downward-sloping ST segment depression of at least 0.1 mV (1 mm) for at least 0.08 second is associated with significant coronary artery narrowing in at least 85 per cent of patients (a sensitivity of 0.85) and that at least 70 per cent of patients with significant narrowing show these changes (a specificity of 0.70) (Roitman et al., 1970; Cahen et al., 1973; Kattus, 1974) (Fig. 7–2). Lesser degrees of ST depression are also associated with a high probability of coronary artery disease, but the changes need to be interpreted in relation to the patient's age, sex, and clinical history (Fig. 7–3). The report of Hollenberg and associates (1985) indicates that ST depression should be standardized to an R-wave voltage of 1.2 mV in V_5 and 0.8 mV in aVF.

ST SEGMENT ELEVATION. Elevation of the ST segment may be an indication of transmural myocardial ischemia (Fortuin and Friesinger, 1970) and is a feature of Prinzmetal's angina (Fig. 7–4). When ST segment elevation occurs in the absence of angina, ventriculography often reveals abnormal ventricular wall motion (Chahine et al., 1976). The finding is relatively common during exercise in patients with previous myocardial infarction and tends to resolve after exercise more slowly than ST segment depression (Wicks et al., 1978). ST elevation during exercise carries a poor prognosis, is most often seen in the right precordial leads (V_1-V_3), and is associated with Q waves (Bruce et al., 1988).

T-WAVE INVERSION. Inversion of the T wave during exercise often accompanies ST segment depression in patients with coronary artery narrowing (Cahen et al., 1973). When T-wave inversion occurs alone, however, it is not a reliable indicator of coronary artery disease, particularly in patients taking cardioactive or psychiatric drugs or in whom the finding occurs during hyperventilation at rest. Occasionally, T waves are inverted at rest but are upright during exercise (Fig. 7–5); this finding occurs almost as frequently in the normal population as it does in patients with coronary artery disease and the mechanism is unknown. Gross increases in T-wave amplitude during exercise may be associated with coronary artery narrowing, but this is another unusual finding that by itself may not mean much. Owing to the relatively frequent occurrence of isolated T-wave changes in normal subjects, they cannot confidently be used in a diagnostic sense.

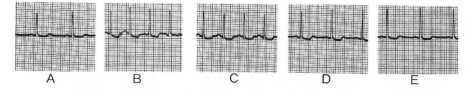

Figure 7–3. Lead V_6 in a 64-year-old female with variable chest pain not consistently related to exercise. *A,* rest; *B,* 500 kpm/min; *C,* maximum exercise; 600 kpm/min; *D,* recovery, 5 min; *E,* recovery, 10 min. There is 1-mm downward-sloping ST depression, which resolves only slowly in recovery. Coronary angiographic results were normal in this patient.

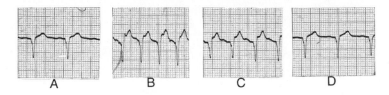

Figure 7–4. Lead V$_5$ in a 58-year-old man assessed 6 months after a transmural myocardial infarction. *A*, rest; *B*, maximum exercise, 1000 kpm/min; *C*, recovery, 1 min; *D*, recovery, 10 min. At rest, there is a Q wave, absent R, and slight elevation of ST segment that increases to 3 to 4 mm in exercise and resolves in recovery.

OTHER CHANGES. Less common changes shown to be associated with significant coronary artery narrowing include U-wave inversion (Cahen et al., 1973), increased R-wave amplitude (Bonoris et al., 1977), ventricular arrhythmias, and reductions in heart rate (sinus node dysfunction, chronotropic incompetence), usually in inferior myocardial ischemia.

TIMING OF CHANGES. The significance of electrocardiographic changes in the diagnosis of coronary artery narrowing is highest when they appear during exercise; if any abnormality occurs only in the recovery period after exercise, the earlier the abnormality appears and the sooner it resolves, the more likely it is to be associated with significant coronary artery narrowing.

INTERPRETATION PROBLEMS. Difficulties in interpretation may arise in a number of situations. First, the measurement of upward-sloping ST depression is made difficult at high heart rates when fusion of the T and P waves occurs and the PQ segment is downward-sloping (see Fig. 7–1). Second, J-point depression and upward-sloping ST depression are common in healthy subjects. Third, ST segment depression may be found in subjects without significant coronary artery narrowing. Sometimes, these changes are due to drug ingestion, hyperventilation, or other conditions, such as mitral valve prolapse (Lobstein et al., 1973), the Wolff-Parkinson-White syndrome (Fig. 7–6) (Gazes, 1969), and vasoregulatory asthenia (Friesinger et al., 1972). The occurrence of exercise-associated ST segment changes in normal females (Cumming et al., 1973) (see Fig. 7–3) has led some observers to question the value of exercise testing for coronary artery disease in females. However, a large and carefully controlled study failed to show that

false-negative responses were more common in females than in males (Weiner et al., 1978).

Diagnostic Interpretation

Although a number of electrocardiographic changes may occur during exercise in patients with diagnosed coronary artery disease, depression of the ST segment is the most common. Early studies sought to establish a criterion of ST depression that might be reproducibly measured to give a reliable indication of significant disease. Agreement was reached on a horizontal or downward-sloping ST depression of 1 mm (0.1 mV) lasting for at least 0.08 second (American Heart Association, 1972) or 0.06 second after the J point. Many subsequent studies used this criterion to identify "positive" or "negative" responses to exercise.

General agreement on other criteria has not been reached, and there is still argument regarding the exercise protocol that should be used to provoke changes. The most commonly performed test likely uses the Bruce treadmill protocol (Bruce and McDonough, 1969). Other workers have preferred a progressive incremental test in which power increases in smaller steps than in the Bruce protocol (Balke and Ware, 1959), and many have used a cycle ergometer. However, these factors are unlikely to account for important differences in diagnostic accuracy among different studies (Wicks et al., 1978). More important is the maximum power used; some investigators use a symptom-limited maximum, and others, a "target" heart rate based on a proportion (usually 85 per cent) of the maximum heart rate predicted on the basis of age (American Heart Association, 1972). Tests in which the patient stopped exercise at a heart rate below this value have been judged "submaximal" and ex-

Figure 7–5. Lead V$_5$ in a 27-year-old male, an elite marathon runner. *A*, rest; *B*, maximum exercise, 2000 kpm/min; *C*, recovery, 10 min. There is T-wave inversion at rest, which becomes upright in exercise.

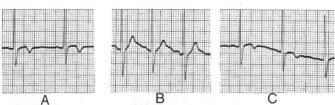

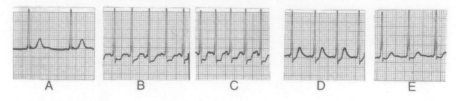

Figure 7–6. Lead V_5 in a 45-year-old male with type A Wolff-Parkinson-White syndrome. *A*, rest; *B*, 900 kpm/min; *C*, maximum exercise, 1000 kpm/min; *D*, recovery, 1 min; *E*, recovery, 5 min. Short PR interval and pre-excitation, with 3-mm horizontal ST depression in exercise. Coronary angiographic results were normal.

cluded from some studies, even though the true maximal heart rate may be significantly reduced in a proportion of patients (Powles et al., 1979). Other differences between reported studies may be due to the electrocardiographic leads used and the times at which recordings are made. Although most ST segment changes are identified in one precordial (V_4 or V_5) lead, the yield is increased by standard 12-lead recordings (Mason et al., 1967). The changes are maximal during maximal exercise or immediately on stopping; delayed recording may miss changes.

Throughout discussions of the diagnostic validity of the exercise electrocardiogram, a number of authorities suggested a move away from the "all or none" usage of positive and negative test results. Rifkin and Hood (1977) demonstrated that likelihood of disease was increased even with 0.5-mm depression of the ST segment and progressively increased with increasing depression. Diamond and Forrester (1979) reviewed previous work to develop values for the probability of angiographic coronary artery disease in subjects with different ages, of both sexes, and with a history of chest pain who exhibited ST segment depression of varying depth. For example, a man aged 45 years with typical anginal pain who shows a 2-mm ST depression has a 99 per cent probability of coronary artery narrowing. This contrasts with an asymptomatic woman of the same age showing the same ST depression, in whom the probability of disease is only 10 per cent. The approach of Diamond and Forrester has been supported by other studies and is helpful in interpreting the results of an exercise test (Figs. 7–7 and 7–8).

Given the variations in protocol and interpretation, a surprising degree of unanimity on the value of exercise tests existed in early reports (Bruce and McDonough, 1969). This suggested that a positive test result would be obtained in most patients with symptoms of coronary artery disease and stimulated a dramatic increase in the use of exercise tests (Blackburn, 1977; McNeer et al., 1978).

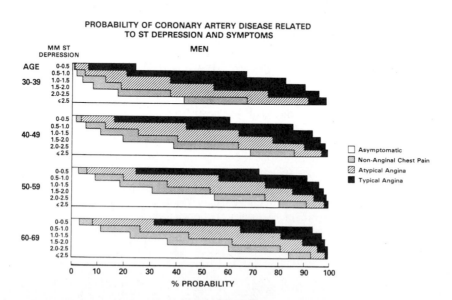

Figure 7–7. Diagram expressing probability of coronary artery disease in males of varying age and symptoms and ST segment depression during exercise. Note that shaded areas do not represent a range; the probability is given by the right-hand limit of a given area: for example, a 65-year-old asymptomatic man with 2-mm ST depression has a 60 per cent probability of coronary disease. (Data from Diamond GA, Forrester JS. Analysis of probability as an aid in the clinical diagnosis of coronary artery disease. N Engl J Med 1979;300:1350–1358.)

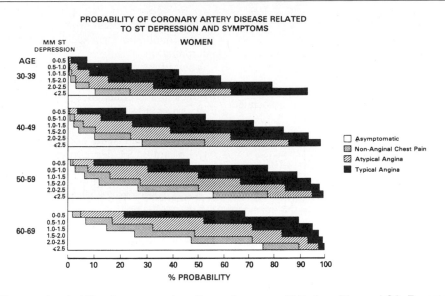

Figure 7–8. Diagram of probability of coronary artery disease in women. (Data from Diamond GA, Forrester JS. Analysis of probability as an aid in the clinical diagnosis of coronary artery disease. N Engl J Med 1979;300:1350–1358.)

SENSITIVITY AND SPECIFICITY. The early reports were followed by an inevitable turn of the tide, set in motion by reports of the high incidence of false-positive test results—ST depression in patients with normal coronary angiographic results—and false-negative results—normal exercise electrocardiograms in patients with coronary narrowing (Froelicher et al., 1973). Subsequent investigations examined the sensitivity and specificity of exercise responses in subjects who underwent coronary angiography. *Sensitivity* in this context is defined as the percentage of patients with "positive" angiograms who show positive electrocardiographic changes. *Specificity* is the percentage of "negative" electrocardiograms in patients with "negative" angiograms. Sensitivity varied between 54 and 85 per cent, and specificity varied between 82 and 100 per cent (Blackburn, 1977). Although the variation was accounted for in part by variations in angiographic criteria (50 per cent or 75 per cent luminal narrowing) and exercise protocols (maximal or submaximal), it was mainly due to differences in the populations under study. It became clear that the predictive value of a positive exercise test result depended on the pretest likelihood of disease, *predictive value* being defined as the ratio of true-positive results to the sum of true-positive and false-positive results in a population.

BAYES' RULE. The Reverend Thomas Bayes presented his rule of conditional probabilities more than two centuries ago (1763), and recently it has often been invoked to establish the predictive accuracy of exercise ST segment depression. The rule allows us to be more precise about the probability of coronary artery disease in a given patient from a knowledge of the incidence of the disease in a population that meets the defined characteristics present in the patient. The characteristics may be defined in terms of coronary risk factors, age, sex, presence of symptoms, or any factors associated with a known prevalence of disease. We also need to know the probability with which subjects with coronary disease show ST segment depression that is similar in degree to that found in the patient. Bayes' rule is defined for coronary artery disease in the following way (Remington and Schork, 1970):

Let the probability (P) of disease (D) if ST depression is found in the electrocardiogram (S) be denoted $P(D/S)$; let the incidence of ST segment depression in diseased subjects ("sensitivity") be denoted $P(S/D)$, and in nondiseased subjects $P(S/\overline{D})$; and let the probability of disease in the population be denoted $P(D)$, and its absence $P(\overline{D})$. Using this notation, "specificity" may be represented $P(\overline{S}/\overline{D})$. Then, the probability of disease in a patient with ST depression is given by the following equation:

$$P(D/S) = \frac{P(D) \times P(S/D)}{[P(D) \times P(S/D)] + [P(\overline{D}) \times P(S/\overline{D})]}$$

An example may make this complex-looking equation simpler to understand. If the incidence of the disease in the population under study is 15 per cent, and if 80 per cent of patients with the disease show ST depression, compared with only 10 per cent of nondiseased subjects, then

$$P(D) = .15$$
$$P(\overline{D}) = 1.0 - .15 = .85$$
$$P(S/D) = .80$$
$$P(S/\overline{D}) = .10$$

The probability that ST depression is associated with disease is given by

$$P(D/S) = \frac{.15 \times .80}{(.15 \times .80) + (.85 \times .10)}$$
$$= .58 \text{ (or 58\%)}$$

The relationships may be readily appreciated intuitively; Bayes' rule states that the probability of disease, given a positive test result, is (1) directly related to the prevalence of disease in the total population and the incidence of positive test results in all cases of the disease and (2) inversely related to the proportion of the population without disease and the proportion of nondiseased showing positive results.

The application of Bayes' rule requires us to know the pretest likelihood (or probability) and the qualities of the test result (sensitivity, specificity) that allow us to calculate the post-test likelihood of coronary artery narrowing given a positive result. We now have access to a large body of information relating to both these factors, but this has been provided by studies of different populations using different tests and different diagnostic criteria. How, then, may we develop criteria applicable to our own needs? An approach advocated by a number of authors is based on the use of likelihood ratios.

LIKELIHOOD RATIO. We may rephrase Bayes' rule to state that the post-test probability (P[D/S]) is related to the pretest probability (P[D]) through a likelihood ratio (LR) for the positive test result. Likelihood ratio is defined as sensitivity divided by (1 − specificity) (or $P[S/D] \div P[S/\overline{D}]$) and thus incorporates the important predictive values for the test results. In the foregoing example, pretest probability is 0.15 and the likelihood ratio is 0.80 ÷ 0.10 or 8; that is, someone with a positive result is eight times as likely to have the disease as someone without one.

The LR ''expresses the odds that a given level of a diagnostic test result would be expected in a patient with (as opposed to one without) the target disorder'' (Sackett et al., 1985). Sackett and colleagues pointed out that likelihood ratios are more stable than values for sensitivity and specificity because they are less affected by variations in prevalence. Another advantage of the LR lies in its power to define the value of adding information to a given test result in order to improve the predictive accuracy. We may calculate the post-test likelihood

of a given result and then use this value as the pretest likelihood for a second test or refinement of interpretation.

The actual calculation of post-test likelihood is simplified by the use of a nomogram, as described by Sackett and colleagues (1985) and shown in Fig. 7–9. An example illustrates its use: the probability of coronary artery disease can be calculated in a 45-year-old man with nontypical chest pain who has 1.5 mm of ST depression at a maximum power output of 70 per cent predicted and a maximum heart rate of 140 beats per minute (b/min) (78 per cent predicted). The prevalence of coronary disease (greater than 70 per cent stenosis of at least one coronary artery) is a function of age and sex (Diamond and Forrester, 1979) and in this example is

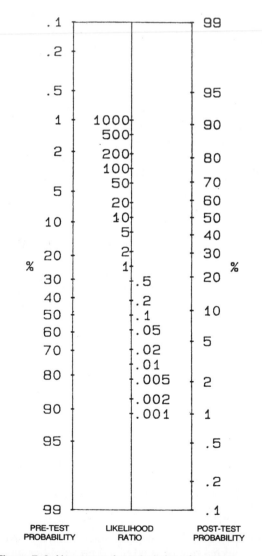

Figure 7–9. Nomogram for calculation of post-test probability from pretest probability and likelihood ratio. (From Sackett DL, Haynes RB, Tugwell P. Clinical Epidemiology. Toronto: Little, Brown & Co.; 1985.)

5.8 per cent; this is the first pretest likelihood and an anchorpoint on the left-hand side of the nomogram. The LR for nontypical angina (Fig. 7–10) is 20; that is, someone who experiences nontypical angina is 20 times more likely to have coronary artery narrowing than is someone of the same age and sex who does not. On the nomogram, a straight line may be drawn from 5.8 per cent through the value for LR (20) in order to obtain a new probability of 55 per cent. This value, the likelihood of coronary artery disease in a man of this age and history, even before the exercise results are obtained, is used as the next pretest likelihood. We may then apply the LR appropriate to the extent of ST depression in the test; at 1.5 mm, the LR is 2, giving a post-test likelihood of 70 per cent (Diamond and Forrester, 1979; Chaitman et al., 1981). Another way to understand the approach is to calculate the relative odds of coronary artery narrowing; thus, the odds of a man of this age having the condition are about 0.06 (5.8:94.2) to 1; with non-anginal chest pain, the odds increase 20-fold to 1.2 (55:45) to 1, and with ST depression to 2.3 (70:30) to 1.

Other Criteria Added to ST Depression

A number of studies have shown that the diagnostic accuracy of exercise results may be improved by the inclusion of several variables measured in the test; these may be either assigned a cutoff value and included in a multivariate analysis (Detry et al., 1985) or used to construct a score, which is then judged positive or negative for disease (Kansal et al., 1983). Because the use of such approaches currently appears to preclude the use of the Diamond and Forrester approach, it is preferable to use data presented in such studies to improve the LR developed on the basis of the large population studies of Diamond and Forrester and Chaitman and colleagues. Thus, the following values need to be viewed skeptically until they are validated in other studies, and readers may prefer to suspend judgment until they have examined the original data for themselves.

STANDARDIZATION OF ST CHANGES FOR R-WAVE VOLTAGE. Hollenberg and co-workers (1985a) showed a considerable reduction in false-positive ST changes by adjusting the depression to standard R-wave voltages of 12 mm in lead V_5 and 8 mm in aVR. Although the extent to which this procedure increases the LR of ST changes given earlier is uncertain, there is a good case for making this correction as an initial step.

MAXIMUM POWER OUTPUT AND MAXIMUM HEART RATE. Several studies have demonstrated that reductions in exercise capacity contribute powerfully to the prediction of coronary artery disease; this is because ST changes occurring at low exercise levels and low heart rates are also occurring at low levels of myocardial oxygen consumption. In the scoring system of Kansal and associates (1983), a maximum heart rate of less than 80 per cent predicted receives a higher

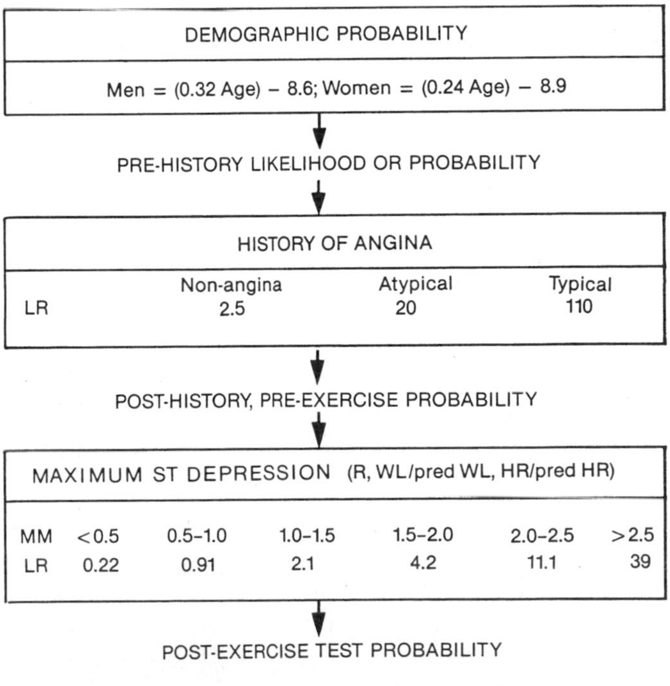

Figure 7–10. A scheme for probability calculation. As detailed in the text, the likelihood of coronary artery disease in the general population is calculated first. Then a likelihood ratio (LR) is applied, according to clinical chest pain classification to obtain pretest probability. Finally the extent of ST depression in mm (MM), corrected for R-wave amplitude (R), workload achieved (WL/pred WL), and maximum heart rate (HR/pred HR), is used to obtain an LR, which is used to derive the post-test probability.

DEMOGRAPHIC PROBABILITY					
Men = (0.32 Age) − 8.6; Women = (0.24 Age) − 8.9					

PRE-HISTORY LIKELIHOOD OR PROBABILITY

HISTORY OF ANGINA					
	Non-angina		Atypical		Typical
LR	2.5		20		110

POST-HISTORY, PRE-EXERCISE PROBABILITY

MAXIMUM ST DEPRESSION (R, WL/pred WL, HR/pred HR)					
MM	<0.5	0.5–1.0	1.0–1.5	1.5–2.0	2.0–2.5	>2.5
LR	0.22	0.91	2.1	4.2	11.1	39

POST-EXERCISE TEST PROBABILITY

weighting than does a 1-mm ST depression, and a treadmill time of less than 8 minutes also received a weighting; inclusion of these variables approximately doubled the LR from ST changes alone. Detry and colleagues (1985) also found that reduction in maximum heart rate to below 147 b/min and power to below 179 W increased the LR of a given ST depression. However, such findings are difficult to incorporate into an approach that recognizes the extent of ST depression as being an important variable. Furthermore, an arbitrary power output is not appropriate unless it is standardized to the predicted power capacity of the subject. An approach advocated by Linderholm and co-workers (1985), and supported by the findings of Hollenberg and colleagues (1985b), is to correct the ST depression by the maximum power expressed as a fraction of predicted; thus, a 1-mm ST depression at 50 per cent predicted maximum power becomes equivalent to a 2-mm depression, carrying a higher LR. In the example above, a 1.5-mm depression at 70 per cent predicted power becomes a 2.1-mm depression with an LR of 10 and a post-test likelihood of 91 per cent. This correction may not completely account for a reduced heart rate, and the data of Hollenberg and associates (1985b) suggested that division by the percentage of predicted maximum heart rate contributes to an improved diagnostic accuracy. It is possible, however, that the application of both corrections may be misleading; a compromise is to correct for the percentage of predicted power and the percentage of predicted heart rate at that power; in the example, a heart rate of 147 b/min is the normal expected heart rate at 70 per cent of maximum power in a male of the given age and stature; the actual heart rate is 140 b/min, or 95 per cent of expected. Thus, the correction in the example would be as follows:

$$\text{Corrected ST} = 1.5/(0.7 \times 0.95)$$
$$= 2.25 \text{ mm}$$

The current practice is to use a probabilistic approach, based on the prevalence data and likelihood ratios developed in large population studies (Diamond and Forrester, 1979; Chaitman et al., 1981), to ST segment depression, corrected R-wave amplitude (Hollenberg et al., 1985a), and maximum power and heart rate achieved in exercise (Linderholm et al., 1985). This is not the only possible approach but one that is based on carefully validated studies. Because the successive use of likelihood ratios assumes that each pretest likelihood is known exactly, likelihood ratio analysis may be criticized for not incorporating the degree of confidence in the estimated probability (Diamond et al., 1980; Diamond and Forrester, 1983). Thus, it is

likely that new epidemiological techniques will be developed to improve the accuracy and reduce the misinterpretation of exercise electrocardiographic changes.

OTHER APPROACHES TO EVALUATION OF ST CHANGES. The application of computer processing to electrocardiographic signals has allowed a more sophisticated and precise analysis of the extent of ST depression; more leads may be scanned, and information gained throughout the test may be used. In the technique described by Hollenberg and colleagues (1980, 1985a), a microprocessor calculates the J-point depression and the ST slope to identify the area under the isoelectric line; this is summed for the whole test and corrected for R-wave amplitude, test duration, and maximum heart rate to obtain a treadmill exercise score. The analysis improved sensitivity over conventional ST depression (1 mm) but was not compared with a quantitative method; thus, it is not clear to what extent the method might increase likelihood ratios. However, increasing scores were shown to be predictive of increasing extent of disease.

In the method of Elamin and co-workers (1982), ST depression is quantified in several leads throughout the test and is regressed against heart rate in order to obtain an ST/HR slope; the maximum value for the slope initially was found to be highly predictive and to accurately separate patients with varying extent of disease. Subsequently the method was confirmed to be superior to simple ST criteria but was less accurate than first thought; Okin and associates (1985) found that an ST/HR slope of greater than 6 mV/b/min was associated with an LR of 26, compared with 1.7 obtained by use of the criterion of 1-mm ST depression; they also found that increasing slope was associated with increasing extent of disease, but with considerable overlap. The same group (Amiesen et al., 1985) reported that false-negative ST/HR slopes are common after infarct and that false-positive results are common in aortic regurgitation with normal coronaries. Neither of these techniques has been shown to be better than the best available alternative (Sheffield, 1985). A multicenter trial led to the raising of further questions regarding the ST/HR approach (Bobbio et al., 1992).

OTHER TECHNIQUES. Thallium scintigraphy has proved to be a powerful noninvasive diagnostic method (Botvinick et al., 1978); thallium behaves as if it were an isotope of potassium and is readily taken up by healthy perfused cardiac muscle. An intravenous injection of thallium-201 is given 30 to 60 seconds before the end of a maximum exercise test, and imaging is performed with a scintillation camera 5 to 10 minutes later and again 3 to 4 hours after injection. This allows the results to be categorized into fixed perfusion defects, reversible perfusion defects, or normal and identifies the arterial territories involved. Many studies have shown that abnormalities are predictive of coronary artery disease and are also helpful in diagnosing multivessel disease (O'Hara et al., 1985). Diamond and colleagues (1980) showed the likelihood of significant disease to be 0.18 with a normal scan, increasing to 1.4 with a fixed defect and 11.6 with a reversible defect. These findings indicate that the method will not help in evaluating patients with a high pretest likelihood, for example, on the basis of a positive exercise test. For this reason Diamond and co-workers (1980) and Hung and associates (1985) suggested an approach that uses thallium to investigate patients with an indeterminate likelihood after exercise testing. Hung and co-workers (1985) showed that LR was 2 for a 1-mm ST depression in exercise and 2 again for the addition of a positive thallium result. The careful analysis of Diamond and associates (1980) should be read so that a clear view of the cost-effectiveness of serial testing for coronary artery disease can be obtained. Several new techniques in cardiac investigation may be carried out during exercise, although in some, the technical difficulties require exercise of only limited muscle mass, such as handgrip. It is likely that further technological development will eventually allow these techniques to be used during conventional exercise tests. These methods include Doppler flow measurement, echocardiography, positron emission tomography, and magnetic resonance imaging (Kuno et al., 1994; Yabe et al., 1994).

ELECTROCARDIOGRAPHIC EFFECTS OF DRUGS

In any patient undergoing exercise testing for the assessment or diagnosis of coronary artery disease, a careful drug history is mandatory. Whenever possible, testing should be carried out several days after drug therapy has been stopped. Because nearly all such patients are taking some drug or other, whether diuretic, tranquilizer, beta blocker, or even digitalis or another cardioactive drug, this may seem the counsel of perfection. However, a strict laboratory ruling demanding cessation of therapy can be successfully carried out, given adequate communication with referring physicians. The importance of this rule becomes self-evident in considerations of the extent to which drugs may lead to false-positive or false-negative electrocardiographic results.

Digoxin therapy is associated with ST depression with exercise in normal subjects and with normal control exercise study results in patients with coronary artery disease (Fig. 7–11), and it increases ST depression in patients with a positive result (LeWinter et al., 1977). This effect may last up to 2 weeks after withdrawal of digoxin. Propranolol and other beta blockers tend to reduce positive ST changes by the reduction in cardiac frequency, blood pressure, and myocardial oxygen consumption (Gianelly et al., 1969) but do not influence the ST depression found at the onset of angina (LeWinter et al., 1977). Calcium channel blocking drugs may reduce the heart rate response to exercise and thus have an effect similar to beta blockade; verapamil is most likely to do so, and diltiazem may also have this effect, although nifedipine may increase heart rate, probably because of a fall in blood pressure. Diuretic therapy is associated with ST segment and T-wave changes that are reversed by potassium replacement; these false-positive results need not be associated with a low serum potassium concentration. Psychiatric drugs may be associated with false-negative and, less commonly, false-positive changes. Phenothiazines increase heart rate, reduce blood pressure, and may also have a myocardial depressant effect (Carlsson et al., 1966; Burda, 1968). Diazepam increases coronary blood flow and may lead to false-negative results in patients with coronary artery disease (Ikram et al., 1973). Lithium carbonate may cause reversible T-wave changes (Demers and Heninger, 1971) and may have a depressant effect on sinus node function (Wellens et al., 1975). Other drugs with central cardiac or peripheral circulatory effects may influence the responses to exercise and, indirectly, the electrocardiogram during exercise. Heavy cigarette smoking may impair performance and coronary oxygen delivery through a reduction in arterial oxygen content (Aronow et al., 1974).

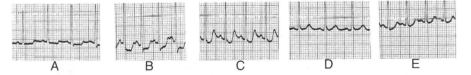

A   B   C   D   E

Figure 7–11. Lead V_6 in a 42-year-old male investigated for chest pain and dyspnea who was being treated with digoxin. Resting tracing was normal. *A,* 500 kpm/min; *B,* maximum exercise, 1200 kpm/min; *C,* recovery, 3 min. There is a 4-mm horizontal ST depression in exercise. Patient was restudied 1 month after withdrawal of digoxin; *D,* 500 kpm/min; *E,* maximum exercise, 1500 kpm/min. No ST changes were found. Exercise thallium scintigraphy was normal. The changes in *B* were interpreted as due to digoxin.

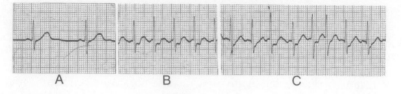

Figure 7–12. Lead V_4 in a 60-year-old male 2 years after a myocardial infarction. *A*, rest; *B*, 500 kpm/min; *C*, 500 kpm/min. The rest appearance is normal; *B* shows a nodal rhythm with ST depression, which progresses to atrial fibrillation. The rhythm reverted to normal within 10 minutes after exercise.

CARDIAC ARRHYTHMIAS IN EXERCISE

Although the ventricular arrhythmias, the most common and potentially the most lethal of the exercise-induced abnormalities, have received the most publicity, nearly all the known arrhythmias may occur during exercise. Atrial abnormalities are uncommon, occurring in fewer than 0.2 per cent of patients undergoing exercise testing (Gooch, 1972). Nodal rhythm and other ectopic atrial rhythms are sometimes provoked by exercise and rarely may precede atrial tachycardia or fibrillation (Fig. 7–12). These arrhythmias usually revert spontaneously after exercise, although atrial fibrillation may persist.

The most common ventricular arrhythmia encountered in exercise is the ventricular premature beat; in a population survey of nearly 800 men, Vedin and associates (1972) found an incidence of 13.5 per cent in subjects with signs of myocardial ischemia compared with 3 per cent of healthy subjects, and the presence of ventricular premature beats was associated with an increased incidence of sudden death during a follow-up period of 5 years. Ventricular premature beats at rest may be suppressed by exercise, or they may occur at low exercise intensities and disappear during heavy exercise; exercise suppression occurs with the same frequency (about 40 per cent) in patients with coronary artery disease as in normal subjects, and in patients with disease, there is no relation between ST segment depression and the occurrence of ventricular premature beats (McHenry et al., 1974). However, exercise-induced ventricular premature beats occurring in runs or at a frequency of greater than 10 per minute are more common in ischemic heart disease (Jelinek and Lown, 1974; Marieb et al., 1990). Goldschlager and associates (1973) emphasized the severe forms of ventricular arrhythmias that may occur after exercise. The induction of ventricular ectopic beats by exercise testing may be used as an alternative to 24-hour ambulatory monitoring (Crawford et al., 1974), although the yield of arrhythmias is not quite as high (Ryan et al., 1975). Coupled premature beats may precede ventricular tachycardia and fibrillation (Fig. 7–13). The reproducibility of exercise-induced ectopic beats is not high enough (Faris et al., 1976) to make exercise testing a reliable method for control of antiarrhythmic drugs (Winkle et al., 1978). Although exercise-induced ventricular ectopic beats are a common manifestation of coronary artery disease, they may also be seen in other cardiac diseases, particularly in mitral valve prolapse (Gooch et al., 1972; Demaria et al., 1976).

ABNORMALITIES OF CONDUCTION

Sinoatrial or atrioventricular (AV) block occurs rarely during exercise. In patients with pre-existing first-degree AV block, the PR interval usually shortens (see Fig. 7–18), but not invariably. Presumably, withdrawal of vagal tone and increased sympathetic activity are the main factors reducing the PR interval in exercise, as occurs in normal subjects. Occasionally, first-degree block may be followed by the Wenckebach phenomenon in recovery. The occurrence of second-degree or third-degree (complete) AV block after exercise in a subject with normal conduction or first-degree block at rest is extremely uncommon (Bakst et al., 1975).

Complete AV block is a relative contraindication to maximum exercise testing. Subjects with congen-

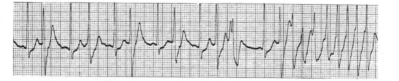

Figure 7–13. Lead V_5 in a 50-year-old male with coronary artery disease. Continuous strip obtained during exercise at 400 kpm/min shows ventricular ectopic beats becoming coupled and leading to ventricular tachycardia, which reverted spontaneously on stopping of exercise.

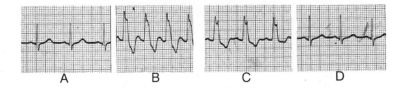

Figure 7–14. Lead V_5 in a 54-year-old male assessed for entry into a postcoronary exercise program. *A,* rest; *B,* maximum exercise, 800 kpm/min; *C,* recovery, 5 min; *D,* recovery, 7 min. Left bundle branch block with a supraventricular tachycardia developed during exercise but resolved with rest.

ital AV block show little or no increase in heart rate during exercise, tending to maintain cardiac output with large increases in stroke volume (Ikkos and Hanson, 1960).

Intraventricular conduction defects may occur during exercise, when they are usually rate related—arising during exercise above a given rate and settling when the rate drops below it in recovery from exercise. Their occurrence is not usually associated with any hemodynamic consequences unless there is coexisting coronary artery disease. Underlying coronary artery disease tends to be more common in patients who develop left bundle branch block (Fig. 7–14) (Vasey et al., 1985) than in those who develop right bundle branch block (Fig. 7–15) (Williams et al., 1988), but the occurrence of intraventricular conduction defects in isolation cannot be taken as a specific indicator of disease. Rate-dependent blocks may precede the occurrence of permanent block (Williams et al., 1988). Pre-existing bundle branch block may not impair exercise performance, but the predictive value of ST segment changes is much reduced in its presence (Whinnery et al., 1977a, 1977b).

Patients with the Wolff-Parkinson-White syndrome may develop ST segment depression during exercise (see Fig. 7–6) (Sharma et al., 1987). Sometimes, normal AV conduction appears during exercise, and ST depression then reverts to normal.

Occasionally, aberrant intraventricular conduction may be seen in exercise, associated with arrhythmias such as atrial fibrillation (Fig. 7–16).

THE ELECTROCARDIOGRAM IN ATHLETES. When standard electrocardiographic criteria are applied to athletes, a high incidence of

abnormalities is found. Some of the changes, especially those associated with rhythm disturbances, ventricular hypertrophy, and abnormalities of repolarization, are identical to those found in patients with organic heart disease, making it important to recognize these normal variants.

RATE AND RHYTHM. Sinus bradycardia with rates of 35 to 45 b/min is an almost universal occurrence in endurance athletes.

Sinus arrhythmia, second-degree AV block, and wandering atrial pacemaker are also frequently seen. At very low sinus rates, subsidiary pacemakers in the junctional tissue may lead to junctional rhythms or junctional escape beats (Fig. 7–17). With exercise or atropine or isoprenaline use, the junctional rhythm reverts to a sinus rhythm.

P WAVE. Increases in the P-wave amplitude and duration, sometimes associated with notching or biphasic waves, have been reported in athletes, with a rightward shift of the P wave vector after exercise (Nakamoto, 1969).

PR INTERVAL. The PR interval is often at the upper limit of normal for the cardiac rate in athletes, and an incidence of first-degree AV block varying between 5 and 30 per cent has been reported (Lichtman et al., 1973). The prolonged PR interval shortens with exercise (Fig. 7–18) or atropine or isoprenaline use.

QRS COMPLEX. Voltage criteria for right and left ventricular hypertrophy are often met in athletes (Nakamoto, 1969). The voltage may increase with exercise. Beckner and Winsor (1954) reported an

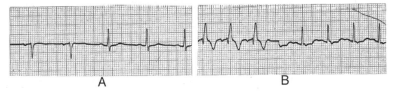

Figure 7–15. Leads V_1 and V_4 in a 63-year-old female with typical angina. *A,* rest; *B,* after exercise, 500 kpm/min, showing right bundle branch block, and associated T-wave inversion. Changes persisted for 1 hour. Coronary angiographic results were normal in this patient.

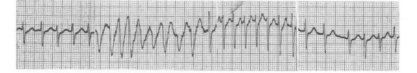

Figure 7–16. Lead V_5 in a 42-year-old male investigated for intermittent idiopathic atrial fibrillation. *A*, rest; *B*, maximum exercise, 1400 kpm/min; *C*, recovery, 1 min; *D*, recovery, 10 min. There was atrial fibrillation throughout, with aberrant conduction in exercise at a rate of 240/min. Normal conduction was re-established shortly after end of exercise. Note that maximum exercise capacity was high normal.

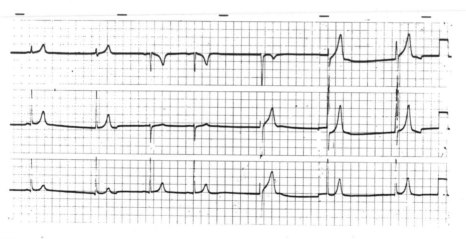

Figure 7–17. Standard resting 12-lead electrocardiogram in a 27-year-old elite marathon runner. Voltage criteria for left ventricular hypertrophy—SV_2 + RV_5 separately measured at 70 mm. There are peaked T waves and high junctional rhythm with escape beats.

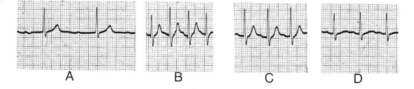

Figure 7–18. Lead V_6 in a 39-year-old male, a regular but not elite marathon competitor. *A*, rest; *B*, maximum exercise, 1900 kpm/min; *C*, recovery, 1 min; *D*, recovery, 10 min. The PR interval is 0.44 second at rest, shortening to 0.16 second in exercise, and lengthening to 0.20 second in recovery.

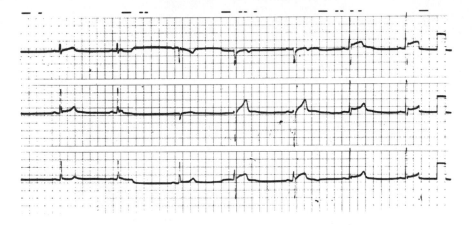

Figure 7–19. Standard resting 12-lead electrocardiogram in a 20-year-old black sprinter showing widespread elevation of ST segments.

incidence of positive criteria for right ventricular hypertrophy in marathon runners of 18 per cent at rest and 43 per cent after exercise. A third (33 per cent) satisfied criteria for left ventricular hypertrophy at rest, and 44 per cent, after exercise. Athletes do not show the ST segment and T-wave "strain" pattern changes associated with pathological left ventricular hypertrophy. Notching and slurring of the QRS complex and incomplete right bundle branch block are common. ST segment elevation or an early repolarization pattern is a common finding in blacks and black athletes (Thomas et al., 1960) (Fig. 7–19), but the finding of ST segment and J-point elevation is also common in white athletes; these changes return to normal after exercise (McKechnie et al., 1967). The early repolarization phenomenon may be confused with pericarditis or myocardial injury.

T WAVE. T-wave amplitude may be increased in athletes at rest and may increase further on exercise; the changes resemble those found in hyperkalemia, but serum potassium is normal (see Fig. 7–17). Biphasic, flattened, or inverted T waves are also seen in athletes. Rose (1969) found a 3.9 per cent incidence of inverted T waves in a large group of college athletes; in our experience, T-wave inversion usually clears during exercise but recurs in recovery (see Fig. 7–5).

SUMMARY

It is important that the electrocardiographic changes seen in athletes are recognized for what they are—the electrical correlates of the trained normal heart. Despite the absence of any other indications of organic heart disease, the findings have often led to athletes' being advised to give up their pursuits, leading to changes in lifestyle and

cardiac "nondisease" neurosis. Of course, athletes are not excluded from congenital cardiac abnormalities; the rare sudden death of an athlete with a previously unrecognized anomalous coronary artery, cardiomyopathy, or even coronary artery disease usually receives widespread publicity and provides ammunition for the antiexercise lobby.

REFERENCES

American Heart Association. Exercise Testing and Training of Apparently Healthy Individuals: A Handbook for Physicians. New York: American Heart Association, 1972.

Amiesen O, Okin PM, Devereux RB, et al: Predictive value and limitations of the ST/HR slope. Br Heart J 1985;53:547–551.

Aronow WS, Cassidy J, Vangrow JS, et al. Effect of cigarette smoking and breathing carbon monoxide on cardiovascular hemodynamics in anginal patients. Circulation 1974;50:340–347.

Bakst A, Goldberg B, Shamroth L. Significance of exercise-induced second degree heart block. Br Heart J 1975;37:948–990.

Balke B, Ware RW: An experimental study of physical fitness of Air Force personnel. US Armed Forces Med J 1959;10:675–688.

Bayes T: An essay towards solving a problem in the doctrine of chances. Philos Trans R Soc Lond Biol 1763;53:370–418.

Beckner GL, Winsor T: Cardiovascular adaptations to prolonged physical effort. Circulation 1954;9:835–846.

Blackburn H. The exercise electrocardiogram in diagnosis. Cardiology 1977;62:190–205.

Blomqvist G. The Frank lead exercise electrocardiogram. A quantitative study based on averaging technic and digital computer analysis. Acta Med Scand 1965;178(Suppl. 440):5–98.

Bobbio M, Detrano R, Schmid JJ, et al. Exercise-induced ST depression and ST/heart rate index to predict triple-vessel or left main coronary disease: A multicenter analysis. J Am Coll Cardiol 1992;19:11–18.

Bonoris PE, Greenberg PS, Christison GW, et al. Evaluation of R wave amplitude changes versus ST-segment depression in stress testing. Circulation 1977;57:904–910.

Botvinick EH, Taradash MR, Sharmes DM, et al. Thallium-201 myocardial perfusion scintigraphy for the clinical classification of normal, abnormal, and equivocal electrocardiographic stress tests. Am J Cardiol 1978;41:43–51.

Bruce RA, Fisher LD, Pettinger M, et al. ST segment elevation with exercise: A marker for poor ventricular function and poor prognosis. Circulation 1988;77:897–905.

Burda CD. Electrocardiographic abnormalities induced by thioridazine (Mellaril). Am Heart J 1968;76:153–156.

Cahen P, Depouilly J, Quard S, et al. Myocardial ischemia during exercises: Electrocardiographic criteria. Data recorded in 553 patients with selective coronarography. Lyon Med 1973;229:969–980.

Carlsson C, Dencker SJ, Grimby G, et al. Noradrenaline in blood-plasma and urine during chlorpromazine treatment. Lancet 1966;1:1208.

Chahine RA, Raizner AE, Ishimori T: The clinical significance of exercise-induced ST-segment elevation. Circulation 1976;54:209–213.

Chaitman BR, Bourassa MG, Davis K, et al: Angiographic prevalence of high-risk coronary artery disease in patient subsets (CASS). Circulation 1981;64:360–367.

Chaitman BR, Bourassa MG, Wagniart P, et al. Improved efficiency of treadmill exercise testing using a multiple lead ECG system and basic hemodynamic exercise response. Circulation 1978;57.71–79.

Crawford M, O'Rourke RA, Ramakrishna N, et al: Comparative effectiveness of exercise testing and continuous monitoring for detecting arrhythmias in patients with previous myocardial infarction. Circulation 1974;50:301–305.

Cumming GR, Dufresne C, Kich L, et al. Exercise electrocardiogram patterns in normal women. Br Heart J 1973;35:1055–1061.

Demaria AN, Amsterdam EA, Vismara LA, et al. Arrhythmias in the mitral valve prolapse syndrome. Ann Intern Med 1976;84:656–660.

Demers RG, Heninger GR: Electrocardiographic T wave changes following lithium carbonate treatment. JAMA 1971;218:381–386.

Detry J-MR, Robert A, Luwaert RJ, et al: Diagnostic value of computerized exercise testing in men without previous myocardial infarction. A multivariate compartmental and probabilistic approach. Eur Heart J 1985;6:227–238.

Diamond GA, Forrester JS. Analysis of probability as an aid in the clinical diagnosis of coronary-artery disease. N Engl J Med 1979;300:1350–1358.

Diamond GA, Forrester JS. Metadiagnosis. An epistemologic model of clinical judgment. Am J Med 1983;75:129–137.

Diamond GA, Forrester JS, Hirsch M, et al. Application of conditional probability analysis to the clinical diagnosis of coronary artery disease. J Clin Invest 1980;65:1210–1221.

Elamin MS, Boyle R, Kardash MM, et al. Accurate detection of coronary heart disease by new exercise test. Br Heart J 1982;48:311–320.

Faris JV, McHenry PL, Jordan JW, et al: Prevalence and reproducibility of exercise-induced ventricular arrhythmias during maximal exercise testing in normal men. Am J Cardiol 1976;37:617–622.

Fletcher GF, Balady G, Froelicher V, et al. Exercise standards: A statement for healthcare professionals from the American Heart Association. Circulation 1995;91:580–615.

Fortuin NJ, Friesinger GC. Exercise-induced electrocardiographic and arteriographic studies in twelve patients. Am J Med 1970;49:459–464.

Friesinger GC, Biern RO, Likar I, et al. Exercise electrocardiography and vasoregulatory abnormalities. Am J Cardiol 1972;30:733–740.

Froelicher VF, Yanowitz FG, Thompson AJ, et al. The correlation of coronary angiography and the electrocardiographic response to maximal treadmill testing in 76 asymptomatic men. Circulation 1973;48:597–604.

Gazes PC. False-positive exercise test in the presence of the Wolff-Parkinson-White syndrome. Am Heart J 1969;78:13–15.

Gianelly RE, Treister BL, Harrison DC. The effect of propranolol on exercise-induced ischemic S-T segment depression. Am J Cardiol 1969;24:161–165.

Goldschlager N, Cake D, Cohn K. Exercise-induced ventricular arrhythmias in patients with coronary artery disease. Am J Cardiol 1973;31:434–440.

Gooch AS. Exercise testing for detecting changes in cardiac rhythm and condition. Am J Cardiol 1972;30:741–746.

Gooch AS, Vicencio F, Maranhao V, et al. Arrhythmias and left ventricular asynergy in the prolapsing mitral leaflet syndrome. Am J Cardiol 1972;29:611–620.

Hollenberg M, Budge WR, Wisnecki JA, et al. Treadmill score quantifies electrocardiographic response to exercise and improves test accuracy and reproducibility. Circulation 1980; 61:276–285.

Hollenberg M, Go M Jr, Massie BM, et al. Influence of R-wave amplitude on exercise-induced ST depression: need for a "gain factor" correction when interpreting stress electrocardiograms. Am J Cardiol 1985a;56:13–17.

Hollenberg M, Zoltick JM, Go M, et al. Comparison of a quantitative treadmill exercise score with standard electrocardiographic criteria in screening asymptomatic young men for coronary artery disease. N Engl J Med 1985b;313:600–606.

Hung J, Chaitman BR, Lam J, et al. A logistic regression analysis of multiple noninvasive tests for the prediction of the presence and extent of coronary artery disease in men. Am Heart J 1985;110:460–468.

Ikkos D, Hanson JJ. Response to exercise in congenital atrioventricular block. Circulation 1960;22:583–590.

Ikram H, Rubin AP, Jewkes RF. Effect of diazepam on myocardial blood flow of patients with and without coronary artery disease. Br Heart J 1973;35:626–630.

Jelinek MV, Lown B: Exercise stress testing for exposure of cardiac arrhythmias. Prog Cardiovasc Dis 1974;16:497–522.

Kansal S, Roitman D, Bradley EL, Sheffield LT. Enhanced evaluation of treadmill tests by means of scoring based on multivariate analysis and its clinical application: A study of 608 patients. Am J Cardiol 1983;52:1155–1160.

Kattus AA. Exercise electrocardiography: Recognition of the ischemic response, false positive and negative patterns. Am J Cardiol 1974;33:721–731.

Kurita A. Significance of exercise-induced junctional ST depression in evaluation of coronary artery disease. Am J Cardiol 40:492–497, 1977.

Lepeschkin E. The U wave of the electrocardiogram. Mod Concepts Cardiovasc Dis 1969;38:39–45.

LeWinter MM, Crawford MH, O'Rourke RA, et al. The effects of oral propranolol, digoxin and combination therapy on the resting and exercise electrocardiogram. Am Heart J 1977;93:202–209.

Lichtman J, O'Rourke RA, Klein A, et al. Electrocardiogram of the athlete. Arch Intern Med 1973;132:763–770.

Linderholm H, Osterman G, Teien D. Detection of coronary artery disease by means of exercise ECG in patients with aortic stenosis. Acta Med Scand 1985;218:181–188.

Lobstein HP, Horwitz LD, Curry GV, et al. Electrocardiographic abnormalities and coronary arteriograms in the mitral click-murmur syndrome. N Engl J Med 1973;289:127–131.

Marieb M, Beller G, Gibson R, et al. Clinical relevancy of exercise-induced ventricular arrhythmias in suspected coronary artery disease. Am J Cardiol 1990;66:172–178.

Mason RE, Likar I, Biern RO, et al. Multiple lead exercise electrocardiography experience in 107 normal subjects and 67 patients with angina pectoris, and comparison with coronary arteriography in 84 patients. Circulation 1967;36:517–525.

McHenry PL, Phillips JF, Knoebel SB: Correlation of computer-quantitated treadmill exercise electrocardiogram with arteriographic location of coronary artery disease. Am J Cardiol 1972;30:747–752.

McHenry PL, Morris SN, Kavalier M. Exercise-induced arrhythmias—recognition, classification, and clinical significance. Cardiovasc Clin 1974;6:245–254.

McKechnie JK, Leary WP, Joubert SM. Some electrocardiographic and biochemical changes recorded in marathon runners. S Afr Med J 1967;41:722–725.

McNeer JF, Margolis JR, Lee KL, et al. The role of the exercise test in the evaluation of patients for ischemic heart disease. Circulation 1978;57:64–70.

Nakamoto K. Electrocardiograms of 25 marathon runners before and after 100 meter dash. Jpn Circ J 1969;33:105–128.

O'Hara M, Lahiri A, Whittington JR, et al: Detection of high risk coronary artery disease by thallium imaging. Br Heart J 1985;53:616–623.

Okin PM, Kligfield P, Amiesen O, et al. Improved accuracy of the exercise electrocardiogram: Identification of three-vessel coronary disease in stable angina pectoris by analysis of peak rate-related changes in ST segments. Am J Cardiol 1985;55:271–276.

Powles ACP, Sutton JR, Wicks JR, et al: Reduced heart rate response to exercise in ischemic heart disease: the fallacy of the target heart rate in exercise testing. Med Sci Sports 1979;11:227–233.

Remington RD, Schork MA. Statistics with Applications to the Biological and Health Sciences. Englewood Cliffs, NJ: Prentice-Hall; 1970.

Rifkin RD, Hood WB Jr. Bayesian analysis of electrocardiographic exercise stress testing. N Engl J Med 1977;297:681–686.

Roitman D, Jones WB, Sheffield LT: Comparison of submaximal exercise ECG test with coronary cineangiocardiogram. Ann Intern Med 1970;72:641.

Rose KD. Relationship of cardiac problems to athletic participation. JAMA 1969;208:2319–2324.

Ryan M, Lown B, Horn H. Comparison of ventricular ectopic activity during 24-hour monitoring and exercise testing in patients with coronary heart disease. N Engl J Med 1975;292:224–229.

Sackett DL, Haynes RB, Tugwell P. Clinical Epidemiology. Toronto: Little, Brown & Co; 1985.

Sandberg L. Studies on electrocardiographic changes during exercise tests. Acta Med Scand 1961;169(Suppl 365):1–117.

Sharma AD, Yee R, Guiraudon G, Klein GJ. Sensitivity and specificity of invasive and noninvasive testing for risk of sudden death in Wolff-Parkinson-White syndrome. J Am Coll Cardiol 1987;10:373–381.

Sheffield LT. The use of the computer in exercise electrocardiography. Pract Cardiol 1978;4:101–108.

Sheffield LT. Editorial: Another perfect treadmill test? N Engl J Med 1985;313:633–635.

Sheffield LT, Roitman D. Stress testing methodology. In: Sonnenblick EH, Lesch M, editors. Exercise and Heart Disease. New York: Grune & Stratton; 1976.

Simoons ML. Optimal measurements for detection of coronary artery disease by exercise electrocardiography. Comput Biomed Res 1977;10:483–499.

Simoons ML, Hugenholz PG. Gradual changes of ECG waveform during and after exercise in normal subjects. Circulation 1975;52:570–577.

Thomas J, Harris E, Lassiter G. Observations on the T wave and ST segment changes in the precordial electrocardiogram of 320 young negro adults. Am J Cardiol 1960;5:468–472.

Vasey C, O'Donnell J, Morris SN, McHenry P. Exercise-induced left bundle branch block and its relation to coronary artery disease. Am J Cardiol 1985;56:892–895.

Vedin JA, Wilhelmsson CE, Wilhelmsen L, et al. Relation of resting and exercise-induced ectopic beats to other ischemic manifestations and to coronary risk factors. Am J Cardiol 1972;30:25–31.

Weiner DA, McCabe BS, Klein MD, et al. ST segment changes post-infarction: Predictive value for multivessel coronary disease and left ventricular aneurysm. Circulation 1978;58:887–891.

Wellens MJ, Cats VM, Duren DR. Symptomatic sinus node abnormalities following lithium carbonate therapy. Am J Med 1975;59:285–298.

Whinnery JE, Froelicher VF Jr, Stewart AJ, et al. The electrocardiographic response to maximal treadmill exercise of asymptomatic men with left bundle branch block. Am Heart J 1977a;94:316–324.

Whinnery JE, Froelicher VF Jr, Longo MR Jr, et al. The electrocardiographic response to maximal treadmill exercise of asymptomatic men with right bundle branch block. Chest 1977b;71:335–340.

Wicks JR, Sutton JR, Oldridge NB, et al: Comparison of the electrocardiographic changes induced by maximum exercise testing with treadmill and cycle ergometer. Circulation 1978;57:1066–1070.

Williams MA, Easterbrooks GA, Nair CK, et al. Clinical significance of exercise-induced bundle branch block. Am J Cardiol 1988;61:346–348.

Winkle RA, Gradman AJ, Fitzgerald JW, et al: Antiarrhythmic drug effect assessed from ventricular arrhythmia reduction in the ambulatory electrocardiogram and treadmill test: comparison of propranolol, procainamide and quinidine. Am J Cardiol 1978;42:473–480.

Yabe T, Mitsunami K, Okada M, et al. Detection of myocardial ischemia by P-31 magnetic resonance spectroscopy during handgrip exercise. Circulation 1994;89:1709–1716.

8

Interpretation of Stage 1 Exercise Test Results

An exercise test is usually one part of a clinical assessment, the results of which are best interpreted by the clinician or by the clinical physiologist in the light of clinical information. This chapter and those that follow discuss interpretation at a series of levels of increasing sophistication by examining data obtained in patients studied according to the staged procedures described in the preceding chapters. In addition to demonstrating the quality of information obtained from each procedure, the examples illustrate points made previously regarding the changes in the adaptations to exercise brought about by structural change.

This chapter reviews factors to be taken into account in the interpretation of a stage 1 incremental exercise test. Additional factors that influence interpretation of stage 2 and stage 3 steady state test results are left for later chapters. Of course, an arbitrary division of this sort is artificial because many of the measurements are common to all the procedures, and the interpretation of physiological changes depends on the same concepts. However, from a practical laboratory point of view, they may be considered separate, and the strengths of each approach are clearly established.

Several problems arise in the interpretation of exercise test results; two are considered in this chapter. First, there is some variation in measurements made at the same workload, even in the same subject. Second, certain factors lead to variation among healthy persons. Such variation reduces the precision with which the extent of an abnormality may be quantified and may cause difficulty in the recognition of minor abnormalities. Variations owing to experimental errors can be kept to a minimum if the test is carefully performed.

As pointed out above, establishing predictions of the exercise responses expected in the average healthy individual is difficult because predictive equations need to be just as precise in older, shorter, or taller individuals as in subjects of average age (30–50 years) and stature (1.6–1.8 m). Unless variables such as age and height are scaled appropriately, the desired precision is not obtained. Our approach cannot be considered ideal, but it is at least based on large numbers of subjects, allowing us to explore all combinations of age and stature and in both sexes; in addition, equations are nonlinear, with parameters that are consistent with theoretical scaling concepts.

MAXIMAL OXYGEN CONSUMPTION VERSUS MAXIMAL POWER OUTPUT

For many years, the index used for characterizing exercise capacity has been the maximal oxygen intake ($\dot{V}O_2$max), usually scaled to body weight ($\dot{V}O_2$max/kg). Many reasons for this approach existed, including a need to standardize different protocols and methods, such as treadmill running and cycling. Well-motivated subjects were able to exercise beyond the point at which a plateau in $\dot{V}O_2$ was observed; this was also observed in animals, in whom the plateau occurred at the same speed as the blood lactate began to increase. Ever since, regular debates have been conducted on whether these findings were due to limitation of oxygen delivery mechanisms or to maximal utilization of oxygen in the muscle mitochondria; perhaps surprisingly, this debate has not yet been resolved. Although some authorities still may argue that a plateau must be observed for the measurement to be accepted as $\dot{V}O_2$max, it is well known that many well-motivated subjects do not show a plateau and that this requirement is difficult to meet in clinical situations. An alternative in fit individuals is to present a series of increasing workloads performed intermittently, each sustained for 6 minutes or as long as possible, and to measure the $\dot{V}O_2$ during the last minute or 30 seconds, in order to find a maximal value (Åstrand and Rodahl, 1977). An alternative approach in an incremental cycle or treadmill protocol is measurement of the peak $\dot{V}O_2$ achieved and acceptance of this value as $\dot{V}O_2$max if it is accompanied by evidence of blood lactate concentration increase (from blood sampling or indirectly from the respiratory exchange ratio or the ventilatory anaerobic threshold) (Wasserman et al., 1987) or by a heart rate that is close to the expected maximum. Because we have adopted a progressive incremental exercise test on a cycle ergometer as a practical approach to exercise testing in healthy individuals and patients with a wide variety of disorders, we use the maximal achieved power output as the measurement of capacity, rather than peak $\dot{V}_{O_2}$ or $\dot{V}_{O_2}max$. This frees us from the concept of a limitation of oxygen consumption; maximal power includes aerobic and anaerobic components, and the measurements of $\dot{V}_{O_2}$, lactate concentration, heart rate, and respiratory exchange ratio are merely physiological observations that may or may not be present and are interpreted in their own right. Furthermore, the measurement of power on a modern cycle ergometer is a good deal more precise than the measurement of $\dot{V}_{O_2}$, and the correlation between power and $\dot{V}_{O_2}$ is extremely close ($r^2 > 95\%$). However, the calculation of a power equivalence for exercise on a treadmill (as in Appendix C, Fig. C–2, for example) is not as precise, and in this situation, the measurement of peak $\dot{V}_{O_2}$ may be required as an index of capacity.

VARIABILITY IN A PATIENT'S RESPONSE TO EXERCISE

It may be difficult to know whether the measurements obtained in a test are representative of the patient's usual or "best" exercise performance. Many factors may influence performance in any one person, but when formally studied in healthy subjects, the variation in performance has been found to be small. Of course, minor variations in performance by athletes may make the difference between winning and losing a race, but the effect is often trivial when related to performance in maximal exercise in patients.

Habituation to repeated maximal exercise tests has been found to lead to a reduction in heart rate response (Davies et al., 1970), but the habituation effect is difficult to separate from a training response. Other studies have shown no appreciable effects when exercise tests of the type described in this book were repeated daily in naive subjects (Jones and Kane, 1979). Anxiety may lead to changes in heart rate and ventilation; these effects may be marked at rest but usually become less during exercise. Shephard (1966) studied the effect of personality in a large group of healthy subjects who exercised on 5 successive days and found that anxious subjects were no more variable in their heart rate and ventilatory responses than were control subjects. However, hysterical subjects overbreathed in the initial studies, and ventilation became less with repeated testing. Although the majority of healthy subjects who are tested on a cycle ergometer have comparable results on 2 successive days, rarely, a subject shows an improved performance on the second occasion. Thus, it is

sometimes necessary to repeat a study on a subject who appears unduly distressed by the test or who exhibits increases in heart rate and ventilation at rest that remain high throughout the test. The question of "malingering" is often brought up in the interpretation of results; however, in our experience, it seldom presents a problem. Objectively, the malingering subject stops exercise without distress and with minimal disturbance of heart rate and ventilation.

A recent heavy meal influences the metabolic response to exercise and leads to an increase in carbon dioxide output and ventilation, but again, the effect is small (Jones and Haddon, 1973) and is easily avoided by ensuring that exercise tests are performed an hour or more after the patient has eaten.

There is a diurnal variation in the heart rate response to exercise, with lowest levels being found in the early morning (Voigt et al., 1967). Most athletes perform better at this time than later in the day (Conroy and O'Brien, 1973). Although this effect is small, tests should be repeated at the same time of day if changes, either spontaneous or owing to treatment, are being studied.

Many drugs are liable to influence heart rate during exercise. Beta adrenergic blockers are the most frequently encountered, and results need to be interpreted with their effects borne in mind.

If an attempt is made to avoid these effects, repeat studies at the same power output carried out on successive days show the following variance in some important factors: oxygen uptake ± 4 per cent, cardiac frequency ± 3 per cent, and ventilation ± 4 per cent (Jones and Kane, 1979). Such variation should be taken into account in the interpretation of results, and on some occasions, a repeat study is required so that a minor abnormality can be identified.

VARIATION IN MAXIMUM EXERCISE PERFORMANCE IN THE HEALTHY POPULATION

It is self-evident that the performance of a small elderly lady cannot be related directly to a standard established in young men attending a college of physical education. Studies in normal subjects have established quantitative effects of various factors, and it is now possible for these factors to be taken into account in interpretations of results, so that a deviation of the observed value from the expected value in the normal population can be quantified more realistically. The major factors, most of which are discussed in Chapter 2, need to be allowed for in the prediction of the expected response in a patient, as discussed in more detail later in this chapter.

We have learned so much about the factors that influence exercise that theoretically we should be able to predict anyone's performance from measurements made at rest. However, some of the measurements are difficult, expensive, and time consuming and are thus really not practical on a routine basis, particularly in subjects who are not usually included in large studies because they are small, elderly, or female. Furthermore, some of the variables that might be used as independent predictors of exercise capacity in healthy individuals are themselves prone to be affected by various diseases and could not be validly applied in a prediction equation. Many studies have quantified factors related to body size, age, and gender, and at least these should be included in any prediction.

The *effect of age* has been extensively studied. It was shown by Robinson (1938) and later by P.-O. Åstrand (1952, 1956) that maximal aerobic power ($\dot{V}O_2$max) increases during childhood to reach a peak in the late teens, which is maintained until the mid-20s and then gradually declines. The early increase is due to the growth of muscle, heart, and lungs, and the later decline is probably mainly due to reductions in muscle strength and metabolic capacity, at least in part because of reductions in daily activity and in age-related changes in the function of the heart (Bruce et al., 1974; Port et al., 1980; Longhini et al., 1995) and cardiovascular system (Vaitkevicius et al., 1993; Seals et al., 1994), the lungs (Guenard et al., 1994; Johnson et al., 1994), the muscles (Murray et al., 1980; Grimby and Saltin, 1983), and the central nervous system (Campbell et al., 1973; Young and Skelton, 1994). The variable most often used to characterize the age-related decline in exercise capacity is the maximal cardiac frequency; although a decline in the intrinsic (totally blocked) heart rate does occur with age (Seals et al., 1994), it seems more likely that the decrease in maximal heart rate merely reflects a reduction in aerobic capacity. Studies of high-inten-sity training in older subjects have shown dramatic increases in maximal exercise capacity (Brown et al., 1990; Makrides et al., 1990), oxygen intake, and maximal heart rate.

When plotted as a function of age, the decline in aerobic capacity appears linear (Fig. 8–1) and less in females than in males. When scaled as a proportional decline, the gender difference lessens, with the decline being approximately 0.7 per cent per year. A more plausible suggestion is that the decline actually lessens with increasing age, as described by a power function (e.g., $age^{-0.5}$). Other measurements made at given levels of power output do not appear to be affected by age, if the effects of sex, size, and habitual activity are allowed for.

Although there are well-marked *differences between males and females* at comparable ages (Åstrand, I., 1960; Jones et al., 1985), these differences largely disappear when other factors, such as size—particularly lean body mass (Cotes et al., 1973)—hemoglobin level, and levels of habitual activity, are taken into account.

The dimensions of muscles, heart, and lungs influence the response of related mechanisms in exercise, necessitating allowance for the *effect of body size*. Weight is usually taken into consideration when the agreed measure of fitness—the maximum oxygen uptake per kilogram of body weight ($\dot{V}O_2$max/kg)—is obtained. The relevance of this factor to the energy cost of everyday activity is clear (Godin and Shephard, 1973), and it should certainly be considered in relation to the patient's occupation. However, it is not directly related to the performance of oxygen transport mechanisms. A low $\dot{V}O_2$max/kg in an obese patient may be due to an increase in weight alone and thus may be a misleading value for "the thin person inside, trying to get out," who may have a high degree of cardio-respiratory "fitness." The size of heart, lungs, and

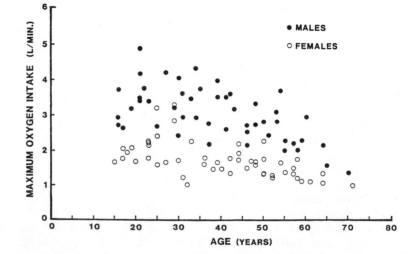

Figure 8–1. Relationship between $\dot{V}O_2$max and age in 100 healthy Canadians (50 men, 50 women).

skeletal muscle may be poorly related to total body weight, which in this situation is a less reliable predictor of cardiorespiratory performance than lean body mass. However, Åstrand and Rodahl (1977) pointed out that the use of $\dot{V}O_2$max/kg is invalid, being itself negatively related to weight even in athletes.

Height is at least as valid an index as weight and in most situations is to be preferred, particularly in children (Gadhoke and Jones, 1969; Godfrey et al., 1971).

Although it is possible that *body surface area* may be a better index than either height or weight, it suffers from the same disadvantages that apply to weight. Cardiologists usually determine the cardiac index by dividing cardiac output by surface area, and although this may be logical for resting measurements, it is of no value for exercise results (Faulkner et al., 1977), in which the increase in cardiac output is related to the increase in oxygen intake, body size having little influence.

Fat-free body weight (lean body mass) is reliably obtained from body weight by correcting for body fat, which is estimated from skinfold measurements (Durnin and Rahaman, 1967) or underwater weighing. Measurement of total muscle mass by the radioactive potassium (^{40}K) method is the most reliable index of lean body mass, but it is a time-consuming and expensive procedure. Cotes and colleagues (1973) showed that measurement of thigh muscle diameter by radiography is an acceptable alternative and precision may be improved by use of computed tomographic scans of the thigh (Mac-Dougall, 1986). Cotes and colleagues (1973) demonstrated a close relationship between lean body mass and cardiac frequency at submaximal oxygen intakes of 1.0 and 1.5 L/min. Thus, an index of lean body mass increases accuracy of the cardiac frequency predicted as the normal value at a given power output. This prediction may be compared with measurements made in a patient.

Radiographic *heart size* was shown to be related to maximum oxygen uptake by Sjöstrand (1960). The measurement is made relatively simply from anteroposterior and lateral radiographs of the chest and is related to the stroke volume during exercise. It has the added advantage that in patients with heart disease, an increase in heart size is accompanied by reductions in cardiac performance and stroke volume. It seems likely that a measurement of heart volume defines the heart rate response in the normal population, but comparative data with other indices are lacking, and it is not clear if the measurement offers an advantage over body size alone.

Total body hemoglobin also is related to maximum oxygen intake (Sjöstrand, 1960). In the method, which is well established in Scandinavian departments of clinical physiology (Sjöstrand, 1948), a tracer amount of carbon monoxide is rebreathed to obtain equilibration with blood. The same information is obtained from an estimate of lean body mass and the blood hemoglobin level.

The *level of habitual physical activity* influences exercise performance by imposing a degree of physical fitness. This is an extremely difficult factor to assess, but a measurement of the physical activity of patients in their everyday life can be obtained through a simple questionnaire, which allows the observer to categorize patients into four groups: sedentary; sedentary with some daily activity; active, through occupation or recreation activity; and trained athlete.

Race-related differences in exercise performance have been suspected for many years. For example, measurements of $\dot{V}O_2$max have shown higher values in Scandinavians than in North Americans (Shephard, 1969). Studies carried out under the auspices of the International Biological Program have examined performance in different ethnic groups in the Caribbean (Edwards et al., 1972; Miller et al., 1972, 1977) and in New Guinea (Cotes et al., 1972). These have shown that there are few race-related differences in exercise performance if allowance is made for variations in size, level of habitual activity, hemoglobin, and altitude of residence.

Pulmonary function measurements such as vital capacity, forced expired volume in one second (FEV_1), lung volumes, and carbon monoxide uptake all show some relationship to exercise performance in the healthy population. However, they are all related to lung size, which is itself related to lean body mass. Although vital capacity may be used as a predictor of maximum oxygen intake in health (Jones et al., 1985), it is no more precise than other measurements more closely related to lean body mass. However, being a measurement of volume, it has the advantage of scaling linearly to power.

NORMAL VALUES FOR STAGE 1 TEST RESULTS

It may seem a relatively simple matter to establish normal values for exercise test results, but the large number of variables that may influence performance makes such studies virtually impossible. Maximal power and oxygen uptake and maximum heart rate have been measured in a variety of populations, providing standards for comparison with test results (Shephard, 1969). However, more complex measurements have been made in smaller numbers of subjects and in more homogeneous groups, leaving some room for argument regarding the normal expected response. For these reasons, "normal" values are given when possible, but in addition, an approach based on the interrelationships among variables is presented, which to a large extent frees us from a reliance on the normal value for any given variable at a given exercise level. Furthermore, faith in normal values may be misplaced for a number of reasons. For example, a "normal" value for ventilation may hide a combination of reduced alveolar ventilation with increased VD/VT ratio. An "abnormally high" ventilation may be accounted for by normal variations, such as increased carbon dioxide output or a high breathing frequency, acting alone or in combination. Many other examples might be used to reinforce the value of taking an integrative approach, rather than referring to a series of normal values to compare with the results obtained in the test. You have turned to this section of the book to obtain equations that predict the normal responses to exercise, possibly for use in your own laboratory. I have done my best to provide these, but first, a number of points regarding such equations in general and our own equations in particular deserve your consideration before you commit them to your computer.

What Is Meant By "Normal"?

The values presented later may be used as a guide to the responses expected in healthy persons. By healthy, we mean free of serious disease, but there are obvious problems in defining this state any more precisely. Some might argue that to be healthy, subjects should meet certain criteria of weight, physical activity, smoking habits, and so on; these criteria may define normality in terms of cultural desirability (Sackett et al., 1985) but taken to an extreme might require standards based on studies of athletes, as the ultimate in "disease-free" subjects. Statistics are provided in order to define the mean and variation for a number of dependent variables that we have to assume have a normal (gaussian) distribution in the population. This does not mean, however, that subjects falling below 2 SD from the mean (or below the 5th centile) are necessarily abnormal or "diseased."

What Use Will Be Made of the Standards?

A number of approaches to normal values are presented for the important variables measured in routine maximal exercise tests. Readers have to decide on the best approach for their own needs; the approach may be different for someone who wishes to assess the fitness of football teams than for someone assessing patients entering a rehabilitation program after an infarct or measuring the capacities of muscles, heart, and lungs of children with cystic fibrosis. Different equations may be needed for each of these applications.

Furthermore, we must be careful not to overemphasize the importance of normal standards in a clinical setting; there may be little relationship between an abnormal result and the presence of a disease or its severity. A potentially important use of exercise testing is in the evaluation of disability, for example, for industrial compensation purposes. Here, as in the application of other measurements, we may not be able to equate a percentage reduction in exercise capacity with a comparable percentage disability. The relationship between impairment and disability is seldom linear (see Fig. 1–1).

Is the Reference Population Used for Deriving the Standards an Appropriate One?

This question is related to the previous questions of normality and utility, but it also raises some additional points. In published reports of exercise in normal subjects, it may be difficult to know how the reference population was recruited. There is often a need to avoid a bias toward the more active members of a community who may tend to volunteer for study. Cumming (1978) emphasized this problem in a survey of exercise test results used to assess children with heart disorders; the exercise capacity of a reference normal population was higher than the exercise capacity in children who were referred for testing and were found on independent evidence to have normal cardiac function. Given this problem, a laboratory director may be advised to choose the reference population with the lowest exercise capacity; this choice tends to lessen the frequency of false-positive results. In assessing whether published standards are applicable to the laboratory, other factors may need to be considered, such as racial differences in hemoglobin content. Also, one may have to question whether measurements made 30 to 40 years ago are still appropriate. More common, as alluded to earlier, may be differences in the activity patterns between the reference population and referred patients; activity data may be given in a report so that this question can be answered and the effect can be allowed for. The effect may be quite gross, for example, if the prediction data were obtained in students attending a gymnastic institute or enrolled in an ice hockey program. Remember that an athlete may have a $\dot{V}O_2$max that is at least 150 per cent that of an untrained person of the same sex, age, and size! This may seem to exaggerate the problem, but the same inference may be drawn from studies of untrained persons who increase their activity for a few weeks by joining a training program; in a recent study in our department (Makrides et al., 1986), a group of men aged 20 to 30 years increased $\dot{V}O_2$max from 2.54 to 3.26 L/min (an increase of 28 per cent), and a group aged 60 to 70 years increased $\dot{V}O_2$max from 1.60 to 2.21 L/min (38 per cent increase) during 12 weeks of training. In arriving at our own prediction equations, we chose the approach of Cumming, by accumulating a large population of subjects referred for exercise testing and judged clinically healthy.

Are Independent Variables Suitably Distributed in the Reference Population?

It is apparent that variation in maximal exercise performance in a healthy population is related to a number of variables that, if possible, should be accounted for in a prediction algorithm. These variables are considered independent variables and as a minimum consist of sex, age, and an index of body mass, of which the simplest is height. Probably, it is best to use data from separate studies of males and females rather than use an equation that assigns a numerical value to gender (usually 0 and 1). If a wide age range is expected, the reference population needs to have an age distribution that is even across the whole age range. Similarly, stature should be evenly distributed. A general point is being made here; the distribution of a variable to be used for prediction purposes, and thus to act independently, should be even across the reference population and not have a normal or gaussian distribution. To caricature the problem, predictions based on a population whose subjects are mostly under 30 years of age may be seriously in error if they are used to predict the responses of a patient aged 70 years. Our large population allowed us to create "cells," containing a range of combinations of age and stature in males and females. The equations were then derived from the mean values in each cell so that the independent effects of age and stature can be quantified.

What Precision May Be Expected for Predictive Equations?

Precision depends on the ability to measure both the independent and dependent variables and on appropriate distributions for the variables in the population. Also, theoretically, the more independent variables we can validly include, the better our predictions should be. If we consider measurement alone (see Chapter 10), it is clear that we cannot hope to be more precise than ± 10 per cent (95 per cent confidence) for predictions of $\dot{V}O_2$max. Also, there may be other factors that have not been considered or that are unknown or impossible to measure. Added to these factors are those related to the methods used in the study. Many normal standards for $\dot{V}O_2$max are derived from treadmill exercise, which is now known to overestimate $\dot{V}O_2$max in cycle ergometer exercise by about 10 per cent.

The conclusion is that for $\dot{V}O_2$max, we consider ourselves fortunate if precision is better than ± 20 per cent. Except for a narrowly defined population, it is probably futile to expect greater precision. Before expressing disappointment with this conclusion, we may recall that even the predictions of simple physiological measurements, such as vital capacity, carry this order of residual variation (Crapo et al., 1981; Cotes, 1993).

THE PREDICTION OF MAXIMUM POWER AND $\dot{V}O_2$

Accurate predictions for the most important variables, those of maximum power output (Wmax) and $\dot{V}O_2$max, paradoxically are the most difficult to find. This is not because of a lack of studies or because the populations have been too small, but because of the difficulty in obtaining generally applicable equations that include all the essential independent variables. Often, linear regression techniques have defined $\dot{V}O_2$max in terms of one independent variable; in a few studies, several variables have been used to improve predictive accuracy in multiple regression equations. I first review some published relationships of this type and then take a different approach that starts with some preconceived notions based on what is known about exercise physiology (Chapter 2).

First, let us consider how we might predict the expected $\dot{V}O_2$max to compare with the $\dot{V}O_2$max measured in a male patient referred for a cardiac disorder. Data are available from large studies in Europe and North America (Shephard, 1969). From these data, we may derive an equation, to describe the gradual fall in $\dot{V}O_2$max with age in males:

$$\text{Males: } \dot{V}O_2\text{max} = 4.2 - (0.032 \times \text{age}) \text{ L/min}$$

$$\text{Females: } \dot{V}O_2\text{max} = 2.6 - (0.014 \times \text{age}) \text{ L/min}$$

Most studies on which this relationship is based were for treadmill exercise, and current opinion favors correction of the value by multiplying by 0.9 if the prediction is for cycle ergometry (Hansen et al., 1984). If the patient is 40 years old, the equation predicts a $\dot{V}O_2$max of 2.92 L/min ($\times$ 0.9 = 2.63). Because we know that body mass influences $\dot{V}O_2$max, this is not a very precise prediction unless our patient has the same mass as the mean mass of the population used to derive the equation. However, perhaps this problem may be overcome by dividing $\dot{V}O_2$max by mass to obtain $\dot{V}O_2$max/kg; an equation derived from several studies is

$$\text{Males: } \dot{V}O_2\text{max} = 60 - (0.55 \times \text{age}) \text{ mL/kg/min}$$

$$\text{Females: } \dot{V}O_2\text{max} = 48 - (0.37 \times \text{age}) \text{ mL/kg/min}$$

For our patient, the value is 38 mL/kg/min; is this value more helpful? Well, not much—if his weight is similar to the mean of the reference population at, say, 75 kg, we obtain a value of 38 × 75 mL/min, or 2.85 L/min. However, his weight may actually represent a degree of obesity if he is short; in this case, we would be overestimating $\dot{V}O_2$max. We may correct for this possibility by looking up the weight expected in a person of his height and age in a table such as that provided by the publishers of the Geigy Scientific Tables; if his height is 165 cm, the expected weight is 69 kg, and thus the expected $\dot{V}O_2$max is 38 × 69, or 2.62 L/min. This assumes that the relationship between height and weight in the reference population was the same as in the policyholders of American and Canadian insurance companies and, given that we cannot expect a high degree of precision from any relationship of this type, may be the best we can do. We should notice also that the last equation has two implicit assumptions: first, that the decline in $\dot{V}O_2$max/kg with age is linear and a constant proportion (0.55/60, or 0.92 per cent) per year, and second, that at any given age the expected $\dot{V}O_2$max is linearly related to weight (at 40 years, 38 mL/kg for any body weight). Longitudinal studies of healthy persons (Åstrand et al., 1973) suggest that the first assumption is a reasonable one, but the value of 0.92 per cent is partly explained by an increase in weight with age (about 0.2 per cent) and partly by a true fall in $\dot{V}O_2$max (0.7 per cent). Studies of athletes show that the $\dot{V}O_2$max/kg is influenced by weight, casting doubt on the second assumption— the heavier the athlete, the lower the $\dot{V}O_2$max/kg. A way round this problem might be provided by an equation that predicted $\dot{V}O_2$max on the basis of height and age; for example, from our own population study (Jones et al., 1985), the following equations were derived for cycle ergometry in males (height is in meters):

$$\text{Males: } \dot{V}O_2\text{max} = 5.41\,\text{ht} - 0.025\,\text{age} - 5.66\,\text{L/min}$$

Equation 1a

$$\text{Females: } \dot{V}O_2\text{max} = 3.01\,\text{ht} - 0.017\,\text{age} - 2.56\,\text{L/min}$$

Equation 1b

These two equations were derived from studies on 100 Canadians, 50 males and 50 females (see Fig. 8–1), with equal representation in five age categories and approximately equal numbers in categories of stature (Jones et al., 1985). A more recent study of similar design was reported by Fairbarn and colleagues (1994) in healthy Canadians, 120 women and 111 men, aged 20 to 80 years. The comparable equations were

$$\text{Males: } \dot{V}O_2\text{max} = 2.3\,\text{ht} - 0.031\,\text{age} + 0.0117\,\text{wt} - 0.332$$

$$\text{Females: } \dot{V}O_2\text{max} = 1.58\,\text{ht} - 0.027\,\text{age} + 0.00899\,\text{wt} + 0.207$$

These equations include weight as a variable and should be compared with the following equations (Jones et al., 1985):

$$\text{Males: } \dot{V}O_2\text{max} = 3.45\,\text{ht} - 0.028\,\text{age} + 0.022\,\text{wt} - 3.76\,\text{L/min}$$

$$\text{Females: } \dot{V}O_2\text{max} = 2.49\,\text{ht} - 0.018\,\text{age} + 0.010\,\text{wt} - 2.26\,\text{L/min}$$

At first sight, the constants used in these equations appear to be similar to those in Equations 2a and 2b, providing similar weighting to the variables, but the equation for males predicts a $\dot{V}O_2$max of 3.03 L/min. Such discrepancies are common when different studies are being compared, and they make the choice of equations difficult because the cause of the differences is not apparent, whether resulting from analytical bias, different weighting in the population of the variables, or differences in habitual activity levels (see below).

If we apply Equation 1a to our subject, we derive a value for our subject (height 1.65 m, age 40 years) of 2.27 L/min. This last equation may fit the experimental data fairly well ($r = 0.769$) and yet be a poor predictor of a person's $\dot{V}O_2$max. Both independent variables (height and age) are taken to influence $\dot{V}O_2$max linearly, and the large constant (5.66) has no physiological meaning and may have an unrealistically large effect on subjects with a low predicted $\dot{V}O_2$max (e.g., related to small stature or high age). For some patient groups in which lean body mass is liable to be reduced, such as those with cystic fibrosis (Lands et al., 1993), measurement by densitometry may be justified in order to determine whether poor exercise capacity may be explained on the basis of loss of muscle or cardiopulmonary impairment. In a study of children with cystic fibrosis, Lands and co-workers (1992, 1993) found close relationships between lean body mass and both leg muscle strength and $\dot{V}O_2$max. Furthermore, the statistical method used to derive equations of this type is one that minimizes the squares of deviations from the mean; for this reason, the relationship may be weighted by high values of the dependent variable and again may not be a good predictor in small or elderly subjects.

Perhaps instead of height, weight, and age, we may use other independent variables that take care of their effects; studies of fat-free body mass (Cotes et al., 1969) and lean thigh volume (Jones et al.,

1985) suggest that these two indices may be used to predict $\dot{V}O_2$max, but precision is not improved, and the techniques are time consuming.

For lean thigh volume (TV) (sum of both thighs in liters):

$$\dot{V}O_2\text{max} = 0.306\,\text{TV} - 1.04\,\text{L/min}$$

Vital capacity (VC) may be a useful predictor in subjects free of lung disease (Jones et al., 1985):

$$\dot{V}O_2\text{max} = 0.74\,\text{VC} - 1.04\,\text{L/min}$$

If our patient's VC is that expected for a healthy person at 4.33 L, predicted $\dot{V}O_2$max is 2.16 L/min.

Comparable equations to Equations 1a and 1b may be derived for maximum power output (in kilopond-meters per minute):

$$\text{Males: Wmax} = 2526\,\text{ht} - 9.08\,\text{age} - 2759$$

$$\text{Females: Wmax} = 950\,\text{ht} - 9.21\,\text{age} - 756$$

For children, these equations are comparable to those of Godfrey and colleagues (1971) in a population of 55 boys and 58 girls aged 6 to 16 years and with a range of height from 1.10 to 1.90 m:

$$\text{Males: Wmax} = 1755\,\text{ht} - 1780$$

$$\text{Females: Wmax} = 1456\,\text{ht} - 1456$$

Having chosen our preferred prediction, we may also want to consider if a reduction in $\dot{V}O_2$max might be explainable on inactivity; studies of healthy subjects have shown significant and quantitative effects of activity on $\dot{V}O_2$max that may help us to allow for this. A recent study of untrained persons attempted to quantify activity by questionnaire on a four-point scale based on exercise during leisure time—less than 1 h/wk (1), 1 to 3 h/wk (2), 3 to 6 h/wk (3), and more than 6 h/wk (4). The results suggested that each point was worth about 5 per cent of $\dot{V}O_2$max; a linear multiple regression equation was derived for males:

$$\dot{V}O_2\text{max} = 2.5\,\text{ht} - 0.023\,\text{age} + 0.019\,\text{wt} + 0.15\,\text{lei} - 2.32\,\text{L/min}$$

For females, the constant (-2.32) was increased to -2.86. The equations provided here were derived from measurements made in a mainly sedentary population consisting of 50 males and 50 females, having an evenly distributed age between 15 and 70 years and an evenly distributed stature (155 to 175 cm in females; 165 to 190 cm in males) (Jones et al., 1985). The values are broadly similar to those obtained by use of the approaches outlined earlier but tend to be lower for smaller subjects, as the reader may judge by calculating values for comparison.

Note that the effect of activity may be very large; based on the mean data, $\dot{V}O_2$max increased from 1.97 L/min in subjects exercising less than 1 h/wk to 3.11 L/min in those exercising more than 6 h/wk (Jones et al., 1985). It is possible, however, that these figures exaggerate this effect through an interaction between inactivity and increasing age. A smaller effect of activity was found by McDonough and colleagues (1970), but a more recent study of a large population drawn from the United States Armed Forces (Vogel et al., 1986) showed a large effect of activity; indeed, two recent studies showed that $\dot{V}O_2$max may be accurately predicted ($r^2 = 0.77$; standard error of the estimate [SEE], 12.7 per cent) from the responses to an activity questionnaire and the measurement of lean body mass (Heil et al., 1995), or in treadmill exercise from a similar questionnaire and age ($r^2 = 0.67$) (Myers et al., 1994).

Use of Nonlinear Equations

The reader may be wondering where this discussion is leading. We have questioned various approaches, including our own, to the prediction of normal values. Given that the precision of most normal values in physiology is seldom better than $\pm$ 20 per cent (2 standard deviations [SDs]), perhaps we should not attempt to improve on these approaches but live with the variability. However, because values of $\dot{V}O_2$max or maximum power may influence clinical decision making, re-examination of the prediction process is important. We may do this by imposing certain restrictions on prediction equations that have a theoretical basis; this leads to the development of a different model on which we base our prediction, which is based on more appropriate scaling methods, outlined in Chapter 2. We may then see how well the predictions work on the basis of published data. Unfortunately, there has been a reluctance to use nonlinear relationships in the past, which means that we cannot compare the equations directly with published studies.

We may start by affirming that, if possible, prediction equations should take account of the effects of stature, age, and gender.

Stature

If we agree that weight may not be an appropriate variable for the prediction of $\dot{V}O_2$max, the equation needs to be based on height. In our own study, quoted earlier, height was a strong prediction variable in a linear regression equation. Unfortunately, most studies of normal exercise capacity have not systematically explored a wide and evenly distributed range of stature; the exceptions are studies of children, such as the recent study of Cooper and Weiler-Ravell (1984), in which the following equations were derived:

$$\text{Boys: } \dot{V}_{O_2}\text{max} = 4.36 \text{ ht} - 4.55 \text{ L/min}$$

$$\text{Girls: } \dot{V}_{O_2}\text{max} = 2.25 \text{ ht} - 1.84 \text{ L/min}$$

These data agree well with the equations derived in our study, as may be seen by comparing these equations with Equations 1a and 1b earlier. However, it may be noted that the linear equations of Cooper and Weiler-Ravell (1984) imply that at heights of less than about 1.3 m, girls show a higher $\dot{V}_{O_2}$max than do boys, an unlikely possibility physiologically. The results of other studies in children are consistent with these conclusions (Cumming and Friesen, 1967; Godfrey, 1974; Cunningham et al., 1984).

As pointed out in Chapter 2, theoretically, $\dot{V}_{O_2}$max is a function of mass to the power 2/3, and thus of height to the power 2. This is borne out by studies of elite athletes in whom $\dot{V}_{O_2}$max is about $0.3 \times \text{wt}^{2/3}$ L/min (Åstrand and Rodahl, 1977); however, in untrained subjects, a higher exponent is found. In our own studies, it was found that $\dot{V}_{O_2}$max varied as a function of height to the power 2.0 to 2.9; arbitrary variation of exponent and constant by trial and error produced equations that fitted the data at least as well as the linear equations derived directly from the data:

$$\text{Males: } \dot{V}_{O_2}\text{max} = 0.83 \times \text{ht}^{2.7}$$

$$\text{Females: } \dot{V}_{O_2}\text{max} = 0.62 \times \text{ht}^{2.7}$$

where height is in meters and $\dot{V}_{O_2}$max in liters per minute. These exponential equations also fitted the mean data of Cooper and Weiler-Ravell, when corrections for age were applied (see below). However, the general validity of the equations required further testing.

Age

A prediction equation such as that above:

$$\dot{V}_{O_2}\text{max} = 5.41 \text{ ht} - 0.025 \text{ age} - 5.66$$

implies that for all heights, the reduction with age is linear and constant; at the age of 40 years, the $\dot{V}_{O_2}$ is (0.025×20) or 0.50 L/min less than that at the age of 20 years, whether the person is tall or short. From what is known of the aging process and from experimental studies, a proportional change with age is more realistic—that $\dot{V}_{O_2}$max declines

by about 0.7 per cent per year. Adding this factor to the height scaling yields the following:

$$\text{Males: } \dot{V}_{O_2}\text{max} = 0.83 \text{ ht}^{2.7} \times (1 - 0.007 \text{ age})$$

$$\text{Females: } \dot{V}_{O_2}\text{max} = 0.62 \text{ ht}^{2.7} \times (1 - 0.007 \text{ age})$$

Maximum values for $\dot{V}_{O_2}$max are seen at around the age of 20 years, and in children, a significant negative influence of age on $\dot{V}_{O_2}$max standardized for stature is not detectable. For this reason, in patients younger than 20 years, this effect is ignored, as in the equations of Cooper and Weiler-Ravell, given above, or in the following exponential equations:

$$\text{Boys: } \dot{V}_{O_2}\text{max} = 0.67 \text{ ht}^{2.7}$$

$$\text{Girls: } \dot{V}_{O_2}\text{max} = 0.48 \text{ ht}^{2.7}$$

When we consider the theoretical scaling relationships presented above and in Chapter 2, the fact that a decline with age cannot be linear in an absolute sense, and that maximum power and aerobic capacity for any given stature and age are higher in men than women (because of a greater mass of muscles, heart, and lungs), it becomes apparent that nonlinear equations have a better chance of describing the expected normal exercise capacity in a population that must include the whole range of statures and ages encountered in a clinical exercise laboratory. Through studies in large numbers of subjects, we derived the following equations that meet both the concepts and the practical requirements:

For maximum power output (kpm/min):

$$\text{Males: } W\text{max} = 2521 \text{ ht}^{1.78} \text{ age}^{-0.46}$$
$$\text{Equation 2a (Fig. 8–2)}$$

$$\text{Females: } W\text{max} = 1775 \text{ ht}^{1.78} \text{ age}^{-0.46}$$
$$\text{Equation 2b (Fig. 8–3)}$$

(Height is in meters, age in years; $r^2 = 0.971$)

For maximum oxygen intake (L/min):

$$\text{Males: } \dot{V}_{O_2}\text{max} = 5.14 \text{ ht}^{1.88} \text{ age}^{-0.49}$$
$$\text{Equation 3a (Fig. 8–4)}$$

$$\text{Females: } \dot{V}_{O_2}\text{max} = 3.55 \text{ ht}^{1.88} \text{ age}^{-0.49}$$
$$\text{Equation 3b (Fig. 8–5)}$$

$$(r^2 = 0.969)$$

Gender

In accounting for the effects of stature and age, we have already identified differences between the

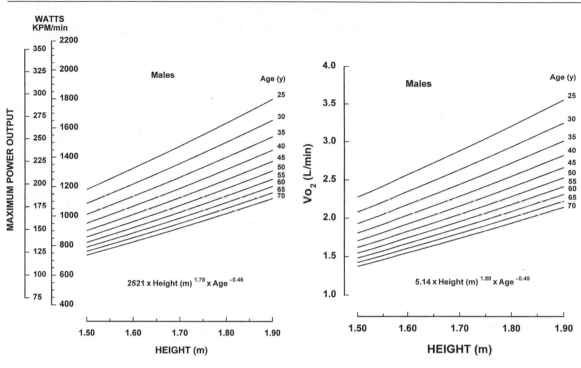

Figure 8–2. Prediction of maximum exercise capacity (cycle ergometer) in males on the basis of height and age.

Figure 8–4. Prediction of oxygen intake at maximum exercise capacity in males on the basis of height and age.

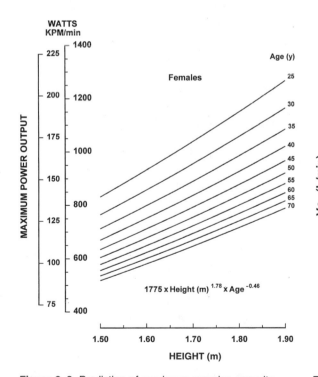

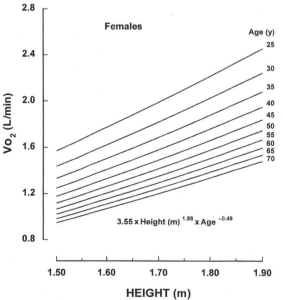

Figure 8–3. Prediction of maximum exercise capacity (cycle ergometer) in females on the basis of height and age.

Figure 8–5. Prediction of oxygen intake at maximum exercise capacity in females on the basis of height and age.

two sexes at any given age and height. To take account of these differences between the sexes, we can either derive separate equations for males and females, as given above, or include a constant correction factor. An equation derived from large surveys of females (Drinkwater et al., 1975):

$$\dot{V}O_2max \ (mL/kg/min) = 48 - 0.37 \ age$$

indicates a lower $\dot{V}O_2max$ compared with males, females showing values that are, on average, 0.8 (48/60) of those in males, but the fall with age is similar at 0.77 per cent (0.37/48) per year. Because adipose fat is higher in females, a prediction based on height rather than on weight might appear to be the answer, but for any given height, lean body mass is about 20 per cent higher in males than in females. The equations above (Eqs. 3a and 3b) suggest a slightly lower proportion (0.69). The current practice is to use separate predictions for males and females; however, if necessary, the equations may be combined and a gender factor included in the equation.

Fitness

The fact that $\dot{V}O_2max$ may be at least 50 per cent higher in athletes than in sedentary persons of the same age and stature and that increases of up to 40 per cent may be achieved in a sedentary subject who takes part in a 3-month program of endurance training suggests that some account of the subject's activity patterns should be taken in a prediction of $\dot{V}O_2max$. One may argue about our ability to do so because, although this factor undoubtedly accounts for at least some of the differences between different studies, we lack precise and practical methods for quantifying the amount of activity a subject takes. The approach based on questionnaire information regarding habitual leisure time activity, described earlier, provides at least a partial solution; this grades activity into four categories (1, 2, 3, or 4). Because the regression equations presented above were validated in a population with a median rating of 2, they may be corrected by 5 per cent for each grade (i.e., multiplied by 0.95, 1.0, 1.05, and 1.10 for categories 1, 2, 3, and 4, respectively). There is no doubt that the factor of 1.10 for subjects exercising for 6 or more hours per week should be much higher (1.2 to 1.3) and in a competitive athlete should be higher still, but we do not have experimental data that allow us to quantify the effects of training more precisely.

Our "model," or exponential, equations may be tested by applying them to the same population that was used to derive the linear equations. Although it may be difficult to establish statistically that these equations are more valid than the linear ones described earlier, they are, theoretically, more attractive and have the advantage that for statures that are far from the median of the population, more realistic predictions are obtained. Similarly, they appear equally valid when they are applied to children as when they are applied to adults.

Measurements at Maximum Exercise

The symptoms and measurements recorded at the maximum power output in the stage 1 test are used to determine the main factors that limit exercise.

Symptoms

The discomfort that accompanies increasing exercise intensity provides the signal for the subject to stop exercise, and subjects vary in their tolerance; this variation is reflected in the variation in maximal scores recorded by the Borg scale; 75 per cent of subjects stop when the sensation is appreciated as "severe" to "very severe" (Borg 5–7); of the remainder, some subjects stop when intensity is "somewhat severe" (4), and some push themselves to "maximal" (10). For reasons that are not readily apparent but perhaps are understandable, the maximal tolerated discomfort declines with age; there is a tendency for taller individuals to accept a higher rating of discomfort, but no difference exists between the genders:

Females
and males: Max dyspnea $= 14.2 \ ht^{0.70} \times age^{-0.34}$

Females: Max leg effort $= 15.6 \ ht^{0.81} \times age^{-0.35}$

Males: Max leg effort $= 17.1 \ ht^{0.81} \times age^{-0.35}$

In subjects with limited ventilatory reserve, dyspnea is usually rated higher than effort, and it is not unusual for dyspnea to be rated 10 at a level of exercise rated only 3 or 4 for leg effort in such patients; however, in respiratory patients, up to 30 per cent are limited by greater leg effort than by dyspnea (Killian, 1992). Patients with angina will usually stop exercise at a rating of 5 or less for chest discomfort; the rating, in relation to the workload, reflects the severity of the coronary disease (Borg et al., 1981).

Cardiac Frequency

Many studies, reviewed by Spiro (1977), have established that the cardiac frequency in maximal exercise bears a linear negative relationship to age, as expressed in the following equation, which is valid for males and females:

$$f_c max = 210 - 0.65 \text{ age b/min (SD} \pm 10)$$

Other equations derived from the studies already quoted are similar but may be preferable because they include subjects in older age groups:

Males
and females: $f_c max = 202 - 0.72$ age
(Jones et al., 1985)

Females: $f_c max = 209 - 0.86$ age
(Fairbarn et al., 1994)

Males: $f_c max = 207 - 0.78$ age
(Fairbarn et al., 1994)

In our own population, the $f_c max$ could be expressed as power functions of both stature and age:

Females: $f_c max = 347 \, ht^{0.24} \times age^{-0.25}$

Males: $f_c max = 362 \, ht^{0.24} \times age^{-0.25}$

If a subject reaches this value, we may conclude that cardiac frequency is limiting: a difficulty arises if the maximal cardiac frequency is recorded 10 to 20 beats below the predicted value—for example, an f_c of 155 b/min in a 60-year-old patient (predicted $f_c max$ 171 b/min). Did the patient reach a cardiovascular limit or not? Other evidence is required, for example, from measurements of ventilation or plasma lactate, to help in this decision.

Oxygen Pulse

The "oxygen pulse" is defined by a rearrangement of the Fick equation:

$$\dot{V}O_2 f_c = V_s (CaO_2 - C\bar{v}O_2)$$

At maximal exercise, the arteriovenous oxygen content difference varies to a relatively minor degree among subjects. Thus, the oxygen pulse reflects stroke volume, and if a maximum value for ($CaO_2 - C\bar{v}O_2$) is assumed at 160 mL/L, a minimum value for stroke volume may actually be calculated from $\dot{V}O_2/f_c$. Normal expected values are related to stature and are smaller in females than in males (Fig. 8–6):

$$\text{Males: } \dot{V}O_2/f_c max = 34.2 \, ht - 44.0 \text{ mL/beat}$$

$$\text{Females: } \dot{V}O_2/f_c max = 19.0 \, ht - 21.4 \text{ mL/beat}$$

However, rather than comparing the value obtained in a patient at maximum exercise, with the value predicted by these equations, it is preferable to calculate an estimated maximum stroke volume. This is because oxygen pulse represents a ratio that has no validity in its own right because the intercept in the relationship between $\dot{V}O_2$ and f_c does not pass through zero. The relationships expressed in the Fick equation are very tight in both healthy subjects and cardiac patients, which allows calculation of V_s from the measured $\dot{V}O_2 max$ and $f_c max$, with a surprising degree of precision. For example, a subject who attains a $\dot{V}O_2 max$ of 3 L/min is predicted to have a cardiac output of 20 L/min, and if $f_c max$ is 175, V_s is estimated to be 114 mL. The derived V_s may then be interpreted in relation to expected values for healthy subjects of the given stature.

Carbon Dioxide Output

$\dot{V}CO_2 max$ in normal subjects reaches values that are similar to $\dot{V}O_2 max$ (Eqs. 2a and 2b) but higher,

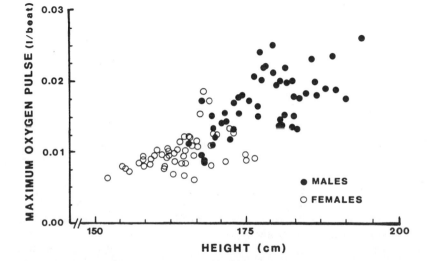

Figure 8–6. Oxygen pulse at maximum exercise ($\dot{V}O_2 max/f_c max$) in healthy males and females.

and in some ways, they represent the sum of aerobic and anaerobic capacities:

$$\text{Males: } \dot{V}_{CO_2}\text{max} = 6.23 \text{ ht}^{1.79} \times \text{age}^{-0.49}$$

$$\text{Females: } \dot{V}_{CO_2}\text{max} = 4.22 \text{ ht}^{1.79} \times \text{age}^{-0.49}$$

$$(\text{Height is in meters, } r^2 = 0.975)$$

Ventilation

In normal subjects, ventilation in maximum exercise reaches 60 to 75 per cent of the maximum voluntary ventilation (MVV), indicating that reserve is still present in the ventilatory capacity.

The ventilation achieved at maximum exercise is not surprisingly related to the subject's height and age:

$$\text{Females: } \dot{V}_E\text{max} = 96 \text{ ht}^{0.92} \times \text{age}^{-0.29}$$

$$\text{Males: } \dot{V}_E\text{max} = 143 \text{ ht}^{0.92} \times \text{age}^{-0.29}$$

but in all subjects is closely related to the maximum carbon dioxide output:

$$\dot{V}_E\text{max} = 10.3 + 26.0 \ \dot{V}_{CO_2}\text{max}$$
$$(r = 0.88 \text{ [Blackie et al., 1991]})$$

It is quite closely related to the subject's VC and FEV_1 (Jones et al., 1985):

$$\dot{V}_E\text{max} = 26.3 \text{ VC} - 34 \text{ L/min } (r = 0.78)$$

$$\dot{V}_E\text{max} = 30.6 \text{ FEV}_1 - 29 \text{ L/min } (r = 0.76)$$

However, such predictions are of little value in interpreting exercise responses; more important is the question of whether ventilation at maximum is close to the voluntary ventilatory capacity, usually estimated from VC or, more commonly, from FEV_1.

The MVV is defined as a ventilation that can be maintained for 4 minutes in an isocapnic test (Freedman, 1970); usually, values some 25 per cent lower than the long-established 15-second maximum breathing capacity are recorded. Freedman (1970) showed that MVV could be predicted from the FEV_1 in normal subjects:

$$\text{MVV} = 129 + 25 \ (\text{FEV}_1 - 4) \text{ L/min}$$

where FEV_1 is expressed in liters.

In patients with very limited ventilatory capacities owing to chronic airway obstruction or diffuse fibrosing alveolitis, a better equation to use is as follows (Spiro, 1977):

$$\text{MVV} = (\text{FEV}_1 \times 20) + 20 \text{ L/min}$$

As a broad guide applicable to all subjects, ventilatory capacity is obtained from the equation $FEV_1 \times 35$ (Clark et al., 1969). However, it must be remembered that the FEV_1 is a forced expiratory maneuver that is influenced by the mechanical characteristics of the respiratory system. In decisions of whether ventilation has reached a limiting value, it may be helpful to analyze ventilation into its components of tidal volume and inspiratory and expiratory flow rates; these components may then be examined in relation to the maximum flow: volume curve (inspiration and expiration) measured at rest. Such an analysis is particularly helpful in patients with severe airflow obstruction or with weak respiratory muscles. In the former, inspiratory flow rates may be relatively well preserved in the presence of gross reductions in expiratory flow, as long as the respiratory muscles are strong. On the other hand, in patients with respiratory muscle weakness, FEV_1 may be relatively well preserved, but the ability to increase inspiratory flow and volume is reduced, and ventilation during exercise is associated with severe dyspnea.

Tidal Volume

In normal subjects, maximal tidal volume is related to vital capacity, as expressed in the following equation:

$$V_T\text{max} = 0.67 \text{ VC} - 0.64 \text{ l BTPS}$$

In a large study in subjects aged 20 to 80 years, Blackie and colleagues (1991) found the respiratory frequency at maximum exercise to be 36.1 ± 9.2 b/min and the ratio of $V_T$max to VC to be 0.53 ± 0.08.

Measurements at Submaximal Power in Stage 1 Tests

Although the measurements at maximal exercise are important in quantifying impairment and identifying possible limiting factors, it is often just as important to examine the evolution of variables in submaximal exercise, especially because many patients stop exercising well below expected maximum values. The results are then used to decide whether variables are abnormal at a given intensity of exercise, thus allowing impairment of specific mechanisms to be identified.

Similar considerations as those reviewed earlier for maximal exercise values apply to the definition of submaximal normal standards, but once data have been obtained in healthy subjects at several levels in incremental exercise tests, several approaches may be taken. The most attractive is to use the data at all exercise loads to describe the evolution of the response to increasing exercise. Because many variables increase linearly with increasing exercise, the normal standard may be described by an intercept and slope of the dependent variable as a function of an independent variable, such as power output, or $\dot{V}O_2$. An important advantage of this approach is that the use of data at all exercise levels reduces error resulting from random biological or technical variation, but a disadvantage is the difficulty of quantifying abnormality in a way that may be easily understood. An attractive alternative is to plot the variables graphically in a way that may be easily presented in a test report form. Another approach is to compare the results at given power outputs or $\dot{V}O_2$; this might appear a logical way of standardizing results, and it has been well argued, particularly by Cotes (1993) and by Spiro and associates (1974), who present standards for heart rate and ventilation at $\dot{V}O_2$ of 0.75, 1.0, and 1.5 L/min. However, in applying such standards, care must be taken that the effects of other major independent variables have been allowed for; for example, heart rate is influenced by stature as well as $\dot{V}O_2$. The tables provided in Appendix D allow readers to apply this type of approach in interpreting results, but for most variables, we use data at all power outputs in the examples that follow.

Oxygen Intake

The increase in oxygen intake with increasing power outputs in an incremental stage 1 test is linear and, in healthy subjects, predictable. For this reason it is possible to predict oxygen intake to within $\pm$ 10 per cent, a precision that is close to that expected when experimental and biological variations are taken into account (Jones and Kane, 1979). In general, the need for oxygen intake measurements is less than might be expected, as long as the exercise is carried out on a well-calibrated ergometer or treadmill. Also, the measurement of ventilation during submaximal exercise is a useful check that the metabolic requirements are normal. An acceptable estimate of oxygen intake at given power (W = kpm/min) is obtained from the following equation:

$$\dot{V}O_2 = 3.5 \text{ wt} + 1.8 \text{ W}$$

where $\dot{V}O_2$ is expressed in milliliters per minute and weight is expressed in kilograms. In this equation, 3.5 wt expresses resting $\dot{V}O_2$, and 1.8 W the increase in $\dot{V}O_2$ per unit increase in power.

Cardiac Frequency

In submaximal exercise, cardiac frequency usually increases linearly with increasing power and $\dot{V}O_2$. The slope of the relationship reflects stroke volume and is dependent in normal subjects on size and fitness; age does not appear to influence the relationship (Spiro et al., 1974). Our practice is to draw a predicted line for a given subject by joining the resting cardiac frequency (zero load) to a point relating maximum predicted power (or predicted $\dot{V}O_2$max) and predicted maximum cardiac frequency (from age). The slope of the subject's response and the displacement from the predicted line may then be examined for the complete exercise test. Because $\dot{V}O_2$max may be predicted from stature and age, and $f_c$max is also related to age, the slope as defined in this way is normally related to stature alone, with a systematic difference between males and females. An alternative approach is to derive cardiac frequency at given power or $\dot{V}O_2$ and to compare the values with normal standards. Normal values for f_c at $\dot{V}O_2$ of 0.75, 1.0, and 1.5 L/min are given by Spiro and associates (1974). Cotes and colleagues (1973) showed that these derived values depend also on body size, measured as fat-free body mass. From these observations, slopes of f_c to power may be derived (Appendix D), yielding another parameter with which the measured values are compared. By combining the Fick equation with the equation relating f_c to $\dot{V}O_2$, it may be shown that the slope of the relationship approximates stroke volume times the arterial oxygen content (Durand and Mensch-Dechene, 1979); if the latter is known or assumed, an estimate of stroke volume may be derived.

Ventilation

The response of ventilation to increasing exercise may usually be separated into two components. At low and moderate loads, below about 50 per cent of $\dot{V}O_2$max, the response is linear in relation to power output

$$\dot{V}E = 8 + 0.0525 \text{ W L/min}$$

and to $\dot{V}O_2$

$$\dot{V}E = 5 + 21.8 \dot{V}O_2 \text{ L/min}$$

where W is in kpm/min, and $\dot{V}O_2$ is in liters per minute. These responses are not significantly influenced by age or stature. With increasing power, $\dot{V}E$ shows a disproportionate increase in relation to W and $\dot{V}O_2$, owing mainly to increases in $\dot{V}CO_2$.

$$\dot{V}E \text{ (L/min)} = 5.4 + 23.9 \dot{V}CO_2$$
$$(r^2 = 0.88; \text{ SEE, } 3.6)$$

In a graphical plot of $\dot{V}E$ versus power or $\dot{V}O_2$, the point of inflexion—the "anaerobic threshold" (AT), or "proportional limit"—is worth identifying because in most instances it indicates an increase in plasma lactate concentration. Unfortunately, the curve of $\dot{V}E$ against $\dot{V}O_2$ is usually smooth, which may make identifying an inflection point difficult, leading to interobserver error in its identification. To obviate this difficulty, a number of groups have devised computerized regression analysis for identification of a change in slope in the relationship between $\dot{V}E$ and $\dot{V}O_2$ (Orr et al., 1982) or $\dot{V}CO_2$ and $\dot{V}O_2$ (V-slope method [Beaver et al., 1986]); the latter method accords with the definition of Wasserman and Sue (1991) for the AT as "the $\dot{V}O_2$ at which $\dot{V}CO_2$ begins to increase at a faster rate at lower work rates . . . a marker of the increased lactic acid production by the exercising muscles." Although we may argue about the literal interpretation of the phenomenon, the identification of an accelerated rate of carbon dioxide output almost invariably indicates an increase in plasma lactate concentration.

The $\dot{V}O_2$ at which the inflexion is expected may be predicted by use of the following equation:

$$\dot{V}O_2 = 2.4\ ht - 0.007\ age - 2.43\ L/min$$

where height is in meters. The point of inflexion occurs at an average $\dot{V}O_2$ of 58 per cent $\dot{V}O_2max$ but occurs at a higher percentage of $\dot{V}O_2max$ in smaller persons and in trained rather than in untrained subjects (Wasserman and Whipp, 1975).

A standardization of the ventilatory response to exercise was suggested by Cotes (1972), who proposed similar indices to those described above for cardiac frequency, obtained by calculating $\dot{V}E$ at oxygen intakes of 0.75, 1.0, and 1.5 L/min ($\dot{V}E$ 0.75, $\dot{V}E$ 1.0, $\dot{V}E$ 1.5). This is a useful procedure when the responses of groups of subjects are compared; results in normal subjects are given in the report by Spiro and associates (1974).

Tidal Volume

Tidal volume shows an increase with increasing exercise toward an asymptote (see Fig. 2–8). This response has been analyzed in terms of two linear functions (Hey et al., 1966; Spiro et al., 1974), but because the response is usually curvilinear (Jones and Rebuck, 1979), there seems little reason to do so.

Standardization, by calculation of V_T at given values of $\dot{V}E$, 20 L/min and 30 L/min (V_T 20, V_T 30), has been suggested by Cotes (1972) and Spiro and associates (1974). As with the other indices described above, I have not found any particular advantage in making these calculations for individual subjects, although they are useful in describing differences between groups (Spiro et al., 1974). An alternative is to relate V_T at any given $\dot{V}E$ to the subject's height (Fig. 8–7).

Systolic Blood Pressure

Normally, systolic blood pressure increases linearly with increasing power and $\dot{V}O_2$ (Sannerstedt, 1967) in normotensive subjects, but the extent of the increase is larger in older than in younger subjects. This behavior may be described in the following equation, in which the increase above resting systolic blood pressure (120 mm Hg) is related to both the increase in power (W, kpm/min) and to age (years):

Systolic BP = 120 + [(2.0 + 0.1 age) × 0.01 W]

Diastolic blood pressure normally changes little

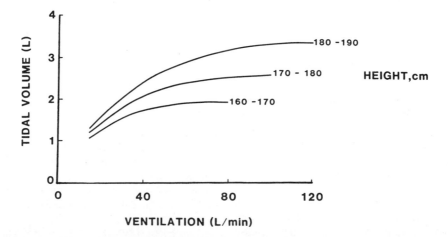

Figure 8–7. Tidal volume during exercise in males and females as a function of height.

with exercise, remaining within ± 10 mm Hg of resting values.

Symptoms

The magnitude of dyspnea and leg effort, quantified by the Borg scale, increases with power output, decreases with increasing height and age, and is greater in females than in males; leg effort is on average greater than dyspnea:

$$\text{Leg effort} = 4.82 + 0.007 \text{ kpm/min} - 0.055 \text{ ht (cm)} + 0.04 \text{ age} + 1.05 \text{ sex}$$

$$\text{Dyspnea} = 4.96 + 0.006 \text{ kpm/min} - 0.50 \text{ age} + 0.96 \text{ sex}$$

where sex is denoted by 1 for males and 2 for females.

The nonlinear increase in the magnitude of both symptoms may be expressed as a function of the predicted maximum power output (MPO), which removes the effects of gender and other variables:

$$\text{Leg effort} - 0.0016 \times \% \text{ MPO}^{1.79}$$

$$\text{Dyspnea} = 0.0014 \times \% \text{ MPO}^{1.86}$$

Almost invariably, the evolution in symptom intensity follows this accelerating but smoothly progressive pattern; when this is seriously disturbed, the validity of the reported intensity may be questioned.

There will always be some skepticism in accepting measurements of subjective symptom intensities, but with a few exceptions, their validity is sufficient for them to be used as a basis for an exercise test report. Personality might be expected to exert a significant effect, but in a recent study, type A individuals were shown to systematically under-rate the intensity of leg effort by only a small amount (Hassmén et al., 1993). More common is an under-rating by individuals who on other evidence are prone to ''deny'' the severity of their illness, such as patients recovering from a myocardial infarction; although they may rate effort and dyspnea very low and stop exercising at a Borg scale of 2 or 3, when asked why they stopped exercise, they usually admit an inability to go on because of muscle fatigue. Occasionally, a subject reports appropriate symptom intensities but then stops exercise, stating an inability to continue and an intensity of 10, but without any outward signs of severe effort; this behavior needs to be treated with the same suspicion as an obvious variability in effort exerted during spirometry.

Prediction of Normal Values for Nonexercise Measurements

For most pulmonary function measurements, internationally agreed-upon standards exist (American Thoracic Society, 1979, 1987, 1986), which most laboratories use to predict the expected normal values. Some of these equations do not conform to plausible scaling concepts and thus should be viewed with some skepticism when they are applied to extremes of stature or age.

Simple Spirometry

Measurements of maximal expired volumes, total (forced vital capacity [FVC]) and in 1 second (FEV_1), provide an indication of breathing capacity and pulmonary impairment. Normal values are predicted on the basis of a surprisingly small nonsmoking population (Crapo et al., 1981):

$$\text{Males:} \quad \text{FVC (L)} = 0.0600 \text{ ht (cm)} - 0.214 \text{ age} - 4.65$$

$$FEV_1 = 0.0414 \text{ ht (cm)} - 0.0244 \text{ age} - 2.19$$

$$\text{Females:} \quad \text{FVC} = 0.0491 \text{ ht (cm)} - 0.0216 \text{ age} - 3.59$$

$$FEV_1 = 0.0342 \text{ ht} - 0.0255 \text{ age} - 1.578$$

Values for children (younger than 16 years) are from Weng and Levison (1969).

Flow-Volume Loop

The addition of maximal inspiratory flow (V_I) to expiratory (V_E) measurements is helpful in identifying patients whose maximum breathing capacity is not well predicted from expiratory flow measurements. Conventionally, values are reported at peak flow and at 25 and 50 per cent of the subject's VC; this method may lead to difficulty in interpretation if VC is reduced for any reason. Normal predictions for expiratory flow are from Knudson and associates (1976): values for 50 per cent of expired VC in adults:

$$\text{Males: } V_E\text{max}_{50} = 0.0684 \text{ ht (cm)} - 0.0366 \text{ age} - 5.541$$

$$\text{Females: } V_E\text{max}_{50} = 0.0268 \text{ ht (cm)} - 0.0289 \text{ age} + 0.6088$$

Normal predictions for inspiratory flow are hard to find; in our laboratory, the following equation was derived from measurements in 900 subjects (sex is rated as follows: males = 1; females = 0):

$$V_{Tmax} = 0.057 \text{ ht (cm)} - 0.04 \text{ age} + 1.75 \text{ sex} - 2.57$$

Carbon Monoxide Uptake

The generally accepted method is the single-breath technique, originally described by Ogilvie and co-workers (1957), subdivided into its alveolar volume (V_A) and transfer factor (D_L/V_A) components. Predicted values are provided by Crapo and Morris (1981):

$$\text{Males: } D_{LCO} = 0.416 \text{ ht (cm)} - 0.219 \text{ age} - 26.34$$

$$D_L/V_A = 7.08 - 0.034 \text{ age}$$

$$\text{Females: } D_{LCO} = 0.256 \text{ ht} - 0.144 \text{ age} - 8.36$$

$$D_L/V_A = 6.58 - 0.025 \text{ age}$$

Values need to be interpreted in the light of false reductions in D_L/V_A in subjects with anemia (divide value by 0.06965 hemoglobin, in grams per deciliter), and in subjects with increased blood carboxyhemoglobin levels resulting from smoking (Cotes, 1993).

Skeletal Muscle Strength

Normal values of muscle strength are needed, but these are difficult to establish for many reasons, the most obvious being a lack of agreement on methods and population selection. In our laboratory, we have measured strength in legs and arms in all subjects coming for exercise tests by use of the method described in Chapter 14, and we have derived equations describing strength in all individuals whose exercise capacity was within 20 per cent of predicted capacity. This has provided a large population (> 1000), which we hope has yielded valid estimates of strength in nondisabled subjects. The derived equations (Hamilton, 1995) are expressed in terms of age (years) and height (ht, meters) with a weighting for gender (S = 0 for females, 1 for males).

1. Bilateral knee extension (kg)

$$\text{Strength} = (42.4 + 17.6 \text{ S}) \text{ ht}^{2.72} \times \text{age}^{-0.39}$$
$$(r^2 = 0.62; \text{SD}, 28.1)$$

2. Bilateral knee flexion

$$\text{Strength} = (21.8 + 9.1 \text{ S}) \text{ ht}^{2.62} \times \text{age}^{-0.39}$$
$$(r^2 = 0.49; \text{SD}, 20.6)$$

3. Arm push

$$\text{Strength} = (70.9 + 52.0\text{S}) \text{ ht}^{1.87} \times \text{age}^{-0.39}$$
$$(r^2 = 0.72; \text{SD}, 29.7)$$

4. Arm pull

$$\text{Strength} = (21.7 + 10.9\text{S}) \text{ ht}^{2.34} \times \text{age}^{-0.18}$$
$$(r^2 = 0.65; \text{SD}, 25.0)$$

Knee extension strength and a combination of all these indices are highly correlated to maximum work capacity in healthy subjects and in patients with cardiorespiratory disorders (Hamilton, 1995) and also contribute to the sensation of effort during exercise in all these groups (Killian, 1992).

Respiratory Muscle Strength

The simplest measurements reflecting respiratory muscle strength are derived from the maximum pressure generated against an occluded mouthpiece at FRC during inspiration (MIP) and expiration (maximum expiratory pressure [MEP]) (Black and Hyatt, 1969). The following equations expressed as cm H_2O were derived in our laboratory in healthy subjects with normal exercise capacity (S = 0 for females, 1 for males):

$$\text{MIP} = (118.4 + 55.2 \text{ sex}) \text{ ht}^{0.859} \times \text{age}^{-0.254}$$
$$(r^2 = 0.42; \text{SD}, 23.9)$$

$$\text{MEP} = (115.6 + 47.4 \text{ sex}) \text{ ht}^{0.600} \times \text{age}^{-0.163}$$
$$(r^2 = 0.43; \text{SD}, 23.9)$$

Maximum inspiratory pressure contributes to the sensation of dyspnea during exercise in healthy subjects and patients with cardiorespiratory disorders (El-Manshawi et al., 1986; Leblanc et al., 1986).

Summary: Interpretation of Stage 1 Test Results

The following is a simple framework that may be used to identify abnormalities in stage 1 test responses. The prediction equations given above are summarized in Appendix D.

1. Predicted maximum power and $\dot{V}O_2max$ are obtained by suitable equations.
2. If $\dot{V}O_2max$ has not been measured, the measured maximum power is converted into an oxygen intake. For the treadmill, this is

conveniently obtained from a graph (Appendix C) (Fig. C–2) or nomogram (Bruce et al., 1973; American College of Sports Medicine, 1986). For the cycle ergometer, oxygen intake is obtained by multiplying power (in kilopond-meters per minute) by 1.8 and adding the resting oxygen intake (3.5 $\times$ weight in kilograms). Oxygen intake may be expressed in terms of $\dot{V}O_2max/kg$ (milliliters per minute per kilogram) or in mets (milliliters per minute per kilogram $\div$ 3.5) and as a percentage of the predicted value. Normal values are expected to lie within $\pm$ 20 per cent of predicted.

3. Predicted maximum cardiac frequency is calculated from the patient's age.

4. The predicted cardiac frequency for submaximal power is derived by interpolation between the resting and the predicted maximum cardiac frequencies.

5. The ventilation at maximum exercise is compared with an estimated ventilatory capacity obtained by multiplying FEV_1 by 35.

6. The ventilation in submaximal exercise is compared with that expected.

7. The pattern of breathing is examined in terms of the maximum tidal volume (VTmax) predicted from the vital capacity and in relation to ventilation.

8. Systolic blood pressure changes are interpreted in view of the normal linear increase with power, corrected for age. A rise of more than 15 mm Hg in diastolic pressure is considered abnormal.

9. Electrocardiographic changes are interpreted using the guidelines presented in Chapter 7. If ST depression has occurred, it is first normalized to standard R-wave voltage, divided by Wmax or $\dot{V}O_2max$ (expressed as a proportion of predicted), and further corrected if heart rate is depressed. Likelihood ratios are then chosen for age and sex and for chest pain history so that the pretest likelihood of coronary artery disease can be obtained. The likelihood ratio appropriate to the corrected ST depression is then used to derive the post-test likelihood of disease.

10. Symptoms are assessed in relation to the objective measurements of performance and to the clinical problem, in terms of the subjective factors that stopped further exercise and to the evolution of symptom severity through the test.

Three examples will be used to illustrate the use of this framework and the same patients' results in stage 2 and stage 3 tests in later chapters.

INTERPRETATION AND REPORTING

In the examples that follow, in this chapter and in Chapter 13, a more-or-less obvious approach is taken to examining the results of an exercise test and providing the referring health professional with a report that may be viewed in relation to other clinical information. In addition to answering clinical questions, a standardized report is also a powerful learning tool that helps to integrate the information into clinical problem solving and improve the effectiveness of this clinical investigation.

The interpretations illustrated in the present chapter are more detailed and structured than are usually required for routine reporting, as exemplified in Chapter 13. Resting data are reviewed first (diagnosis, drugs, pulmonary function, muscle strength, electrocardiogram), followed by the maximum power output, limiting symptoms and symptom evolution during the complete test, metabolic measurements ($\dot{V}O_2$, $\dot{V}CO_2$, respiratory exchange ratio), cardiovascular responses (maximum heart rate and heart rate in relation to $\dot{V}O_2$, blood pressure, rhythm and electrocardiogram), and respiratory responses ($\dot{V}E$ in relation to power, $\dot{V}O_2$ and $\dot{V}CO_2$, pattern of breathing [VT and f_b], and arterial oxygen-saturation). Changes following exercise may then be indicated (symptoms, electrocardiographic, spirometric). The conclusion and clinical implications may then be outlined.

SUMMARY

The Stage 1 test is useful as a screening procedure, providing a simple, rapid, and noninvasive means of establishing whether cardiopulmonary responses to exercise are normal. However, its usefulness is not limited to this purpose alone; quantitative information regarding the severity of cardiac or respiratory malfunction is also obtained, which may contribute to clinical assessment.

Example 1

```
Name:                                    Referring Physician:
Sex : M                                  Family Physician:
Age :  49.0 yr.
Ht  : 175.0 cm.                          Reason for Test: Variable chest pain
Wt  :  86.0 kg.
(% of ideal Wt : 130)
Medications:
```

Pulmonary Function & (% predicted)		Gas Exchange & (% predicted)		Muscle Function	
VC 5.5 l (114)	Vemax. 8.5 l/sec.(105)	DLCO 32.0 ml/min/mmHg			1 2 3 4 5 6
FEV1 4.5 l (116)	Ve50 6.1 l/sec.(102)	KCO 4.90 (91)		LEG flex --- --- --- --- --- 48	
FEV1/VC 82 %	Ve25 3.1 l/sec.(104)	VA 6.5 l (101)		ext --- --- --- --- --- 60	
Change in post-	Vimax. 6.5 l/sec.(124)			ARM flex --- --- --- --- --- 58	
exercise FEV1	Vi50 6.0 l/sec.(125)	Hb 15.4 G/dl		ext --- --- --- --- --- 52	
0%	Vi25 5.7 l/sec.(135)			MIP-110 MEP-140 GRIP- 0 N	

EXERCISE RESPONSE

KPM	rest	100	200	300	400	500	600	700	800	900	1000	1100	1200	1300	1400	1500	MECHANICAL
VO2	0.45	0.71	0.78	0.82	0.92	1.13	1.29	1.51	1.74	1.97	2.15	2.25	2.45	2.65	2.82	3.01	
VCO2	0.36	0.55	0.61	0.64	0.74	0.91	1.08	1.28	1.50	1.72	2.05	2.27	2.52	2.82	3.10	3.39	METABOLIC
RER	0.80	0.77	0.78	0.78	0.80	0.81	0.83	0.85	0.86	0.87	0.95	1.01	1.03	1.06	1.10	1.13	
HR	88	92	97	103	110	115	120	126	133	140	148	155	163	172	180	189	
SysBP	130	140		140		150		160		180		190		210		210	CARDIAC
DiaBP	80	80		80		80		85		85		90		90		90	
Ve	15.0	20.0	23.5	27.0	31.2	35.0	40.5	45.0	51.5	56.0	62.0	68.0	79.5	90.0	100.0	110.0	
Vt	1.50	1.70	1.70	1.71	1.85	1.97	2.05	2.17	2.31	2.50	2.60	2.71	2.95	3.02	3.06	3.14	RESPIRATORY
Fb	10	12	14	16	17	18	20	21	22	22	24	25	27	30	33	35	
SaO2	97.0	96.5	96.3	96.0	95.5	95.5	96.0	95.0	96.5	97.0	97.2	97.5	97.3	97.5	97.0	97.0	
Chest																	
Breath								0.5		1.0		2.0		4.0		7.0	SYMPTOMS
Effort						0.5		1.0		2.0		4.0		6.0		9.0	

```
       SYMPTOMS:       Leg Effort    Breathing          Heart Rate (bpm)      Ventilation (l/min)
Maximal           10        10            10
Very,Very Severe   9         9             9
                   8         8             8
Very Severe        7         7             7
                   6         6             6
Severe             5         5             5
Somewhat Severe    4         4             4
Moderate           3         3             3
Slight             2         2             2
Very Slight        1         1             1
Nothing at all     0         0             0
                     25 50 75 100   25 50 75 100
                     KPM % Predicted  KPM % Predicted
```

For Leg Effort and Breathing, lines are 75th & 25th percentiles.   For Heart Rate and Ventilation, lines are predicted values.

Max. work: 1500 (133% pred) kpm   Max. ventilation: 110 (81% pred) l/min   Max. HR 189 (113% pred)

Example 1

Resting Data

The patient was referred for investigation of variable chest pain, not consistently related to exertion (nonanginal). He is slightly overweight (130 per cent of ideal weight). No drugs were being taken. Spirometric results are normal, with a normal ventilatory capacity (MVC = $FEV_1 \times 35$ = 142 L/min). Carbon monoxide uptake is normal, indicating normal pulmonary gas exchange capacity. Respiratory muscle strength and skeletal muscle strength measurements are all in the high-normal range. Cardiovascular variables and the electrocardiogram are normal.

Maximum Power Output

The patient achieves 1500 kpm/min (133 per cent of maximum predicted power).

Symptoms

The patient's exercise capacity is limited by severe leg muscle effort, which prevents the pedaling rate from being maintained. The intensities of leg muscle effort and dyspnea are those expected in relation to the percent of predicted Wmax; he does not experience chest discomfort.

Metabolism

$\dot{V}O_2$max is 3.01 L/min (115 per cent of predicted). The increase in $\dot{V}O_2$ in relation to submaximal power outputs is appropriate (about 170 mL/min for each 100-kpm/min increment). $\dot{V}CO_2$ increases in relation to $\dot{V}O_2$ at low power, but the increase is disproportionate at power outputs greater than 1000 kpm/min (anaerobic threshold at 2.0 L/min $\dot{V}O_2$).

Cardiovascular Responses

Heart rate reaches a maximum of 189 b/min (113 per cent of predicted); at all power outputs, f_c increases normally in relation to $\dot{V}O_2$. At a maximum $\dot{V}O_2$ of 3 L/min, cardiac output is predicted to be 20 L/min; calculated stroke volume is thus 106 mL. Blood pressure increases normally, reaching 210/90 mm Hg; the systolic increase from 130 at rest to 210 is that expected for this age (5.3 mm Hg/100 kpm/min). The electrocardiograph shows J-point depression, with less than 0.5-mm depression of the ST segment at maximum. These electrocardiographic changes are associated with a likelihood ratio of only 0.22 and a post-test probability of about 2 per cent (pretest probability is 4.2 per cent in a 40-year-old man, 10 per cent in a person with nonanginal chest pain).

Respiratory Responses

Ventilation increases normally in relation to power and $\dot{V}CO_2$. Maximal $\dot{V}E$ is 110 L/min, 77 per cent of MVC. The pattern of breathing is normal, with a maximum tidal volume of 3.14 L (57 per cent of VC). Arterial oxygen saturation is maintained in the normal range throughout exercise.

Recovery

Symptoms settle rapidly after exercise. Spirometric values do not change. Electrocardiographic changes revert within 3 minutes of recovery.

Conclusion

This man's exercise capacity is in the high-normal range, and the symptoms experienced and exercise responses are normal. Usual cardiovascular maximal responses were observed, associated with a normal anaerobic threshold, normal cardiac stroke volume, and no increase in the likelihood of coronary artery disease. Although the responses of this subject in stage 2 and 3 studies are used in Chapter 11, such studies are not clinically indicated, because the results would be within the normal expected responses.

Example 2

```
Name: Patient: R. Q.                    Referring Physician:
Sex : F                                 Family Physician:
Age : 35.0 yr.
Ht  : 165.0 cm.                         Reason for Test: Dyspnea, ? EIB
Wt  : 70.0 kg.
(% of ideal Wt : 116)
Medications:
```

Pulmonary Function & (% predicted)			Gas Exchange & (% predicted)		Muscle Function							
VC 3.5 l (93)	Vemax. 4.5 l/sec.(73)		DLCO 20.5 ml/min/mmHg				1	2	3	4	5	6
FEV1 2.4 l (75)	Ve50 3.0 l/sec.(61)		KCO 4.20 (74)		LEG flex	---	---	---	---	---	23
FEV1/VC 69 %	Ve25 1.6 l/sec.(63)		VA 4.9 l (94)		ext	---	---	---	---	---	40
Change in post-	Vimax. 4.0 l/sec.(102)				ARM flex	---	---	---	---	---	46
exercise FEV1	Vi50 3.8 l/sec.(100)		Hb 13.1 G/dl		ext	---	---	---	---	---	40
108%	Vi25 3.5 l/sec.(106)				MIP- 70 MEP- 90 GRIP- 0 N						

EXERCISE RESPONSE

KPM	rest	100	200	300	400	500	600		MECHANICAL
VO2		0.40	0.55	0.76	0.93	1.16	1.25		
VCO2		0.35	0.50	0.71	0.89	1.22	1.37		METABOLIC
RER		0.88	0.91	0.93	0.96	1.05	1.10		
HR		115	120	132	150	165	182		
SysBP		110		125		135	140		CARDIAC
DiaBP		75		80		80	80		
Ve		15.0	24.0	31.0	38.0	42.0	56.0		
Vt		0.84	1.31	1.35	1.41	1.60	1.58		RESPIRATORY
Fb		18	18	23	27	26	35		
SaO2		96.0	96.0	96.0	95.0	95.0	94.0		
Chest									
Breath			0.5	2.0	3.0	5.0	7.0		SYMPTOMS
Effort				1.0	2.0	4.0	5.5		

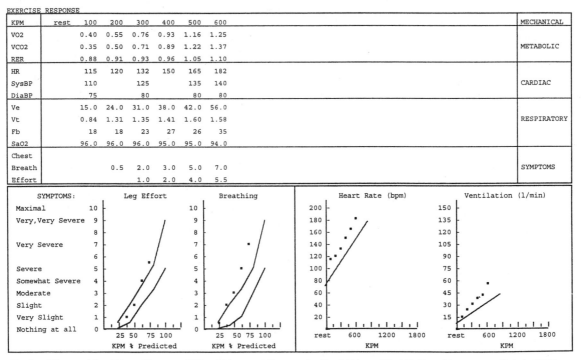

For Leg Effort and Breathing, lines are 75th & 25th percentiles.   For Heart Rate and Ventilation, lines are predicted values.

Max. work: 600 (70% pred) kpm   Max. ventilation: 56 (50% pred) l/min   Max. HR 182 (102% pred)

Example 2

Resting Data

The patient was referred for progressive exercise induced dyspnea; she had had asthma symptoms several years previously. Her weight is average (116 per cent of ideal weight). No drugs were being taken. Spirometry and flow-volume loop show minimal expiratory air flow limitation, and estimated MVC is 84 L/min. Carbon monoxide intake is slightly reduced at 73 per cent of predicted, indicating possible mild impairment of pulmonary gas exchange capacity. Respiratory muscle strength and skeletal muscle strength are normal. Cardiovascular variables are normal, and electrocardiogram also normal.

Maximum Power Output

She achieves 600 kpm/min (70 per cent of maximum predicted power).

Symptoms

The patient's exercise capacity is limited by severe dyspnea. The intensity of dyspnea is increased at all workloads, and leg muscle effort is a little greater than expected at high power output; she does not experience chest discomfort.

Metabolism

$\dot{V}O_2$max is 1.25 L/min (78 per cent of predicted). $\dot{V}O_2$ in submaximal power outputs is appropriate. $\dot{V}CO_2$ increases out of proportion to $\dot{V}O_2$ at power outputs greater than 400 kpm/min (anaerobic threshold at a $\dot{V}O_2$ of 1.0 L/min).

Cardiovascular Responses

Heart rate reaches a maximum of 182 b/min (102 per cent of predicted); at all power outputs, f_c is high in relation to power and $\dot{V}O_2$. At a maximum $\dot{V}O_2$ of 1.25 L/min, cardiac output is predicted to be 11 L/min; calculated stroke volume is thus 62 mL. Blood pressure increases in the low-expected range, reaching 140/80 mm Hg. The electrocardiogram shows no changes in exercise.

Respiratory Responses

Ventilation is high in relation to power and $\dot{V}O_2$; only part of the increase is accounted for by increases in $\dot{V}CO_2$. The pattern of breathing shows a maximum tidal volume of 1.6 L (46 per cent of VC). Arterial oxygen saturation does not change during exercise.

Recovery

Symptoms are slow to resolve. Spirometry values show a small increase in FEV_1, suggesting a minor degree of variability in air flow, but no exercise-induced bronchoconstriction.

Conclusion

This patient's exercise capacity is moderately reduced, but she is limited by severe and excessive dyspnea. Dyspnea is accounted for by an increase in $\dot{V}E$, accompanied by an increase in f_b. Maximum cardiovascular responses were reached, with results suggesting a cardiac stroke volume that is low in relation to body mass. There was evidence of lactate accumulation, but the increases in $\dot{V}E$ were greater than expected for the increase in $\dot{V}CO_2$ alone and suggest that V_D/V_T and/or $\dot{V}A$ are increased. Although no arterial oxygen desaturation occurred, impaired pulmonary gas exchange may have been masked by hyperventilation, as suggested by the impairment of carbon monoxide uptake. Disability is not severe, but the results suggest impaired cardiac and pulmonary function not consistent with an initial diagnosis of exercise-induced asthma; a stage 3 study to document cardiac and gas exchange functions is indicated; the results are detailed in Chapter 11.

Example 3

```
Name: Patient: A. B.                    Referring Physician:
Sex : F                                 Family Physician:
Age : 41.0 yr.
Ht  : 155.0 cm.                         Reason for Test: Post Mitral Valvotomy
Wt  : 51.0 kg.
(% of ideal Wt : 93)
Medications: Beclovent, Ventolin
```

Pulmonary Function & (% predicted)

VC	3.0 l (95)	Vemax.	2.5 l/sec.(45)	
FEV1	0.9 l (33)	Ve50	0.5 l/sec.(11)	
FEV1/VC	30 %	Ve25	0.2 l/sec.(8)	
Change in post-		Vimax.	2.2 l/sec.(52)	
exercise FEV1		Vi50	2.1 l/sec.(55)	
0%		Vi25	2.2 l/sec.(62)	

Gas Exchange & (% predicted)

DLCO	21.0 ml/min/mmHg	
KCO	5.10	(92)
VA	4.1 l	(89)
Hb	13.5 G/dl	

Muscle Function

	1	2	3	4	5	6
LEG flex	---	---	8	---	---	---
ext	---	---	16	---	---	---
ARM flex	---	---	14	---	---	---
ext	---	---	17	---	---	---

MIP- 35   MEP- 40   GRIP-   0 N

EXERCISE RESPONSE

KPM	rest	100	200	300	400	500		
VO2		0.38	0.51	0.75	0.94	1.12		MECHANICAL
VCO2		0.32	0.44	0.66	0.82	1.01		METABOLIC
RER		0.84	0.86	0.88	0.87	0.90		
HR		100	115	130	142	155		
SysBP		110		125		135		CARDIAC
DiaBP		60		65		65		
Ve		12.0	18.0	22.0	28.0	34.0		
Vt		0.74	0.91	1.05	1.20	1.15		RESPIRATORY
Fb		16	20	21	23	30		
SaO2		90.0	90.0	91.0	91.0	90.0		
Chest								
Breath			2.0	3.0	5.5	8.0		SYMPTOMS
Effort	1.0	1.5	2.0	4.0	6.0			

For Leg Effort and Breathing, lines are 75th & 25th percentiles.   For Heart Rate and Ventilation, lines are predicted values.

Max. work: 500 (74% pred) kpm   Max. ventilation: 34 (36% pred) l/min   Max. HR 155 (89% pred)

Example 3

Resting Data

The patient, who has symptoms of chronic bronchitis and a previous history of valvotomy for mitral stenosis, was referred for the evaluation of exertional dyspnea. She was slightly underweight (93 per cent of ideal weight). Inhaled steroids and betamimetics were being taken. Spirometry shows evidence of severe air flow limitation, both inspiratory and expiratory, and estimated MVC is 38 L/min. Carbon monoxide uptake is normal, indicating normal pulmonary gas exchange capacity. Respiratory muscle strength (MIP) is low. Leg muscle strength is also less than predicted. Cardiovascular variables and the electrocardiogram are normal.

Maximum Power Output

The patient achieves 500 kpm/min (74 per cent of maximum predicted power).

Symptoms

Her exercise capacity is limited by severe dyspnea. The intensity of dyspnea is greatly increased, and leg muscle effort is slightly increased to greater-than-expected values, at most workloads.

Metabolism

$\dot{V}O_2$max is 1.12 L/min (85 per cent of predicted). $\dot{V}O_2$ in submaximal power outputs is appropriate to the power output. $\dot{V}CO_2$ increases normally in relation to $\dot{V}O_2$, without evidence of an anaerobic threshold.

Cardiovascular Responses

Heart rate reaches a maximum of 155 b/min (only 89 per cent of predicted); at submaximal power outputs, f_c increases normally in relation to $\dot{V}O_2$. At a maximum $\dot{V}O_2$ of 1.12 L/min, cardiac output is predicted to be 10.6 L/min; calculated stroke volume is thus 68 mL. Blood pressure increases in the low-expected range, reaching 135/65 mm Hg. The electrocardiographic results do not show any changes during exercise.

Respiratory Responses

Ventilation increases normally in relation to power, $\dot{V}O_2$, and $\dot{V}CO_2$, reaching a maximum of 34 L/min, which is close to estimated MVC. The pattern of breathing shows a limited V_T, as expected from spirometry, but the maximum tidal volume of 1.15 L is greater than resting FEV_1. Arterial oxygen saturation is slightly reduced at rest but does not decrease during exercise.

Recovery

Spirometry values are unchanged.

Conclusion

This patient's moderate disability and severe dyspnea are related to air flow limitation and to mild respiratory muscle weakness; cardiac function and pulmonary gas exchange appear to be normal, and no evidence of lactate accumulation is present. It is unlikely that important information would be gained from steady state stage 2 or 3 tests. However, the normal $\dot{V}E$ in a patient with air flow limitation this severe may mask the combination of underventilation (low $\dot{V}A$, high $PaCO_2$) and increased V_D/V_T. A study with blood sampling would identify this combination and would also assess other gas exchange indices (PaO_2 and alveolar-arterial PO_2 difference). This study is included in Chapter 11.

REFERENCES

Adams FH, Linde LM, Miyake H. The physical working capacity of normal schoolchildren. I. Calif Pediatrics 1961;28:55–64.

American College of Sports Medicine. Guidelines for exercise testing and prescription, 3rd ed. Philadelphia: Lea & Febiger; 1986.

American Thoracic Society. ATS Statement: Snowbird workshop and standardization of spirometry. Am Rev Respir Dis 1979;119:831–838.

American Thoracic Society. ATS Statement: Evaluation of impairment/disability secondary to respiratory disorders. Am Rev Respir Dis 1986;133:1205–1209.

American Thoracic Society. ATS Standards for the diagnosis and care of patients with chronic obstructive pulmonary disease (COPD) and asthma. Am Rev Respir Dis 1987;136:225–244.

Åstrand I. Aerobic work capacity in men and women with special reference to age. Acta Physiol Scand 1960;49(Suppl 169):1–92.

Åstrand I, Åstrand P-O, Hallbäck I, Kilbom A. Reduction in maximal oxygen uptake with age. J Appl Physiol 1973;35:649–654.

Åstrand P-O. Experimental Studies of Physical Working Capacity in Relation to Sex and Age. Copenhagen: Munksgaard; 1952.

Åstrand P-O. Human physical fitness, with special reference to sex and age. Physiol Rev 1956;36:307–335.

Åstrand P-O, Rodahl K. Physical work capacity. In: Anonymous, editor. Textbook of Work Physiology: Physiological Bases of Exercise, 2nd ed. New York: McGraw-Hill International Editions; 1977, pp 289–330.

Åstrand P-O, Rodahl K. Textbook of Work Physiology, 2nd ed. New York: McGraw-Hill Book Co.; 1977.

Beaver WL, Wasserman K, Whipp BJ. A new method for detecting anaerobic threshold by gas exchange. J Appl Physiol 1986;60:2020–2027.

Black LF, Hyatt RE. Maximal respiratory pressures: Normal values and relationship to age and sex. Am Rev Respir Dis 1969;99:696–702.

Blackie SP, Fairbarn MS, McElvaney NG, et al: Normal values and ranges for ventilation and breathing pattern at maximal exercise. Chest 1991;100:136–142.

Borg G, Holmgren A, Lindblad I. Quantitative evaluation of chest pain. Acta Med Scand 1981; 664(Suppl):43–45.

Brown AB, McCartney N, Sale DG. Positive adaptations to weight-lifting training in the elderly. J Appl Physiol 1990;69:1725–1733.

Bruce RA, Fisher LD, Cooper MN, Gey GO. Separation of effects of cardiovascular disease and age on ventricular function with maximal exercise. Am J Cardiol 1974;34:757–763.

Bruce RA, Kusumi F, Hosmer D. Maximal oxygen intake and nomographic assessment of functional aerobic impairment in cardiovascular disease. Am Heart J 1973;85:546–562.

Campbell MJ, McComas AJ, Petito F. Physiological changes in ageing muscles. J Neurol Neurosurg Psychiatry 1973;36:174–182.

Clark TJH, Freedman S, Campbell EJM, et al. The ventilatory capacity of patients with chronic airways obstruction. Clin Sci 1969;36:307–316.

Conroy RTWL, O'Brien M. Diurnal variation in athletic performance. J Physiol 1973;234:52P–53P.

Cooper DM, Weiler-Ravell D. Gas exchange response to exercise in children. Am Rev Respir Dis 1984;129:S47–S48.

Cooper DM, Weiler-Ravell D, Whipp BJ, Wasserman K. Aerobic parameters of exercise as a function of body size during growth in children. J Appl Physiol 1984;56:628–634.

Cotes JE. Response to progressive exercise: A three index test. Br J Dis Chest 1972;66:160–184.

Cotes JE. Lung Function, 5th Ed. Oxford: Blackwell Scientific Publications; 1993.

Cotes JE, Adam JER, Anderson HR, et al. Lung function and exercise performance of young adult New Guineans. Hum Biol Oceania 1972;1:316–317.

Cotes JE, Berry G, Burkinshaw L, et al. Cardiac frequency during submaximal exercise in young adults; relation to lean body mass, total body potassium and amount of leg muscle. Q J Exp Physiol 1973;58:239–250.

Cotes JE, Davies CTM, Edholm OG, et al. Factors relating to the aerobic capacity of 46 healthy British males and females, ages 18 to 28 years. Proc R Soc Lond [Biol] 1969;174:91–114.

Crapo RO, Morris AH. Standardized single breath normal values for carbon monoxide diffusing capacity. Am Rev Respir Dis 1981;123:185–189.

Crapo RO, Morris AH, Gardner RM. Reference spirometric values using techniques and equipment that meet ATS recommendations. Am Rev Respir Dis 1981;123:659–664.

Cumming GR. Maximal exercise capacity of children with heart defects. Am J Cardiol 1978;42:613–619.

Cumming GR, Friesen W. Bicycle ergometer measurement of maximal oxygen uptake in children. Can J Physiol Pharmacol 1967;45:937–946.

Cunningham DA, Paterson DH, Blimkie CJR, Donner AP. Development of cardiorespiratory function in circumpubertal boys: A longitudinal study. J Appl Physiol 1984;56:302–307.

Davies CTM. Measuring the fitness of a population. Proc R Soc Med 1969;62:1171–1174.

Davies CTM, Tuxworth W, and Young IM. Physiological effects of repeated exercise. Clin Sci 1970;39:247.

Drinkwater BL, Horvath SM, Wells CL. Aerobic power of females, ages 10 to 68. J Gerontol 1975;30:385–394.

Durand J, Mensch-Dechene J. Relation theoretique entre le debit cardique et la consommation d'oxygene au cours de l'exercice. Bull Eur Physiopath Resp 1979;15:977–998.

Durnin JVGA, Rahaman MM. The assessment of the amount of fat in the human body from measurements of skinfold thickness. Br J Nutr 1967;21:681–689.

Edwards RHT, Miller GJ, Hearn CED, et al. Pulmonary function and exercise responses in relation to body composition and ethnic origin in Trinidadian males. Proc R Soc Lond [Biol] 1972;181:407–420.

El-Manshawi A, Killian KJ, Summers E, Jones NL. Breathlessness during exercise with and without resistive loading. J Appl Physiol 1986;61:896–905.

Fairbarn MS, Blackie SP, McElvaney NG, et al. Prediction of heart rate and oxygen uptake during incremental and maximal exercise in healthy adults. Chest 1994;105:1365–1369.

Faulkner JA, Heigenhauser GF, Shork A. The cardiac output-oxygen uptake relationship of men during graded bicycle ergometry. Med Sci Sports 1977;9:143–147.

Freedman S. Sustained maximum voluntary ventilation. Respir Physiol 1970;8:230–244.

Gadhoke S, Jones NL. The responses to exercise in boys aged 9–15 years. Clin Sci 1969;37:789–801.

Godfrey S. Exercise Testing in Children. Philadelphia: WB Saunders Co.; 1974.

Godfrey S, Davies CTM, Wozniak E, et al. Cardiorespiratory response to exercise in normal children. Clin Sci 1971;40:419–431.

Godin G, Shephard RJ. Body weight and the energy cost of activity. Arch Environ Health 1973;27:289–293.

Grimby G, Saltin B. The ageing muscle. Clin Physiol 1983; 3:209–218.

Guenard H, Emeriau JP, Manier G. Cardiorespiratory aging and muscular exercise. Sci Sport 1994;9:185–188.

Hamilton AL. Sensory Limitations to Voluntary Muscular Performance. Hamilton, Ontario: McMaster University, 1995, PhD Thesis.

Hansen JE, Sue DY, Wasserman K. Predicted values for clinical exercise testing. Am Rev Respir Dis 1984;129:S49–S55.

Hassmén P, Ståhl R, Borg G. Psychophysiological responses to exercise in type A/B men. Psychosom Med 1993;55:178–184.

Heil DP, Freedson PS, Ahlquist LE, et al. Nonexercise regression models to estimate peak oxygen consumption. Med Sci Sports Exerc 1995;27:599–606.

Hey EN, Lloyd BB, Cunningham DJC, et al. Effects of various respiratory stimuli on the depth and frequency of breathing in man. Respir Physiol 1966;1:193–205.

Johnson BD, Badr MS, Dempsey JA. Impact of the aging pulmonary system on the response to exercise. Clin Chest Med 1994;15:229–246.

Jones NL, Ehrsam R. The anaerobic threshold. In: Terjung RL, editor. Exercise and Sports Science Reviews, Vol 10. Philadelphia: Franklin Institute; 1982, pp 49–83.

Jones NL, Haddon RWT. Effect of a meal on cardiopulmonary and metabolic changes during exercise. Can J Physiol Pharmacol 1973;51:445–450.

Jones NL, Kane JW. Quality control of exercise test measurements. Med Sci Sports 1979;11:368–372.

Jones NL, Makrides L, Hitchcock C, et al. Normal standards for an incremental progressive cycle ergometer test. Am Rev Respir Dis 1985;131:700–708.

Jones NL, Rebuck AS. Tidal volume during exercise in patients with diffuse fibrosing alveolitis. Bull Eur Physiopath Resp 1979;15:321–327.

Killian KJ. Symptoms limiting exercise. In: Jones NL, Killian KJ, editors. Breathlessness. The Campbell Symposium. Burlington, Canada: Boehringer-Ingelheim; 1992, pp 132–142.

Knudson RJ, Slatin RC, Lebowitz MD, Burrows B. The maximal expiratory flow-volume curve (normal standards, variability and effects of age). Am Rev Respir Dis 1976;113:587–610.

Lands LC, Gordon C, Bar-Or O, et al. Comparison of three techniques for body composition analysis in cystic fibrosis. J Appl Physiol 1993;75:162–166.

Lands LC, Heigenhauser GJF, Jones NL. Analysis of factors limiting maximal exercise performance in cystic fibrosis. Clin Sci 1992; 83:391–397.

Lands LC, Heigenhauser GJF, Jones NL. Respiratory and peripheral muscle function in cystic fibrosis. Am Rev Respir Dis 1993;147:865–869.

Leblanc P, Bowie DM, Summers E, et al. Breathlessness and exercise in patients with cardiorespiratory disease. Am Rev Respir Dis 1986;133:21–25.

Longhini C, Ganau A, Vaccari M, et al. The response of the aging heart to regular physical exercise: An echo and Doppler study. Acta Cardiol 1995;50:13–16.

MacDougall JD. Morphological changes in human skeletal muscle following strength training and immobilization. In: Jones NL, McCartney N, McComas AJ, editors. Human Muscle Power. Champaign, IL: Human Kinetics Publishers; 1986, pp. 269–285.

Makrides L, Heigenhauser GJF, Jones NL. High-intensity endurance training in 20- to 30- and 60- to 70-year-old healthy men. J Appl Physiol 1990;69:1792–1798.

Makrides L, Heigenhauser GJF, McCartney N, Jones NL. Physical training in young and older healthy subjects. In: Sutton JR, Brock RM, editors. Sports Medicine for the Mature Athlete. Indianapolis: Benchmark Press; 1986.

Maritz JS, Morrison JF, Peter J, et al. A practical method of estimating an individual's maximum oxygen intake. Ergonomics 1961;4:97–122.

Miller GJ, Cotes JE, Hall AM, et al. Lung function and exercise performance of healthy Caribbean men and women of African ethnic origin. Q J Exp Physiol 1972;57:325–341.

Miller GJ, Saunders MJ, Gilson RJC, et al. Lung function in healthy boys and girls in Jamaica in relation to ethnic composition, test exercise performance, and habitual physical activity. Thorax 1977;32:486–496.

Murray MP, Gardner GM, Mollinger LA, Sepic SB. Strength of isometric and isokinetic contractions: Knee muscles of men aged 20–86. Phys Ther 1980;60:412–419.

Myers J, Do D, Herbert W, et al. A nomogram to predict exercise capacity from a specific activity questionnaire and clinical data. Amer J Cardiol 1994;73:591–596.

Ogilvie CM, Forster RE, Blackmore WS, Morton JW. A standardised breath-holding technique for the clinical measurement of diffusing capacity of the lung for carbon monoxide. J Clin Invest 1957;36:1–17.

Orr GW, Green HJ, Hughson RL, Bennett GW. A computer linear regression model to determine ventilatory anaerobic threshold. J Appl Physiol 1982;52;1349–1352.

Port S, Cobb FR, Coleman E, Jones RH. Effect of age on the response of the left ventricular ejection fraction to exercise. N Engl J Med 1980;303:1133–1137.

Robinson S. Experimental studies of physical fitness in relation to age. Arbeitsphysiol 1938;4:251–323.

Sackett DL, Haynes RB, Tugwell P. Clinical Epidemiology: A Basic Science for Clinical Medicine. Boston: Little, Brown & Co.; 1985.

Sannerstedt R. Hemodynamic response to exercise in patients with arterial hypertension. Acta Med Scand 1967; 180(Suppl) 458:699–706.

Seals DR, Taylor JA, Ng AV, Esler MD. Exercise and aging: Autonomic control of the circulation. Med Sci Sports Exerc 1994;26:568–576.

Shephard RJ. Initial "fitness" and personality as determinants of the response to a training regimen. Ergonomics 1966;9:3–16.

Shephard RJ. Endurance Fitness. Toronto: University of Toronto Press; 1969.

Sjöstrand T. A method for the determinations of the total hemoglobin content of the body. Acta Physiol Scand 1948;16:211.

Sjöstrand T. Functional capacity and exercise tolerance in patients with impaired cardiovascular function. In: Gordon BL, editors. Clinical Cardiopulmonary Physiology. New York: Grune & Stratton; 1960.

Spiro SG. Exercise testing in clinical medicine. Br J Dis Chest 1977;71:145–172.

Spiro SG, Juniper E, Bowman P, et al. An increasing work rate test for assessing the physiological strain of submaximal exercise. Clin Sci Mol Med 1974;46:191–206.

Vaitkevicius PV, Fleg JL, Engel JH, et al. Effects of age and aerobic capacity on arterial stiffness in healthy adults. Circulation 1993;88:1456–1462.

Vogel JA, Patton JF, Mello RP, Daniels WL. An analysis of aerobic capacity in a large United States population. J Appl Physiol 1986;60:494–500.

Voigt ED, Engel P, Klein H. Daily fluctuations of the performance-pulse index. Ger Med Mon 1967;12:394–395.

Wasserman K. The anaerobic threshold measurement to evaluate exercise performance. Am Rev Respir Dis 1984; 129(Suppl)1:S35–S40.

Wasserman K, Hansen JE, Sue DY, et al. Principles of Exercise Testing and Interpretation. Philadelphia: Lea & Febiger; 1987.

Wasserman K, Sue D. Impact of integrative cardiopulmonary exercise testing on clinical decision making. Chest 1991; 99:981–992.

Wasserman K, Whipp BJ. Exercise physiology in health and disease: State of the art. Am Rev Respir Dis 1975;112:219–249.

Weng T-R, Levison H. Standards of pulmonary function in children. Am Rev Respir Dis 1969;99:879–894.

Young A, Skelton DA. Applied physiology of strength and power in old age. Int J Sport Med 1994;15:149–151.

9

Conduct of Stages 2, 3, and 4 Exercise Tests

In contrast to the stage 1 procedure in which the workload is incremented at the end of each minute, workloads in the stage 2, 3, and 4 tests are sustained for several minutes in order to allow metabolism and the cardiac and respiratory responses to reach a "steady state" that is maintained for as long as is needed for all the recordings to be made. Initially this protocol was chosen in the belief that a steady state was essential for valid estimation of cardiac output and pulmonary gas exchange variables, but it has been shown that most measurements may be made in a relatively unsteady state as long as blood samples are taken and related measurements are made simultaneously. For example, cardiac output measurements are similar if related to the oxygen intake measured at the same time (McKelvie et al., 1987; Campbell et al., 1989). Also, there are practical reasons for retaining the protocol because the measurements often are complex and time consuming.

Central to both stage 2 and stage 3 tests is the measurement of oxygenated mixed venous P_{CO_2} ($P\bar{v}_{CO_2}$) by rebreathing. In the stage 2 procedure, the measurement is used in conjunction with other noninvasive measurements in order to estimate cardiac output, alveolar and dead space ventilation, and changes in blood lactate concentration. In the stage 3 test, $P\bar{v}_{CO_2}$ is used with arterial P_{CO_2} (Pa_{CO_2}) to calculate cardiac output. In the stage 4 test, a central venous catheter is introduced percutaneously, and mixed venous blood is sampled in order to obtain direct measurements of mixed venous oxygen and carbon dioxide. This technique is usually reserved for clinical problems that require measurement of pulmonary artery pressures; because the methods used are well established in cardiac catheterization laboratories, I do not describe them in any detail. Before the test procedures are detailed, a brief account of my reasons for adopting the measurement of $P\bar{v}_{CO_2}$ may be helpful.

The changes in cardiac output and pulmonary gas exchange, which emphasize the need for practical methods for their measurement during exercise, were reviewed in Chapter 2.

MEASUREMENT OF CARDIAC OUTPUT

The standard method for cardiac output measurement, against which other methods have usually been judged, is the direct Fick method, in which the Fick principle is applied to measurements of oxygen intake and the arteriovenous oxygen content difference. The method requires central venous and peripheral arterial blood sampling, and a high degree of accuracy in the associated analytical measurements is difficult to achieve. Central venous and arterial catheterizations are also necessary in the dye dilution and thermodilution methods of cardiac output measurement; furthermore, the dilution curves become less reliable in heavy exercise.

In the "foreign gas" methods for cardiac output, the uptake of a soluble gas by the lungs is measured during steady state inhalation rebreathing. Acetylene was widely used for many years (Grollman, 1929) but was almost completely abandoned in favor of the direct Fick method; recently, it has regained popularity in exercise physiology (Pugh, 1964; Winsborough et al., 1980; Smyth et al., 1984; Hsia et al., 1995). Nitrous oxide has also been successfully applied in exercise, either in a steady state method (Becklake et al., 1962) or in rebreathing (Rigatto, 1967; Ayotte et al., 1970). No blood sampling is required. Probably the main drawbacks of these methods are (1) the need for specific analyzers and (2) the difficulty in measuring mean alveolar gas concentrations in any subject with poor alveolar mixing.

THE INDIRECT FICK CARBON DIOXIDE METHOD

Methods based on the measurement of carbon dioxide may be noninvasive, are easily repeatable, and are technically simple and reliable. The same analyzer is used in the measurement of all three terms in the Fick equation. Several methods are available that have been widely used in subjects at rest and during exercise. All use the lung as a tonometer, and the assumption is made that the P_{CO_2} in alveolar gas is the same as that in the pulmonary capillary blood. The approach was popular at the beginning of the century (Plesch, 1909) but later fell into disfavor, mainly because sufficient accuracy could not be obtained with instruments available at the time. The advent of rapid and accurate physical gas analyzers led to a reintroduction of the method (Collier, 1956; Defares, 1958), which was soon followed by its application to exercise physiology (Ashton and McHardy, 1963; Jernérus et al., 1963; Faulkner et al., 1968). Although the rebreathing principle may also be used for estimating mixed venous P_{O_2} (Denison et al., 1971), the accompanying severe transient hypoxemia makes it unsuitable for routine use. A number of methods have been described that fall into three groups according to the respiratory maneuver used to obtain an estimate of mixed venous P_{CO_2} or cardiac output: prolonged expiration; rebreathing from a bag containing a low or zero concentration of carbon dioxide; and rebreathing from a bag containing gas having a P_{CO_2} in excess of $P\bar{v}_{CO_2}$.

Although these methods are all based on the same principle—the application of the Fick principle to carbon dioxide—they differ widely in the measurements used to obtain the Fick equation variables:

$$\dot{Q}tot = \frac{\dot{V}_{CO_2}}{C\bar{v}_{CO_2} - Ca_{CO_2}}$$

$\dot{V}_{CO_2}$ may be measured in a steady state or during rebreathing; $C\bar{v}_{CO_2}$ is derived from $P\bar{v}_{CO_2}$, estimated by extrapolation of the rise in $P_{ET_{CO_2}}$ during a long expiration or rebreathing; Ca_{CO_2} is derived from Pa_{CO_2}, which is either measured or estimated from $P_{ET_{CO_2}}$ in the steady state or during rebreathing.

THE DISSOCIATION CURVE OF CARBON DIOXIDE IN WHOLE BLOOD

Contents of carbon dioxide are derived from pressures by use of some form of the carbon dioxide dissociation curve; even in this respect, there have been differences between the different methods. The differences account for one potential source of variation or error. Initially, a slope of 0.45 mL/dL/mm Hg was assumed for the carbon dioxide dissociation curve, or a standard curve was used, but these were found to be inadequate. The complexities of the curve rival those of the oxygen dissociation curve, and for this reason, the greatest accuracy is obtained from the most exact description of the curve that is available. At the time a carbon dioxide rebreathing method was being developed, McHardy (1967) reviewed previous work on the curve from the standpoint of its application to the measurement of cardiac output in exercise. From first principles, the content of carbon dioxide in plasma at given pH may be derived from

P_{CO_2} and the Henderson-Hasselbalch equation, with the solubility of carbon dioxide being assumed. The content in whole blood may then be derived by application of factors that describe the influence of hemoglobin content, oxygen saturation, and pH. McHardy pointed out that Peters and colleagues (1924) had shown that the curve was linearized by expressing both content and pressure as logarithms, and he constructed tables and a graph to express arteriovenous content differences in terms of pressure differences for a hemoglobin of 15 g/dL, a pH of 7.4, a venous oxygen saturation of 100 per cent (during rebreathing pulmonary capillary blood is assumed to be fully saturated), and an arterial oxygen saturation of 95 per cent. McHardy went on to show that the content differences so derived could then be corrected for different hemoglobin concentrations and arterial oxygen saturations (Loeppky et al., 1983). This left the effect of pH (Visser, 1960) unaccounted for; at that time, the method was bloodless, and the small effect of changes in pH was ignored. Later, Godfrey (1970) presented equations that incorporated a correction for the effect of acid-base changes, as assessed by measurements of base excess, on the slope of the $\log_e P_{CO_2}$:$\log_e C_{CO_2}$ curve. Studies that have compared calculations based on the McHardy equations, equations given in previous editions of this book, and the equations of Godfrey have demonstrated differences in derived contents (Paterson and Cunningham, 1976) that are accounted for by slight differences in constants and inappropriate rounding off of some factors. The equations have been reviewed in view of these studies, and the following approach is suggested.

In a bloodless test, in which hemoglobin and arterial oxygen saturation are known or may be safely assumed, the pressures may be converted into contents by applying the following equation, which describes McHardy's tabular data (1967) for a hemoglobin value of 15 g/dL and an S_{O_2} of 100 per cent:

$$\log_e C_{CO_2} = [0.396 \times \log_e P_{CO_2}] + 2.38$$

Arterial and venous carbon dioxide contents are separately calculated, and the content difference is then corrected for differences in hemoglobin from 15 g/dL or in arterial S_{O_2} from 100 per cent, as detailed later in the chapter. An alternative is to use arterial and mixed venous P_{CO_2} to calculate the content difference, using relationships that assume arterial S_{O_2} to be 95 per cent; this calculation may be performed with McHardy's graph (see Chapter 2), or with the equation

$$C\bar{v} - a_{CO_2} = 10.38 (P\bar{v}_{CO_2}^{0.396} - Pa_{CO_2}^{0.396})$$

If arterial pH has been measured and corrected for, the McHardy equations may be solved from first principles by use of a computer program; the equations are listed in Appendix B, Table B–1. Alternatively, Godfrey's equations (1974) may be used to correct the slope of the logarithmic carbon dioxide dissociation curve for changes in base excess. However, a small difference between these two approaches remains owing to the use of a different solubility coefficient of carbon dioxide in plasma at 37°C (0.0307, compared with 0.030). A more complete equation is provided by Douglas and co-workers (1988).

MEASUREMENT OF MIXED VENOUS $P\bar{v}CO_2$

Several methods have been used to obtain $P\bar{v}CO_2$ indirectly, without blood sampling. The reader is referred to the original descriptions for details of the methods; the brief descriptions below indicate the relative complexity of each and outline our reasons for adopting one technique for routine use in preference to the others.

Gas Analysis During a Single Expiration

In this method, used by Kim and co-workers (1966) to derive a "true" $P\bar{v}CO_2$ (the PCO_2 of pulmonary venous blood with low oxygen saturation), expired gas is rapidly analyzed at the mouth by a respiratory mass spectrometer for oxygen and carbon dioxide concentrations. PCO_2 is plotted against the instantaneous respiratory exchange ratio (R), which progressively falls during expiration, owing to the difference between the rates at which oxygen leaves and carbon dioxide enters alveolar gas. The PCO_2 corresponding to the steady state R obtained before the long expiration is assumed to be equal to arterial PCO_2, and the PCO_2 at an R of 0.32 is taken to be $P\bar{v}CO_2$. Thus, the method is based on the fact that for every unit volume of oxygen taken

up by the hemoglobin of venous blood, a 0.32 volume of carbon dioxide is evolved without a change in PCO_2. Thus, at an R of 0.32, the oxygenated PCO_2 in pulmonary capillary blood is equal to the PCO_2 in deoxygenated pulmonary arterial blood. However, in order for the measurement of R at the mouth to reflect the instantaneous mean alveolocapillary R, ventilation and perfusion in the lung must be ideally matched, and alveolar emptying during expiration must be uniform. It is doubtful if these conditions exist in healthy subjects, and it is certain that they do not exist in patients with cardiac or pulmonary disease. Although well validated in anesthetized dogs (Hainsworth et al., 1981), the method cannot be recommended for use in clinical exercise testing, based on current evidence (Inman et al., 1985).

Rebreathing from a Bag Containing a Low Concentration of Carbon Dioxide in Oxygen (Exponential Method)

This process is the basis of several methods that use the exponential rise in PCO_2 toward an asymptote (the equilibrium PCO_2, $PEqCO_2$) to calculate $P\bar{v}CO_2$ for subsequent use in the Fick equation (Fig. 9–1). They may be termed "exponential" or "extrapolation" methods in order to distinguish them from the "equilibration" method in which the equilibrium PCO_2 is measured. In the earliest descriptions of this approach, the end-tidal PCO_2 of each breath during rebreathing and before recirculation (15 seconds) was plotted against the end-tidal PCO_2 of the preceding breath; a straight line drawn through the points was extrapolated to a line of identity (Fig. 9–2; method A) (Defares, 1958; Jernérus et al., 1963). This value is the PCO_2 at which no carbon dioxide is added to the lung/bag and thus is equal to oxygenated $P\bar{v}CO_2$. Godfrey and Wolf (1972) compared the accuracy and precision of $P\bar{v}CO_2$ measured by this extrapolation method with that measured by the equilibrium method and found

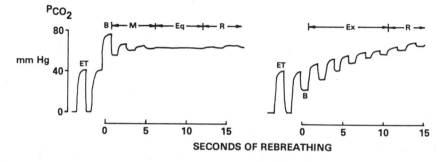

Figure 9–1. Records of PCO_2 during rebreathing in exercise, showing typical records obtained with the equilibrium method *(left)* and the exponential method *(right)*. ET = end-tidal PCO_2 before rebreathing; B = initial bag concentration; M = mixing between bag and lungs in equilibrium method; Eq = equilibrium "plateau"; Ex = "exponential" rise in PCO_2 toward asymptote; R = recirculation.

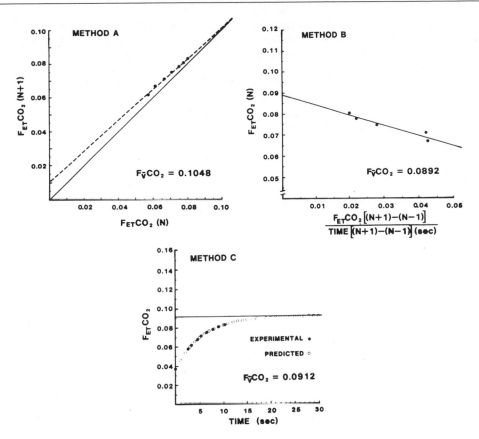

Figure 9–2. Three methods of analysis for the exponential method, using data from the same rebreathe; note the variation in derived $P\bar{v}CO_2$. The computer-derived best fit curve (c), solved for t = 20 sec, was found to be the most precise. (Reprinted from da Silva GA, et al. Measurement of mixed venous CO_2 pressure by rebreathing during exercise. Respir Physiol 1985;59:379–392, with permission from Elsevier Science.)

a larger variation between duplicate estimates using the extrapolation method. The variability is reduced by ensuring that the subject breathes at a constant frequency and by using a statistical method to calculate the asymptote of the exponential rise in end-tidal P_{CO_2}. A computer program allows an iterative technique to be applied to log ($P\bar{v}CO_2$ − $P_{ET}CO_2$), which hunts for the value of $P\bar{v}CO_2$ that will minimize the variance of the points around the least squares regression line (Heigenhauser et al., 1978). With this method, the variance of repeated measurements was 2.7 per cent, and the $P\bar{v}CO_2$ obtained was always within ± 10 per cent of that derived by the equilibration method (Heigenhauser and Jones, 1979). The method was refined further by da Silva and associates (1985); after computer analysis and curve fitting (see Fig. 9–2, method C), the P_{CO_2} at 20 seconds is obtained by extrapolation (Jones and Rebuck, 1973) and may be used as $P\bar{v}CO_2$. This method has been successfully used to assess the cardiac output responses in stage 1 tests applied to healthy subjects and to patients with cardiac disease (McKelvie et al., 1987; Campbell et al., 1989).

Instead of using rebreathing to estimate $P\bar{v}CO_2$, which is then used in the Fick equation with steady state measurements of carbon dioxide output and arterial P_{CO_2}, Farhi and co-workers (1976) took a different approach; they devised an elegant technique to measure all the Fick equation variables during rebreathing. Briefly, this method uses a measured volume of air or high oxygen concentration for rebreathing; deep breaths lead to an initial fall in end-tidal P_{CO_2}, which then climbs back as carbon dioxide accumulates in the bag at a measured rate; rebreathing is continued for about 15 seconds after the control (pre-rebreathing) $P_{ET}CO_2$ has been reached. The carbon dioxide output for the few breaths that $P_{ET}CO_2$ takes to climb back to the control value is calculated, together with the average $P_{ET}CO_2$ during this time, taken to be equal to mean P_aCO_2. The asymptote of the exponential rise in $P_{ET}CO_2$ for the complete rebreathing period is taken to be the equilibrium P_{CO_2}, ($P_{Eq}CO_2$). A standard carbon dioxide dissociation curve is used to obtain $C\bar{v}CO_2$ and C_aCO_2 from $P_{Eq}CO_2$ and P_aCO_2, respectively.

The method described and well validated by Winsborough and colleagues (1980) is similar in some respects to the method of Farhi and associates, except that it uses a two-stage procedure. Instead of calculating an asymptote for the rise in P_{ETCO_2} during rebreathing in the first stage, a second stage is used for obtaining an equilibrium of carbon dioxide between the rebreathing bag and the lungs. The cardiac output is calculated from the rate of rise in P_{ETCO_2} toward this equilibrium. In this way, the method may be considered a combination of the exponential and equilibration methods.

The exponential (extrapolation) methods all share two main advantages over the equilibration method: (1) the choice of the initial breathing bag volume and carbon dioxide concentration is simple and (2) rebreathing is less uncomfortable, particularly at high levels of exercise. However, they have a major disadvantage in being relatively more dependent on uniform lung emptying. Thus, although they may be preferable in healthy subjects at high exercise loads, the exponential methods are less applicable to patients with cardiopulmonary disease. If the advantages outweigh the disadvantages for a given application, our recommendation is the method described by da Silva and co-workers (1985), which is relatively simple to perform and yields reliable results (McKelvie et al., 1987).

Rebreathing from a Bag Containing a High Concentration of Carbon Dioxide in Oxygen (Equilibration Method)

If rebreathing is carried out with a bag at a P_{CO_2} sufficiently higher than $P\bar{v}_{CO_2}$, the gas in the bag mixes with alveolar gas, and the P_{CO_2} decreases to reach an equilibrium (see Fig. 9–1). At this point, the subject breathes in and out of the bag, but the P_{CO_2} remains constant, indicating that alveolar P_{CO_2} is equal to oxygenated $P\bar{v}_{CO_2}$. Good equilibration is obtained if the bag volume is carefully chosen to obtain rapid mixing between the bag and alveolar gas and if the initial carbon dioxide concentration is also chosen appropriately. Satisfactory equilibration may be obtained even in patients with severe ventilation-perfusion disturbances in the lungs; this is because poorly ventilated areas that might equilibrate slowly already contain gas with a composition close to that of mixed venous blood.

In this method, $\dot{V}_{CO_2}$ is measured in a steady state before rebreathing, and arterial P_{CO_2} is measured or estimated from the steady state end-tidal P_{CO_2} measurements. Mixed venous P_{CO_2} is obtained from the equilibrium P_{CO_2}, and blood carbon dioxide contents are derived by use of a standard carbon dioxide dissociation curve. The Fick equation may then be solved for cardiac output.

When this method was first used during exercise,

the calculated values for cardiac output were systematically low, particularly at high power outputs, when the discrepancy was as high as 10 per cent (Jones et al., 1967). This was because values for the rebreathing equilibrium P_{CO_2} led to overestimation of $P\bar{v}_{CO_2}$. When arterial blood was sampled during rebreathing and an appropriate allowance was made for the lung-to-artery circulation time, P_{aCO_2} was found to be lower than the equilibrium gas phase P_{CO_2}. Because the blood was being sampled "downstream" from the lungs, the alveolar-to-blood P_{CO_2} difference became known as the "downstream difference." Later studies confirmed the difference and allowed an empirical correction to be derived (Jones et al., 1969). Other studies in which pulmonary artery blood was sampled showed that an "upstream" difference also existed (Denison et al., 1969). Because these studies suggested that there was incomplete equilibration of carbon dioxide, either between alveolar gas and pulmonary capillary blood or between the plasma and the red cell, they created a lively discussion, which is concisely summarized in an editorial debate in the *Journal of Applied Physiology* (Forster, 1977; Gurtner, 1977). Early on, some reports appeared to show that allowance for the "downstream difference" was not necessary in calculating cardiac output (Godfrey et al., 1971), and Scheid and Piiper, in a series of publications, have argued that it is explained on technical rather than physiological grounds (for a summary see Scheid and Piiper, 1980). However, there were important differences between the methods described here and those of Godfrey and co-workers (1971), and Scheid and Piiper (1980) have not shown that the effect is absent in exercising humans. Several reports that tested the validity of rebreathing cardiac output measurements are in agreement that the correction should be made (Paterson et al., 1976; Reybrouck, 1978; Wolfe et al., 1978; Van Herwaarden et al., 1980; Paterson et al., 1976, 1982; Mahler et al., 1985a, 1985b; McElvaney et al., 1989).

Thus, although the finding and its cause remain controversial, we continue to believe that a correction needs to be applied to the rebreathing equilibrium P_{CO_2} value to derive $P\bar{v}_{CO_2}$ for the calculation of cardiac output during exercise. At rest, the effect appears to be absent, and no correction is needed (Davis et al., 1978).

Patterns of Equilibration During Rebreathing

The method used to obtain a carbon dioxide equilibration reading during rebreathing uses a 5-L anesthesia bag containing a mixture of carbon dioxide guessed to contain a P_{CO_2} higher than $P\bar{v}_{CO_2}$ but not so high as to hinder rapid equilibration or to cause distress. In practice, the carbon dioxide con-

Table 9–1. SUGGESTED INITIAL BAG CO₂ CONCENTRATIONS REQUIRED TO OBTAIN REBREATHING CO₂ EQUILIBRIUM				
Power Output		O₂ Uptake (L/min)	End-Tidal Pco₂ (mm Hg)	Bag CO₂ Concentration (%)
(kpm/min)	(watts)			
300	50	1	30	10.5
			40	11.5
600	100	1.5	30	11.0
			40	12.0
900	150	2.2	30	12.0
			40	13.0
1200	200	3.0	30	13.0
			40	14.0

centration required is usually between 9 and 15 per cent carbon dioxide in oxygen, with higher concentrations being required in heavy exercise when P$\bar{v}$CO₂ is high. An educated guess may be made by reference to an empirical recipe (Table 9–1). The volume of the rebreathing mixture is 1.5 to 2 times the subject's tidal volume.

For starting rebreathing, a tap at the mouthpiece is switched at the end of a normal expiration and rebreathing is continued (a) until an equilibrium is recognized by inspection of the record or (b) for 15 seconds; there is no point in continuing beyond this time because of recirculation. Four main patterns in the carbon dioxide recording may be obtained during rebreathing (Fig. 9–3):

1. Pattern A. The Pco₂ rises continuously and steeply, owing to evolution of carbon dioxide from mixed venous blood, indicating that the initial bag Pco₂ is too low for an equilibrium to be obtained.

2. Pattern B. A transient equilibrium occurs for one complete breathing cycle only (in-out-in), followed by a relatively steep rise in Pco₂ that occurs too early to be explained by recirculation. This pattern indicates a

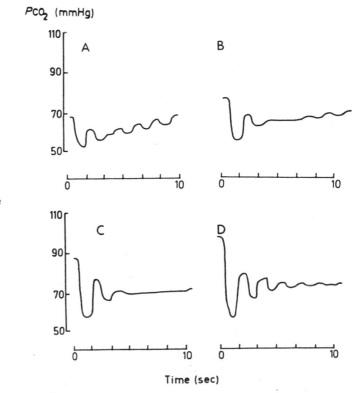

Figure 9–3. Records of Pco₂ during the rebreathing of four mixtures of increasing CO₂ concentration to show the equilibration patterns that may occur.

transient equilibration between the bag and alveolar gas, before alveolar gas has reached equilibrium with mixed venous P_{CO_2}, so that on the next expiration into the bag the P_{CO_2} has risen.

3. Pattern C. A constant P_{CO_2} is reached and is maintained for several breaths until recirculation occurs to raise $P\bar{v}_{CO_2}$ after 9 to 20 seconds (Sowton et al., 1968).

4. Pattern D. The initial P_{CO_2} is so high or the bag volume is so large that an equilibrium is not obtained before recirculation.

Pattern C indicates an ideal equilibrium pattern; if this is obtained during the first attempt, further rebreathing is not required. If pattern A or B is obtained, the procedure is repeated with a higher bag carbon dioxide concentration; if pattern D is obtained, a lower bag carbon dioxide concentration is used. Unless the pattern suggests that the initial bag carbon dioxide concentration was highly inappropriate, subsequent concentrations are increased or decreased by increments of 2 per cent carbon dioxide.

If an equilibrium "plateau" is not obtained, an estimate may be made by the extrapolation of a line joining the points for expired P_{CO_2} at 8 and 12 seconds of rebreathing to that at 20 seconds (Fig. 9–4). This value is within ± 2 mm Hg of the equilibrium value (Jones and Rebuck, 1973).

Occasionally, large brief changes in carbon dioxide are seen in the rebreathing record that are usually due to complete emptying of the bag, collapse of the neck of the bag (remedied by a wire cage or spiral), leakage, or transient blockage of the analyzer sample line.

PROCEDURES FOR STAGE 2, STAGE 3, AND STAGE 4 TESTS

Measurements are made in the steady state at rest and at a minimum of two power outputs chosen according to the results obtained from a preliminary stage 1 procedure. A preceding stage 1 test is important for a number of reasons. First, it establishes power outputs at which the patient may be safely tested in a steady state. Second, it prepares the patient for a test that is potentially uncomfortable (rebreathing, blood sampling), by (a) demonstrating to the patient that he or she can perform the test and (b) serving as a basis for explanation of the additional procedures in detail. Third, it allows measurements made during a steady state to be placed in the context of the total exercise response obtained from the stage 1 test. Usually, in stage 2 and stage 3 tests, power outputs of one third and two thirds of the maximum achieved during a stage 1 test are used.

In the stage 3 procedure, an intra-arterial catheter is placed or preparations for capillary blood sampling are made 20 to 30 minutes before the study is carried out. The same timing applies to the central venous catheterization in stage 4 studies.

Equipment

The following equipment is needed for these tests:

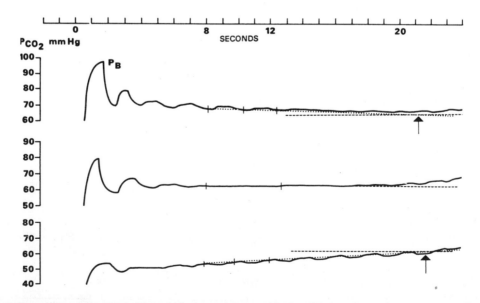

Figure 9–4. P_{CO_2} during rebreathing. The middle trace shows an ideal equilibrium, the upper is too high, and the lower is too low. Extrapolation of the lines joining the end-expiratory values between 8 and 12 seconds of rebreathing intersect at the same point, at 20 to 22 seconds (indicated by arrows) in each example.

- Calibrated cycle ergometer
- Respiratory valve assembly, including rebreathing bag and tap
- Expired gas mixing chamber
- Ventilation measurement by dry gas meter (inspired), Tissot spirometer (expired), or integrated pneumotachograph
- One-lead electrocardiograph
- Carbon dioxide analyzer with sampling lines and switching circuitry for sampling at the lips and in mixed expired gas
- System for mixing carbon dioxide and oxygen for rebreathing gas mixtures
- Oxygen analyzer for mixed expired gas analysis
- Multichannel recorder, with six channels of basic information—time, electrocardiograph, ventilation, mixed expired and end-tidal carbon dioxide, rebreathing carbon dioxide, and mixed expired oxygen
- Blood sampling facilities and blood gas electrode system (for stage 3 tests)

Stage 2 Procedure

In a busy exercise laboratory performing stage 2 and stage 3 tests, weekly quality control studies are carried out to check the operation of the total system. The responses of the carbon dioxide and oxygen analyzers are also documented regularly so that differences in analytical delays may be allowed for.

For stage 2 and stage 3 studies, if a preliminary stage 1 procedure has been carried out, only one electrocardiograph lead is required; an electrode should be placed in the V_5 position, with an independent electrode on the sternum or forehead to reduce interference from muscle artefact. The subject is seated on the ergometer, and the positions of the saddle, handlebars, and respiratory valve are adjusted. The oxygen and carbon dioxide analyzers are calibrated through deflections obtained for standard gases; our habit is to use two channels for carbon dioxide, with the gain adjusted to achieve adequate reading accuracy—at least 1 mm of paper for 1 mm Hg of pressure. One channel is used for mixed expired and end-tidal gas (0 to 7 per cent carbon dioxide), and another channel is used in a higher range (6 to 13 per cent carbon dioxide) for rebreathing; three calibration gases are used for each channel; carbon dioxide mixtures in air are used for the low-range channel, but owing to the interference by oxygen of infrared carbon dioxide analysis in rebreathing, carbon dioxide mixtures in 40 per cent oxygen are used for the higher range. Two standard gases are usually used for calibrating the oxygen analyzer, in addition to air.

Resting measurements are made after 5 to 10 minutes of breathing through the respiratory circuitry; there is little point in extending these observations over a longer period to achieve a perfect steady state at rest. The two exercise power outputs usually are performed without a break between. In each state (rest and exercise), cardiac frequency, end-tidal P_{CO_2}, and oxygen and carbon dioxide concentrations in expired gas are monitored for establishment of a steady state in these variables. Variations of less than $\pm$ 5 beats in cardiac frequency, and of less than $\pm$ 0.1 per cent in expired carbon dioxide and oxygen concentrations, indicate an adequate steady state. Measurements of all the variables are made during the first minute after achievement of a steady state. In a stage 3 test, a blood sample is taken at this time. At the end of the minute and after an examination of the data to ensure that the steady state has been maintained, the rebreathing bag is prepared for the measurement of mixed venous P_{CO_2}. The breathing tap is turned at the end of an expiration so that the subject breathes in a full tidal volume from the rebreathing bag, which is almost emptied; the subject is encouraged to take several rapid deep breaths in order to ensure good mixing between the gas in the bag and that in the lungs. The fluctuation of carbon dioxide content in gas sampled at the mouth is examined to establish whether an adequate tracing has been obtained, and once an equilibrium pattern has been recognized, or after 15 seconds of rebreathing, the tap is turned to allow the subject to breathe room air again. Rebreathing may be repeated if the initial rebreathing is unsatisfactory, after at least 30 seconds has passed so that any accumulated carbon dioxide has been excreted. Once an adequate rebreathing phase has been completed, the cycle ergometer is adjusted for the next stage of the test. At the end of the highest power output, it is usually wise to allow the subject to perform loadless pedaling for a few minutes, and in a patient with known ischemic heart disease, the electrocardiogram is monitored for 10 minutes after the test.

At the end of the test, the gas analyzers are recalibrated.

Recordings

During the test, the following data are obtained (Fig. 9–5), which provide the basis for subsequent calculations:

- From the timer channel of the recorder, the paper length (in centimeters) for 1 minute
- From the electrocardiograph, the paper length for 5 RR intervals
- Paper deflection for 1 L of ventilation (the volume factor)

STAGE II TEST ROUTINE

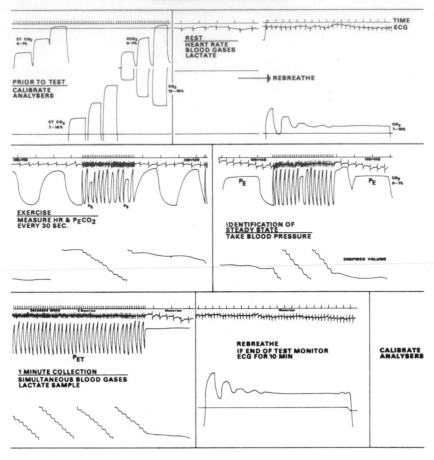

Figure 9–5. Examples of recording made during an exercise test (one third actual size).

- Cumulative deflection for ventilation during the steady state period, either inspiration or expiration, depending on the instrument used
- Carbon dioxide calibration curve, and deflections for mixed expired, end-tidal, and equilibrium rebreathing gases
- Oxygen calibration curve and deflections for mixed expired gas

Calculations

1. Cardiac frequency is measured as outlined for the stage 1 test.
2. Ventilation is measured as in the stage 1 test. Because oxygen intake and carbon dioxide output are measured in a stage 2 test, both expired and inspired ventilation must be known. Also, by convention, ventilation is usually expressed as expired ventilation in this test. If inspired ventilation has been measured, $\dot{V}_E$ is calculated using the Haldane correction, which is based

on the fact that negligible amounts of nitrogen are absorbed and excreted.

$$\dot{V}_E \times F_{EN_2} = \dot{V}_I \times F_{IN_2}$$

$$\dot{V}_E = (\dot{V}_I \times F_{IN_2}) \div F_{EN_2}$$

Similarly, if only $\dot{V}_E$ is measured, $\dot{V}_I$ is calculated. There is some controversy regarding the correction because small amounts of nitrogen may be exchanged in the lungs (Cissik et al., 1972), but in practice, the correction is still valid.

F_{IN_2} and F_{EN_2} are obtained by subtracting the sum of inspired oxygen and carbon dioxide and expired oxygen and carbon dioxide concentrations, respectively, from 1.0:

$$F_{IN_2} = 1.0 - (0.2093 + 0.0003)$$
$$= .7904$$
$$F_{EN_2} = 1.0 - (F_{EO_2} + F_{ECO_2})$$

Two values for ventilation are derived. The first

represents the volume changes in the lungs during breathing, and it is calculated for the conditions that exist in the lungs—that is, at body temperature (37°C) and ambient pressure and saturated with water vapor (BTPS). The second is used to calculate the quantities of oxygen and carbon dioxide exchanged in milliliters per minute (or millimoles per minute), and because these represent metabolic equivalents, they are calculated at standard temperature (0°C) and pressure (760 mm Hg).

a. To calculate $\dot{V}_E$ (BTPS) from $\dot{V}_E$ (ATP) we need to know, additionally, the ambient temperature (T_A°C) and pressure (P_B mm Hg), and the ambient humidity (per cent). Ambient temperature in °C is converted to absolute temperature (°K) by adding 273. The percentage of humidity is converted to ambient water vapor pressure (P_{H_2O}, A) by fractional multiplication of the saturated water vapor pressure at the ambient temperature obtained from a table or an equation; for example, 60 per cent humidity at 20°C (P_{H_2O}, A of fully saturated gas = 17.5 mm Hg) represents 17.5 × 0.6 or 10.5 mm Hg of water vapor pressure. Then

$$\dot{V}_E \text{ (BTPS)} = \dot{V}_E \text{ (ATP)} \times \frac{273 + 37}{273 + T_A}$$
$$\times \frac{P_B - P_{H_2O}, A}{P_B - 47}$$

b. To calculate $\dot{V}_I$ (STPD) and $\dot{V}_E$ (STPD), the following equations are used:

$$\dot{V}_I \text{ (STPD)} = \dot{V}_I \text{ (ATP)} \times \frac{273}{273 + T_A}$$
$$\times \frac{P_B - P_{H_2O}, A}{760}$$

$$\dot{V}_E \text{ (STPD)} = \dot{V}_E \text{ (ATP)} \times \frac{273}{273 + T_A}$$
$$\times \frac{P_B - P_{H_2O}, A}{760}$$

3. Breathing frequency is measured as described for the stage 1 test.
4. Tidal volume is derived by dividing $\dot{V}_E$ (BTPS) by breathing frequency.
5. Expired carbon dioxide concentration is derived from the recorder deflections and the carbon dioxide calibration curve. The P_{CO_2} of mixed expired and of end-tidal gases is calculated by multiplying by barometric pressure (P_B), assuming a water vapor pressure of 47 mm Hg in alveolar gas. The equation used varies

according to whether the sampled gas is cooled and/or passed through a dryer before being analyzed. If expired carbon dioxide is saturated with water vapor at 37°C and this temperature and humidity are maintained in the analyzer, then

$$P_{CO_2} = P_B \times F_{CO_2}$$

If the gas is dried before analysis, this becomes

$$P_{CO_2} = (P_B - 47) \times F_{CO_2}$$

Usually, in practice, the gas is analyzed at a temperature somewhere between the body and the room: a correction using water vapor pressure in the analyzer may then be applied. Usually, such corrections are so small that they may be ignored.

6. Mixed expired oxygen concentration (F_{EO_2}) is derived from the mixed expired oxygen deflection and the calibration curve.
7. Oxygen intake is calculated from the volume of oxygen inspired minus the volume of oxygen expired:

$$\dot{V}_{O_2} = (\dot{V}_I \times F_{IO_2}) - (\dot{V}_E \times F_{EO_2})$$

where $\dot{V}$ is expressed at STPD (see above).
8. Carbon dioxide output is calculated similarly to oxygen intake:

$$\dot{V}_{CO_2} = \dot{V}_E \text{ (F}_{ECO_2}) - \dot{V}_I \text{ (0.0004)}$$

(The second term is small and is usually ignored.)
9. The respiratory exchange ratio is calculated:

$$R = \dot{V}_{CO_2} \div \dot{V}_{O_2}$$

10. Mixed venous P_{CO_2} is derived from the rebreathing equilibrium P_{CO_2}. The record of carbon dioxide during rebreathing is carefully examined to ensure that the criteria for equilibration have been satisfied; if not, an extrapolation procedure is used, as detailed above. An empirical equation is applied to the equilibrium P_{CO_2} (P_{EqCO_2}) to correct for an alveolar-to-arterial P_{CO_2} difference as follows:

$$P_{\bar{v}CO_2} = 0.76 \ P_{EqCO_2} + 11$$

11. Arterial P_{CO_2} may be derived from P_{ETCO_2} if the subject has normal lung function—practically defined as normal spirometry plus a horizontal expired alveolar P_{CO_2} record at rest. A number of factors influence the P_{ETCO_2}-to-Pa_{CO_2} difference in normal subjects, which may be allowed for using an empirical equation:

$$PaCO_2 = 5.5 + 0.90 \; PETCO_2 - 0.0021 \; VT$$

For this equation to be valid, the performance of the carbon dioxide analyzer must be known; the requirements have been detailed (Jones et al., 1979).

Additional Data Obtained in Stage 3 Tests

The following information is obtained for a stage 3 procedure:

- Arterial PCO_2 and PO_2
- Arterial pH
- Arterial plasma lactate concentration

Additional Calculations Made in Stage 3 Tests

1. The dead space:tidal volume (VD/VT) ratio is calculated from the Bohr equation:

$$VD/VT = \frac{PaCO_2 - PECO_2}{PaCO_2 - PICO_2}$$

(Usually $PICO_2$ is considered to be zero.)

Conventionally, VD/VT is corrected for apparatus dead space (VD app), the volume of dead space air between the lips and the respiratory valve separating inspired from expired flow, in the following way:

$$VD = VT \frac{PaCO_2 - PECO_2}{PaCO_2 - PICO_2} - VD \; app$$

This value is divided by VT to obtain the "corrected" VD/VT. There are two controversies regarding the calculation. First, if alveolar dead space is large and VD app is also large (>100 mL), an error is introduced, owing to the inspiration of gas having a high PCO_2 that remains in apparatus dead space at the end of an expiration; the Bohr equation assumes that the dead space contains inspired air (zero carbon dioxide). The error does not lead to a normal calculated dead space in a subject with increased VD/VT, but if there is reason to make a rigorous calculation, suitable equations have been derived by Singleton and associates (1972). The second controversy surrounds the temperature of alveolar gas during exercise. Blood gases are usually measured in electrodes kept at 37°C; if central body temperature differs from this value, an error may be made. Practically, temperature does not increase enough to correct for this effect in subjects undertaking short-duration work in ambient temperatures around 20°C. A correction is needed in long-duration exercise or in high environmental temperature. This effect of temperature changes on the calculation of VD/VT has been well examined by Harris and colleagues (1976).

2. Alveolar PO_2 is derived from the alveolar air equation:

$$PAO_2 = PIO_2 - PaCO_2 \left(FIO_2 + \frac{1 - FIO_2}{R} \right)$$

3. Cardiac output is calculated by applying the Fick principle to carbon dioxide:

$$\dot{Q}_T = \dot{V}CO_2 \div (C\bar{v}CO_2 - CaCO_2)$$

where $(C\bar{v}CO_2 - CaCO_2)$ is derived from $P\bar{v}CO_2 - PaCO_2$ through the carbon dioxide dissociation curve. This derivation may be made graphically (McHardy, 1967) or by using the following equation, which expresses the carbon dioxide dissociation curve as a linear log:log function, as follows:

$$\log_e CCO_2 = 0.396 \log_e PCO_2 + 2.38$$

This equation is for blood 100 per cent saturated with oxygen, normal hemoglobin concentration (15 g/100 mL), and pH of 7.3 to 7.5; if these assumptions do not hold, corrections are needed for the most accurate calculation of $\dot{Q}tot$.

a. Correction for arterial oxygen desaturation. Mixed venous PCO_2 measured by rebreathing is oxygenated $P\bar{v}CO_2$; if arterial desaturation is present, the arterial carbon dioxide content for a given PCO_2 is higher and thus venoarterial carbon dioxide is less. The factor (McHardy, 1967) used for correcting arteriovenous content differences for this effect is

$$C\bar{v} - aCO_2 - [(95 - SaO_2) \times 0.064]$$

b. Correction for hemoglobin concentration. Increased hemoglobin concentration increases the amount of carbon dioxide carried by blood for a given PCO_2 difference. The factor (McHardy, 1967) is

$$C\bar{v} - aCO_2 - [(15 - Hb) \\ \times 0.015 \; (P\bar{v}CO_2 - PaCO_2)]$$

In both a and b, $C\bar{v} - aCO_2$ refers to the uncorrected measurement.

c. Correction for acid-base changes. A change in pH at a given PCO_2 changes the slope of the carbon dioxide dissociation curve. If pH has been measured, the $C\bar{v} - aCO_2$ difference may be calculated by use of equations presented in Appendix B.

4. The venous admixture ($\dot{Q}_{VA}/\dot{Q}_{tot}$) ratio is obtained by first converting P_{AO_2} and Pa_{CO_2} into corresponding oxygen contents—Cc'_{O_2} and Ca_{O_2}; $C\bar{v}_{CO_2}$ is derived by subtracting the arteriovenous oxygen content difference ($\dot{V}_{O_2} \div \dot{Q}_{tot}$) from Ca_{O_2}. The following equation is then solved:

$$\dot{Q}_{VA}/\dot{Q}_{tot} = (Cc'_{O_2} - Ca_{O_2}) \div (Cc'_{O_2} - C\bar{v}_{O_2})$$

Additional Procedures for Stage 3 and Stage 4 Tests: Blood Sampling

Arterial Catheter

Although indwelling Riley or Cournand needles can be used for sampling arterial blood during exercise, a small polyethylene or polytetrafluoroethylene (Teflon) catheter is better because it is less likely to cause trauma or become dislodged during arm movements. The brachial or radial artery is used. If the radial artery is chosen, it is wise to precede the catheterization by a simple test to ensure that the ulnar artery is capable of supplying the total blood flow to the hand. This is carried out by compressing both arteries for a short period while the patient exercises his or her hand, which becomes blanched; the ulnar compression is then released, and the skin of the whole hand flushes rapidly if the ulnar collateral supply is adequate.

The catheter can be inserted by the Seldinger technique or with an internal needle. In the Seldinger method, an 18-gauge thin-walled Riley needle is first placed in the artery (Bernéus et al., 1954). Although arterial puncture is a well-established procedure in cardiorespiratory physiology, some details of the technique are worthy of mention. First, the artery is precisely located by palpation, and anesthesia of the site is obtained by infiltrating 1 mL of local anesthetic down to the artery. The Riley needle with the obturator half-inserted is then passed through the skin and advanced toward the artery at an angle of about 60 degrees to the surface by a series of small jabbing movements. If the artery is very superficial or mobile, it may be stabilized by the index and middle fingers of one hand. On entry of the needle into the artery, blood escapes around the obturator, which may then be gently pushed home, and the needle may be advanced up the artery for 2 to 3 cm; the obturator is removed, and a free flow of blood should be obtained. If blood is not obtained even with the needle tip at sufficient depth, the needle may have passed through both walls of the artery; the obturator is removed and the needle is slowly withdrawn until a brisk flow is obtained; then the obturator is re-placed. If blood is not obtained on withdrawal, the lateral angle of the needle is slightly changed and the needle then reintroduced. It is important that the needle be well placed in the artery. A flexible nylon or coiled steel guidewire is then introduced through the needle. When the guidewire tip is 15 to 20 cm up the artery, the needle is withdrawn over it and replaced by a shaped polyethylene or Teflon catheter attached to a tap; this should pass into the lumen easily, and the guide is then withdrawn. The catheter is filled with heparin-saline solution and taped to the skin, and the puncture site is covered with gauze and a bandage.

Short Teflon catheters that fit closely over a needle are also available. The needle and catheter are placed in the artery, and when a free flow of blood is obtained, the needle is held and the catheter is pushed over it into the artery. The most convenient size is 18 gauge.

The catheters should be filled with a dilute solution of heparin-saline (1000 IU heparin to 500 mL saline) after each sample but may also be continuously flushed with saline under pressure. When the study is complete, the catheter is withdrawn, and the artery is compressed for at least 10 minutes, after which time the compression may be slowly released. The puncture site should be observed for a full minute afterward to ensure that no leakage is occurring; occasionally, compression is required for 20 to 30 minutes. After compression, it is wise to bandage the site for the rest of the day. If these rules are followed, hematomas rarely form. However, occasionally, a delayed hematoma may appear, leading to extensive skin discoloration 48 to 72 hours after the procedure, but it is usually painless and clears without sequelae. Sometimes, arterial puncture is followed by a degree of arterial spasm, identified by diminution in the pulse below the puncture site. However, this is almost invariably relieved within a few minutes by application of heat. Finally, the tips of some fingers may be tender for 1 to 2 days after the procedure; the reason for this phenomenon is not clear, but it is probably due to platelet emboli.

Venous Catheter

Blood samples for P_{CO_2}, pH, and plasma lactate concentration may be obtained from a superficial vein of the warmed hand (Harrison and Galloon, 1965). A catheter similar to those used for arterial sampling is placed in a vein on the back of the hand or just above the wrist. The hand is kept warm throughout the study by use of a hair dryer blowing into a plastic chamber that fits over the handlebar of the cycle ergometer, by keeping the temperature at about 45°C, or by wrapping an electric heating pad around the hand. The adequacy of arterialization can be checked by measuring the blood P_{O_2} while the subject is breathing 100 per cent oxygen; if a P_{O_2} of more than 400 mm Hg is obtained, the blood is adequately arterialized. A P_{O_2} of more than 80 mm Hg while air is being breathed may also be taken as evidence of arterialization. This method gives acceptable values for arterial P_{CO_2} and pH; P_{O_2} is always underestimated.

Capillary Blood Sampling

Small samples of arterialized capillary blood may be obtained from the fingertip or earlobe. Although sampling from either site is not painful, the earlobe has the advantage of being out of the patient's line of vision. In this technique, a small amount of vasodilating cream, such as Finalgon (Boehringer-Ingelheim), is placed on the earlobe, and when sufficient vasodilation has been obtained, the lobe is cleaned and swabbed with alcohol. A small cork is placed behind the earlobe, and a deep horizontal stab is made with a small pointed scalpel blade in the center of the lobe. During sampling, the site should be kept dry in order to enhance drop formation and avoid the possibility of contamination by sweat. The best site for fingertip puncture is the side of the middle finger midway in the thickness of the fingertip and just behind the tip, a position close to the digital artery.

Whichever site is used, the capillary blood should be collected into a long capillary tube or into the cup of a heparinized disposable intravenous catheter. If a sample tube of this size (volume of 125 μL or more) is used and flow is brisk enough to fill it within 30 seconds, the measurements of P_{CO_2}, pH, P_{O_2}, and lactate are close to arterial values (McEvoy and Jones, 1975). However, if flow is not brisk or if manipulation of the earlobe is required, then the capillary P_{CO_2} may be a few millimeters of mercury low. It is helpful to have the operator make a written comment at the time of sampling for later evaluation on the adequacy of flow and time taken to fill the capillary tubing.

"Float" Catheterization of the Right Heart

This simple procedure can be used to obtain pulmonary arterial pressures and blood samples. A nylon catheter (O.D. 0.8 mm) 100 cm long is introduced into the median cubital vein through a wide-bore needle or plastic catheter or by use of the Seldinger technique. A pressure transducer or electrocardiograph electrode is attached to indicate the position of the tip, and the catheter is slowly advanced until it is in the pulmonary artery. The electrocardiograph is monitored continuously. As with classic right heart catheterization, ectopic beats may occur when the tip of the catheter passes into

the right ventricle. If ectopic beats occur, the catheter should be withdrawn a few inches and reintroduced. Usually, it floats into an adequate position within 10 minutes. Blockage can be prevented by continuous flushing with dilute heparin-saline solution.

Right-sided heart catheterization also may be performed by use of the balloon catheters of Swan and associates (1970), which are, however, of larger external diameter (1.2 mm) and are more difficult to introduce percutaneously. Accurate measurement of pulmonary artery pressure requires careful calibration and attention to critical damping.

Precautions Against Hepatitis B

Any laboratory in which blood is handled requires a policy for the identification of hepatitis B carriers. The high infectivity of this agent has led to outbreaks in renal and intensive care units, emergency departments, and operating theaters that have been associated with appreciable mortality. Unfortunately, even when reasonable precautions are taken (e.g., gloves, masks), hepatitis B remains a laboratory hazard. High-risk subjects (drug addicts, patients with a history of jaundice, hospital personnel) preferably should be screened for hepatitis B antigen before a blood study is carried out. Technologists who handle blood frequently should be offered hepatitis B vaccine. Similar precautions are required for patients infected with the human immunodeficiency virus.

REFERENCES

Ashton CH, McHardy GJR. A rebreathing method for determining mixed venous P_{CO_2} during exercise. J Appl Physiol 1963;18:668–671.

Ayotte B, Seymour J, McIlroy M. A new method for measurement of cardiac output with nitrous oxide. J Appl Physiol 1970;28:863–866.

Becklake MR, Varvis CJ, Pengelly LD, et al. Measurement of pulmonary blood flow during exercise using nitrous oxide. J Appl Physiol 1962;17:579–586.

Bernéus B, Carlsten A, Holmgren A, et al. Percutaneous catheterization of peripheral arteries as a method for blood sampling. Scand J Clin Lab Invest 1954;6:217–221.

Campbell RD, McKelvie RS, Heigenhauser GJF, Jones NL. Estimation of cardiac output by CO2 rebreathing during incremental exercise in patients with coronary artery disease. Am J Noninvasive Cardiol 1989;3:147–153.

Cissik JH, Johnson RE, Rokosch DK. Production of gaseous nitrogen in human steady state conditions. J Appl Physiol 1972;32:155–159.

Collier CR. Determination of mixed venous CO_2 tensions by rebreathing. J Appl Physiol 1956;9:25–29.

da Silva GA, El-Manshawi A, Heigenhauser GJF, Jones NL. Measurement of mixed venous CO_2 pressure by rebreathing during exercise. Respir Physiol 1985;59:379–392.

Davis CC, Jones NL, Sealey BJ. Measurements of cardiac output in seriously ill patients using a CO_2 rebreathing method. Chest 1978;73:167–172.

Defares JG. Determination of $P\bar{v}CO_2$ from the exponential CO_2 rise during rebreathing. J Appl Physiol 1958;13:159–164.

Denison D, Edwards RHT, Jones G, et al. Direct and rebreathing estimates of the O_2 and CO_2 pressures in mixed venous blood. Respir Physiol 1969;7:326–334.

Denison D, Edwards RHT, Jones G, et al. Estimates of the CO_2 pressures in systemic arterial blood during rebreathing on exercise. Respir Physiol 1971;11:186–196.

Douglas AR, Jones NL, Reed JW. Calculation of whole blood CO_2 content. J Appl Physiol 1988;65:473–477.

Farhi LE, Nesarajah MS, Olszowka AJ, et al. Cardiac output determination by a simple one-step rebreathing technique. J Respir Physiol 1976;28:141–159.

Faulkner JA, Julius S, Conway J. Comparison of cardiac output determined by CO_2 rebreathing and dye-dilution methods. J Appl Physiol 1968;25:450–454.

Forster RE. Can alveolar PCO_2 exceed pulmonary end-capillary CO_2? No. J Appl Physiol 1977;42:326–328.

Godfrey S. Manipulation of the indirect Fick principle by a digital computer program for the calculation of exercise physiology results. Respiration 1970;27:513–532.

Godfrey S. Exercise Testing in Children. Philadelphia: WB Saunders Co.; 1974.

Godfrey S, Wolf E. An evaluation of rebreathing methods mixed venous PCO_2 during exercise. Clin Sci 1972;42:345–353.

Godfrey S, Katzenelson R, Wolfe E. Gas to blood PCO_2 differences during rebreathing in children and adults. Respir Physiol 1971;13:274–282.

Grollman A. The determination of the cardiac output of man by the use of acetylene. Am J Physiol 1929;88:432–445.

Gurtner GH. Can alveolar PCO_2 exceed pulmonary end-capillary CO_2? Yes. J Appl Physiol 1977;42:324–326.

Hainsworth R, Mohammed MMJ, Wood LM. Evaluation using dogs of a method for estimating cardiac output from a single breath. J Appl Physiol 1981;50:200–203.

Harris EA, Seelye ER, Whitlock RML. Gas exchange during exercise in healthy people. Clin Sci Mol Med 1976;51:335–344.

Harrison EM, Galloon S. Venous blood as an alternative to arterial blood for the measurement of carbon dioxide tensions. Br J Anaesthesiol 1965;37:13–18.

Heigenhauser GF, Faulkner JA, Dixon RW Jr. Estimation of cardiac output by the CO_2 rebreathing method during tethered swimming. J Appl Physiol 1978;44:821–824.

Heigenhauser GF, Jones NL. Comparison of two rebreathing methods for the determination of mixed venous partial pressure carbon dioxide during exercise. Clin Sci 1979;56:433–437.

Hsia CCW, Herazo LF, Ramanathan M, Johnson RL. Cardiac output during exercise measured by acetylene rebreathing, thermodilution, and Fick techniques. J Appl Physiol 1995;78:1612–1616.

Inman MD, Hughson RL, Jones NL. Comparison of cardiac output during exercise by single-breath and CO_2 rebreathing methods. J Appl Physiol 1985;58:1372–1377.

Jernérus R, Lundin G, Thomson D. Cardiac output in healthy subjects determined with a CO_2 rebreathing method. Acta Physiol Scand 1963;59:390–399.

Jones NL, Campbell EJM, Edwards RHT, et al. Alveolar to blood PCO_2 difference during rebreathing in exercise. J Appl Physiol 1969;27:356–360.

Jones NL, Campbell EJM, McHardy GJR, et al. The estimation of carbon dioxide pressure of mixed venous blood during exercise. Clin Sci 1967;32:311–327.

Jones NL, Rebuck AS. Rebreathing equilibration of CO_2 during exercise. J Appl Physiol 1973;35:538–541.

Jones NL, Robertson DG, Kane JW. Difference between end-tidal and arterial PCO_2 in exercise. J Appl Physiol 1979;47:954–960.

Kim TS, Rahn H, Farhi LE. Estimation of true venous and arterial PCO_2 by gas analysis of a single breath. J Appl Physiol 1966;21:1338–1344.

Loeppky JA, Luft UC, Fletcher ER. Quantitative description of whole blood CO_2 dissociation curve and Haldane effect. Respir Physiol 1983;51:167–181.

Mahler DA, Matthay RA, Snyder PE, et al. Determination of cardiac output at rest and during exercise by carbon dioxide rebreathing method in obstructive airway disease. Am Rev Respir Dis 1985a;131:73–78.

Mahler DA, Matthay RA, Snyder PE, et al. Volumetric responses of right and left ventricles during upright exercise in normal subjects. J Appl Physiol 1985b;58:1818–1822.

McElvaney GN, Blackie SP, Morrison NJ, et al. Cardiac output at rest and in exercise in elderly subjects. Med Sci Sports Exerc 1989;21:293–298.

McEvoy JDS, Jones NL. Arterialized capillary blood gases in exercise studies. Med Sci Sports 1975;7:312–315.

McHardy GJR. Relationship between the difference in pressure and content of carbon dioxide in arterial and venous blood. Clin Sci 1967;32:299–309.

McKelvie RS, Heigenhauser GJF, Jones NL. Measurement of cardiac output in unsteady state exercise with a CO_2 rebreathing technique. Chest 1987;92:777–782.

Paterson DH, Cunningham DA. Comparison of methods to calculate cardiac output using the CO_2 rebreathing method. Eur J Appl Physiol 1976;35:223–230.

Paterson DH, Cunningham DA, Plyley MJ, et al. The consistency of cardiac output measurement (CO_2 rebreathe) in children during exercise. Eur J Appl Physiol 1982;49:37–44.

Peters JP, Bulger HA, Eisenman AJ. Studies of the carbon dioxide absorption curve of human blood. J Biol Chem 1924;58:769–771.

Plesch J. Hemodynamische Studien. A Exp Path Therap 1909;6:380–618.

Pugh LGCE. Cardiac output in muscular exercise at 5,800 m (19,000 ft.). J Appl Physiol 1964;19:441–447.

Reybrouck T, Amery A, Billiet L, et al. Comparison of cardiac output determined by a carbon dioxide-rebreathing and direct Fick method at rest and during exercise. Clin Sci 1978;55:445–452.

Rigatto M. Mass spectrometry in the study of the pulmonary circulation. Bull Physiopathol Respir 1967;3:473–486.

Scheid P, Piiper J. Blood/gas equilibrium of CO_2 in lungs: A critical review. Respir Physiol 1980;39:1–31.

Singleton GJ, Olsen CR, Smith RL. Correction for mechanical dead space in the calculation of physiological dead space. J Clin Invest 1972;51:2768–2772.

Smyth RJ, Gledhill N, Froese AB, Jamnik VK. Validation of noninvasive maximal cardiac output measurement. Med Sci Sports Exerc 1984;16:512–515.

Sowton E, Bloomfield D, Jones NL, et al. Recirculation time during exercise. Cardiovasc Res 1968;4:341–345.

Swan HJC, Ganz W, Forrester J, et al. Catheterization of the heart in man with use of a flow-directed balloon-tipped catheter. N Engl J Med 1970;283:447–451.

Van Herwaarden CLA, Binkhorst RA, Fennis JFM, van't Laar A. Reliability of the cardiac output measurement with the indirect Fick principle for CO_2 during exercise. Pflugers Arch 1980;385:21–23.

Visser BF. Pulmonary diffusion of CO_2. Phys Med Biol 1960;5:155–166.

Winsborough M, Miller JN, Burgess DW, et al. Estimation of cardiac output from rate of change of alveolar carbon dioxide pressure during rebreathing. Clin Sci 1980;58:263–270.

Wolfe LA, Cunningham DA, Davis GM, Rosenfeld H. Relationship between maximal oxygen uptake and left ventricular function in exercise. J Appl Physiol 1978;44:44–49.

10

Quality Control in Exercise Studies

A number of points have been made in the preceding chapters regarding the care required in the conduct of exercise tests—for example, attention to comfortable saddle height, proper skin preparation for electrodes, multipoint calibration of analyzers, and precision in measurement. Many errors and mistakes may go undetected at the time unless routines are followed to keep them to a minimum.

It is a good idea to include all the relevant details of the test on the beginning of the recorder output chart—the patient's name, age, height, and weight; date; names of observers; and ambient (laboratory) temperature and barometric pressure. The record should also be used to note blood pressure, symptoms, and any event that may be needed in the interpretation.

Although quality control is not a topic that gets much of an airing in the scientific literature, anyone who has compared the accuracy of measurements made in different laboratories has found a surprising degree of variation. Cotes and Woolmer (1962) circulated a cylinder of gas to a number of British laboratories and obtained a variation in oxygen concentration that, at its worst, might have led to as much as a 25 per cent error in the measurement of oxygen intake. We have described our own experience in comparisons among four Ontario laboratories contributing to a collaborative study (Jones and Kane, 1979), which was similar in showing wide variations in oxygen intake and other variables but which also suggested that the variation could be minimized by carefully followed procedures.

CHECKS PERFORMED AT TIME OF TEST

1. The carbon dioxide analyzer is calibrated at the start and on completion of a test, using at least three gases in the range of 0 to 7 per cent and three in the range of 7 to 13 per cent if rebreathing is to be performed. If more than one sample line is used, calibration should be carried out for each. The calibration gases are best presented as step changes, so that the analyzer response characteristics may be examined.

2. Oxygen analyzers are set up with 100 per cent nitrogen as zero and 100 per cent oxygen. Air should read 20.93 per cent $\pm$ 0.03 per cent, and it is wise to check the analyzer further by using one of the carbon dioxide calibrating gases containing about 16 per cent oxygen. It may be necessary to document the delay of the analyzer, if it is a slowly responding instrument.

3. Analysis of reference gases is made with the Lloyd-Haldane or Scholander technique. Either of these methods may be used to analyze expired gas collections made in a Tissot spirometer or Douglas bags and to analyze calibrating gas mixtures. Although the "certified" gas mixtures obtained from medical gas manufacturers are usually accurate, they should always be checked. An important check is that air is analyzed accurately (oxygen, 20.93 per cent $\pm$ 0.03 per cent; carbon dioxide, 0.04 per cent $\pm$ 0.02 per cent); gas samples are not analyzed until this has been verified. Persistently low ($<$ 20.90 per cent) oxygen readings indicate that the apparatus or reagents require attention. Repeatability of analysis to within $\pm$ 0.03 per cent is also necessary.

4. Blood gas analysis is checked. Blood gas electrodes are notoriously prone to unsuspected error and are therefore set up by use of calibrating gases that have partial pressures close to those expected in the samples. Tonometry should be performed regularly, and electrodes should measure the known P_{CO_2} to within $\pm$ 1.5 mm Hg and P_{O_2} to within $\pm$ 2 mm Hg. Whenever possible, two blood samples should be taken and analyzed once each; this is preferable to duplicate analysis of one sample.

5. Complete, microprocessor-controlled exercise testing systems are now widely used in exercise testing laboratories. Built into such a system should be a convenient calibration procedure that at least establishes precision

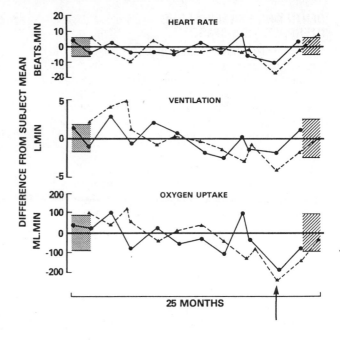

Figure 10–1. Results of exercise studies (600 kpm/min) in two subjects taken over a 25-month period. Each measurement is expressed as a deviation from an average over the whole period. The shaded blocks represent ± 1 SD for each subject. The consistent reduction in all measurements on one occasion *(arrow)* resulted in the identification of ergometer malfunction.

of ventilation and gas analysis modules; if a breath-by-breath system is being used, the calibration needs to incorporate tests of response times of analyzers, washout characteristics of mixing chambers, and inertial properties of flow meters. The specifications of such systems are outlined in Chapter 14; because they are sometimes capable of providing results that appear plausible yet may be in serious error (Matthews et al., 1987), it is very important to routinely obtain data to verify accuracy. For this reason, a mechanical gas mixing system, such as that described by Huszczuk and co-workers (1990), is well worth the extra investment.

PERIODIC CHECKS

1. Ergometer calibration should be performed. Two methods may be used, mechanical and biological. The standard calibration, which should be carried at least once a year, is obtained by driving the pedals with an electric or air-driven motor and measuring the torque produced (Cumming and Alexander, 1968).
2. The calibration and linearity of dry gas meters should be checked every 6 months, using a constant-volume piston in addition to a check at high flow rates.

3. The respiratory circuit, valves, and taps should be checked for leaks once a week.
4. Most variables are closely reproducible from time to time in a given subject. Thus, a useful periodic test of the complete exercise testing system is the repeated study of laboratory staff (Fig. 10–1). Once this is made a routine, it is simple to carry out every week; results are calculated by another member of the team without reference to previous results. This procedure is especially important for automated exercise systems because it is virtually the only way to test the complete system in operation (Jones, 1984). Values obtained at a given power output in a steady state should lie within the limits listed in Table 10–1.

Table 10–1. LIMITS OF VARIATION IN VALUES OBTAINED BY REPEATED STUDY OF THE SAME SUBJECT AT A GIVEN POWER OUTPUT IN A STEADY STATE (±1 SD)

Variable	Limit %
Oxygen intake	±5.1
Carbon dioxide output	6.2
Ventilation	5.0
Cardiac frequency	4.7
Mixed venous P_{CO_2}	2.7
Cardiac output	8.9

IDENTIFYING ERRORS AT THE INTERPRETATION STAGE

It is wise to have a high index of suspicion in approaching exercise test results, particularly when complex measurements (stage 2 and stage 3 tests) have been made, and not to make a clinically important interpretation without examining the record to ensure that the findings are valid. Following are a few examples of the ways in which errors may be identified at this stage.

1. Low values of $\dot{V}E$ in a stage 1 test, particularly if they are accompanied by low cardiac frequency, suggest that the power outputs are lower than indicated, perhaps owing to a fault in the ergometer. In steady state tests, this is shown also by low values for $\dot{V}O_2$ and $\dot{V}CO_2$.
2. Respiratory exchange ratios below 0.7 or above 1.2 call for an examination of gas calibration curves and analyses.
3. An abnormal cardiac output or VD/VT ratio should prompt an examination of the carbon dioxide measurements. The gradation from $PECO_2$ to $PETCO_2$ to $P\bar{v}CO_2$ should be present. If $PETCO_2$ is close to $PECO_2$, the analyzer may be responding slowly, or the sampling lines to the analyzer may be of differing lengths. Too low a cardiac output may be due to a poor rebreathing maneuver with a delayed equilibration or to an error in $PaCO_2$—usually associated with too low a VD/VT. If the cardiac output is high, an inadequate (phase reversal) pattern may have been used for $P\bar{v}CO_2$.
4. Analyzer malfunction may occur. Oxygen analyzers, especially fuel cells, have a tendency to age; furthermore, the complexities of their manufacture are prone to result in variable performance and longevity. Usually, this may be recognized by values for $\dot{V}O_2$ that are low in relation to power.

OTHER SOURCES OF ERROR

Errors occasionally occur for several other reasons.

1. *Gas meter.* Errors occurring at high flow rates or owing to slipping of the potentiometer are easily recognized if ventilation is also measured by a spirometer.
2. *Leakage of valves.* The most common source is the main two-way valve at the mouth. This may be recognized by a biphasic pattern in the dry gas meter or Tissot spirometer readings and by failure of the tidal gas carbon dioxide tracing to fall to zero in inspiration.
3. *Incorrect ergometer setting.* This is usually recognized by an inappropriate oxygen intake, which may also be an indication that the ergometer needs to be calibrated.
4. ***Contamination of an expired gas sample with a high oxygen concentration mixture.*** This is liable to occur after rebreathing and is recognized by high values for the respiratory exchange ratio. It should not occur if criteria for a steady state are observed.
5. ***Contamination of a blood sample with air.*** This is likely to occur with capillary blood samples, particularly if flow is poor. It leads to falsely low PCO_2 and high PO_2 values and causes inappropriately low values for the dead space-tidal volume ratio and the alveolar-arterial PO_2 difference.

REFERENCES

Cotes JE, Woolmer RF. A comparison between 27 laboratories of the results of analysis of an expired gas sample. J Physiol 1962;163:36P–37P.

Cumming GR, Alexander WD. The calibration of bicycle ergometers. Can J Physiol Pharmacol 1968;46:917–919.

Huszczuk A, Whipp BJ, Wasserman K. A respiratory gas exchange simulator for routine calibration in metabolic studies. Eur Respir J 1990;3:465–468.

Jones NL. Evaluation of a microprocessor-controlled exercise testing system. J Appl Physiol 1984;57:1312–1318.

Jones NL, Kane JW. Quality control of exercise test measurements. Med Sci Sports 1979;11:368–372.

Matthews JI, Bush BA, Morales FM. Microprocessor exercise physiology systems vs a nonautomated system: A comparison of data output. Chest 1987;92:696–703.

11

Interpretation of Stage 2 Test Results: Integration Between Measurements and Mechanisms

In the interpretation of noninvasive, or "bloodless," steady state test results, we may make use of the linkage between measurements, which frees us to some extent from reliance on expected values for any given measurement. Because each measurement contributes to the calculation of more than one variable, errors and biological variation are reduced. Furthermore, we may use the linkage between oxygen and carbon dioxide transport mechanisms, outlined previously, to increase precision in the expected response, again freeing us from reliance on "normal values." Finally, even though we may seldom use the approach to solve a problem, because blood sampling and analysis are now commonplace, it is important to grasp the physiological concepts and reasoning, if only because they provide one basis for quality control. In this chapter, I describe the bloodless approach, leaving the interpretation of stage 3 test results for Chapter 12. The reader will soon appreciate that the distinction between stage 2 and stage 3 tests is almost nonexistent with regard to interpretation; in a stage 2 test, several important variables are estimated and limits are assigned; in the stage 3 test, these variables are measured (McKelvie and Jones, 1989).

In a stage 2 test, the following measurements are usually obtained at rest and at two levels of power:

- Power, W (watts)
- Oxygen intake, $\dot{V}O_2$
- Carbon dioxide output, $\dot{V}CO_2$
- Respiratory exchange ratio, R
- Cardiac frequency, f_c (beats [b]/min)
- Ventilation, $\dot{V}E$
- Tidal volume, VT
- Breathing frequency, f_b (breaths/min)
- Mixed expired carbon dioxide pressure, P_{ECO_2}
- End-tidal carbon dioxide pressure, P_{ETCO_2}
- Mixed venous carbon dioxide pressure, $P\bar{v}CO_2$

A guide to the expected responses is provided in Appendix D, obtained from published studies (Higgs et al., 1967; Spiro et al., 1974; Harris et al., 1976). This chapter presents an approach to interpretation based on integration and linkage between these simple noninvasive measurements.

POWER AND OXYGEN INTAKE

Oxygen intake is linearly related to power; at given power, $\dot{V}O_2$ measured in a steady state is higher than that measured in a progressive incremental (unsteady state) test, such as the stage 1 procedure, owing to the kinetics of the $\dot{V}O_2$ response to a step change in W. The steady state response is expressed by

$$\dot{V}O_2 = 0.3 + 0.002\ W$$

where $\dot{V}O_2$ is measured in liters per minute (L/min) and W in kilopond-meters per minute (kpm/min) (McKelvie et al., 1987; Campbell et al., 1989). The slope of the relationship is similar in subjects of all ages (Gadhoke and Jones, 1969; Lands et al., 1992), but the intercept of the line is directly related to body size (Cotes et al., 1969).

This relationship between W and $\dot{V}O_2$ expresses the "efficiency" of work and is influenced by a number of factors. First, the slope is steeper for work performed with smaller muscle groups, for example, in arm ergometry. Second, the complexity of the task may influence the relationship; thus, $\dot{V}O_2$ at the same treadmill setting may fall with repeated studies in subjects unaccustomed to the test. An extreme example is seen in wheelchair ergometry, in which $\dot{V}O_2$ at a given W is as much as fivefold higher in subjects performing the task for the first time, compared with that in experienced subjects (Wicks et al., 1977). Third, some patients may exhibit a higher metabolic demand at a given power—for example, thyrotoxicosis (Massey et al., 1967) and severe airway obstruction (Jones et al., 1971; Spiro et al., 1974). In such conditions, there appears to be a parallel shift in the relationship; that is, the intercept (or resting $\dot{V}O_2$) increases, rather than the slope. The oxygen intake is used as the metabolic equivalent of power, and other variables may be related to it rather than to power alone.

OXYGEN INTAKE AND CARDIAC FREQUENCY

Cardiac frequency is linearly related to $\dot{V}O_2$ in most subjects during exercise. The two variables are related by the Fick equation

$$\dot{Q} = f_c \times V_s = \dot{V}O_2 \div (CaO_2 - C\bar{v}O_2)$$

thus

$$\dot{V}O_2 \div f_c = V_s \times (CaO_2 - C\bar{v}O_2)$$

The term $(\dot{V}O_2 \div f_c)$ is known as the oxygen pulse and from the equation may be seen to equal the product of the arteriovenous oxygen content difference and stroke volume (V_s). Because the limits of the arteriovenous difference at a given oxygen uptake are narrow, the oxygen pulse mainly gives information regarding stroke volume. These relationships may be explored graphically in a diagram (Fig. 11–1), similar to that of Margaria (see Fig. 2–14). Oxygen pulse measurements have to be interpreted in relation to the oxygen intake (see Fig. 11–1) and to the subject's stature, as indicated previously.

Measurement of the oxygen pulse has two main uses. First, in a given subject studied over a period of time, changes in oxygen pulse generally reflect changes in cardiac stroke volume, V_s. Second, the measurement allows limits to be placed on V_s; thus, a normal oxygen pulse is usually compatible with normal V_s, even if the widest limits of the arteriovenous difference are used to stress the relationships above; the examples given later in the chapter amplify this point.

RELATIONSHIPS BETWEEN MEASUREMENTS AND MECHANISMS IN CARBON DIOXIDE EXCRETION

The carbon dioxide "transport line" has been introduced previously to show that it may be used to explore the linkage between mechanisms as they adapt to an increase in carbon dioxide output in exercise, much as Barcroft's analysis may be applied to oxygen transport. The equations that describe the transport line may be linked in sequence and may be expressed diagrammatically by use of four graphs, each of which occupies one quadrant of a four-quadrant figure.

A FOUR-QUADRANT DIAGRAM FOR USE IN THE INTERPRETATION OF TESTS

1. Mixed expired PCO_2 expresses the ventilatory response to an increase in carbon dioxide output.

$$PECO_2 = \frac{\dot{V}CO_2 \times 0.863}{\dot{V}E}$$

This relationship is described by a graph's having carbon dioxide output as the abscissa and $PECO_2$ as the ordinate, and in which a family of isopleths for ventilation is drawn.

Notice that for a given $\dot{V}CO_2$ (1 L/min) shown by the dotted lines in Figure 11–2, doubling ventilation (from 45 to 90 L/min) leads to a halving of $PECO_2$ (from 20 to 10 mm Hg).

2. Total expired ventilation ($\dot{V}E$) has two components—alveolar ventilation ($\dot{V}A$) and dead space ventilation ($\dot{V}D$). The mixed

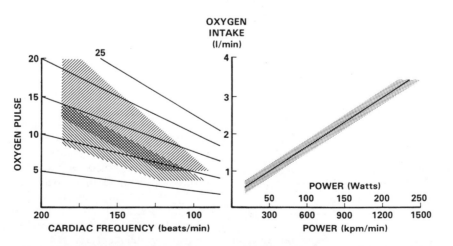

Figure 11–1. *Right,* Oxygen intake (mean ± 1 SD) for steady-state exercise (cycle ergometer). *Left,* heart rate responses for males (////) and females (\\\\\); ± 1 SD from the mean. (Data from Higgs BE, et al. Changes in ventilation, gas exchange and circulation during exercise in normal subjects. Clin Sci 1967;32:329–337.)

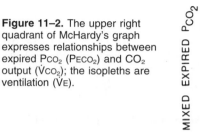

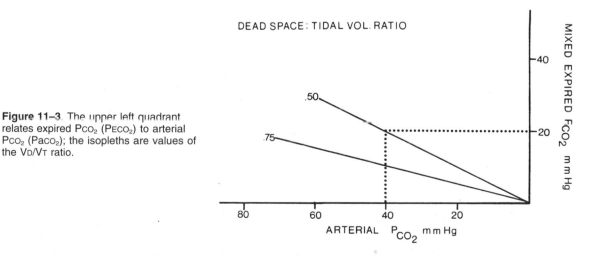

Figure 11–2. The upper right quadrant of McHardy's graph expresses relationships between expired P_{CO_2} (P_{ECO_2}) and CO_2 output ($\dot{V}_{CO_2}$); the isopleths are ventilation ($\dot{V}_E$).

expired P_{CO_2} at any given carbon dioxide output is related to $\dot{V}_A$ and to the $\dot{V}_D/\dot{V}_T$ ratio through the following series of equations:

$$\dot{V}_A = \frac{\dot{V}_{CO_2} \times 0.863}{Pa_{CO_2}}$$

and

$$\dot{V}_D/\dot{V}_T = \frac{Pa_{CO_2} - P_{ECO_2}}{Pa_{CO_2}}$$
(Bohr's equation)

Thus, at a given $\dot{V}_{CO_2}$, $\dot{V}_A$ influences both Pa_{CO_2} and the absolute difference between Pa_{CO_2} and P_{ECO_2}. Therefore, a low P_{ECO_2} may be due to an increase in $\dot{V}_A$ or $\dot{V}_D/\dot{V}_T$, or both.

From Bohr's equation

$$P_{ECO_2} = Pa_{CO_2} (1 - V_D/V_T)$$

or

$$P_{ECO_2} = \frac{\dot{V}_{CO_2} \times 0.863}{\dot{V}_A} (1 - V_D/V_T)$$

we may construct a graph having P_{ECO_2} as the ordinate and Pa_{CO_2} as the abscissa, and in which isopleths of V_D/V_T ratio are drawn.

In the example shown in Figure 11–3, P_{ECO_2} is 20 mm Hg, Pa_{CO_2} is 40 mm Hg, and V_D/V_T is 0.5. Notice that the higher the value for V_D/V_T, the greater the difference between Pa_{CO_2} and P_{ECO_2}, but also that for a given V_D/V_T ratio, this difference becomes

Figure 11–3. The upper left quadrant relates expired P_{CO_2} (P_{ECO_2}) to arterial P_{CO_2} (Pa_{CO_2}); the isopleths are values of the V_D/V_T ratio.

smaller if Pa_{CO_2} falls, that is, if alveolar ventilation increases.

3. The process of carbon dioxide carriage by blood is described by the dissociation curve relating carbon dioxide content to carbon dioxide pressure. Because both venous and arterial blood is being examined, there are logical and mathematical arguments for expressing this process as the relationship between the venoarterial pressure *difference* and the venoarterial content *difference:*

$$(C\bar{v}_{CO_2} - Ca_{CO_2}) = f(P\bar{v}_{CO_2} - Pa_{CO_2})$$

where f is a function of the carbon dioxide dissociation curve. The advantage of this approach, introduced by McHardy (1967), is that absolute carbon dioxide content need not be derived from the separate values of $P\bar{v}_{CO_2}$ and Pa_{CO_2}, thereby simplifying graphical plotting of data (Fig. 11–4).

This relationship may be plotted with Pa_{CO_2} as the abscissa, and the venoarterial carbon dioxide content difference may be plotted as the ordinate. The carbon dioxide dissociation curve may then be used to construct a series of curved lines, which are isopleths of $P\bar{v}_{CO_2}$. The lines are constructed for an arterial oxygen saturation of 95 per cent and a mixed venous oxygen saturation of 100 per cent, so that the curves, which have been derived for blood with a hemoglobin content of 15 g/100 mL, may be

used for oxygenated $P\bar{v}_{CO_2}$ measured by rebreathing. Deviations from this arterial oxygen saturation or hemoglobin content influence the relationships, and corrections are made to the carbon dioxide content difference to allow for them.

The example shows that for a Pa_{CO_2} of 40 mm Hg and $P\bar{v}_{CO_2}$ of 60 mm Hg, the carbon dioxide content difference is 8.4 mL/100 mL.

4. At any carbon dioxide output, the venoarterial content difference is governed by the cardiac output. This is expressed mathematically by use of the Fick principle

$$\dot{Q}tot = \frac{\dot{V}_{CO_2}}{C\bar{v}_{CO_2} - Ca_{CO_2}}$$

and is expressed graphically by plotting $\dot{V}_{CO_2}$ as the abscissa and $(C\bar{v}_{CO_2} - Ca_{CO_2})$ as the ordinate, with isopleths of $\dot{Q}tot$ radiating from their intersection (Fig. 11–5).

Each of these four relationships describes a portion of the carbon dioxide transport system. We may now combine the four graphs to obtain a single figure that allows us to solve the equations, given data obtained in an exercise test (Fig. 11–6).

In the example used previously to illustrate the construction of the diagram, all the values necessary to calculate V_D/V_T, $\dot{V}_A$, and $\dot{Q}tot$ were given: that is, $\dot{V}_{CO_2}$, $P_{E_{CO_2}}$, Pa_{CO_2}, and $P\bar{v}_{CO_2}$. The main function of the diagram is exploration of the limits of these interrelated variables when Pa_{CO_2} is not measured. Therefore, in the examples that follow,

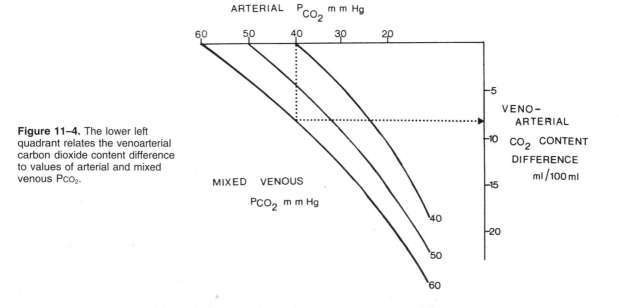

Figure 11–4. The lower left quadrant relates the venoarterial carbon dioxide content difference to values of arterial and mixed venous P_{CO_2}.

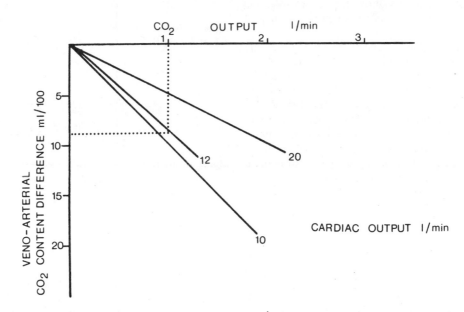
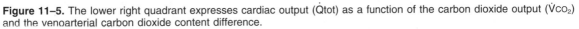

Figure 11–5. The lower right quadrant expresses cardiac output (Q̇tot) as a function of the carbon dioxide output (V̇co₂) and the venoarterial carbon dioxide content difference.

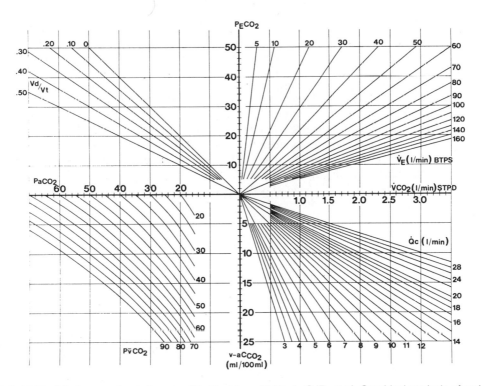

Figure 11–6. McHardy's four-quadrant diagram. (Modified from McHardy GJR, et al. Graphical analysis of carbon dioxide transport during exercise. Clin Sci 1967;32:289–298.)

the data are analyzed initially without benefit of the blood measurements, to allow the reader to judge the value of the measurements taken in the stage 2 and stage 3 tests.

Briefly, the measurements that are made in the stage 2 test and entered in the equations above consist of $\dot{V}CO_2$, $PECO_2$, and $P\bar{v}CO_2$; $\dot{V}CO_2$ is the metabolic load, and $P\bar{v}CO_2$ and $PECO_2$ are interrelated through alveolar ventilation and the VD/VT ratio, the blood carbon dioxide dissociation curve, and the cardiac output. This fact allows the interaction between mechanisms to be explored and limits to be assigned to each; often, the limits so defined are narrow enough for a conclusion to be drawn. When measurements of arterial PCO_2 are available, all the equations may be solved, and the diagram may then be used to interpret the interplay between mechanisms. An alternative to measured $PaCO_2$ is an estimate derived from end-tidal PCO_2; however, this estimate may be valid only if pulmonary function is normal.

Finally, changes in $P\bar{v}CO_2$ reflect changes in the amount of carbon dioxide stored during exercise. This fact is used to analyze the metabolic (aerobic-anaerobic) responses to exercise in the following discussion.

THE INDIRECT ESTIMATION OF LACTATE PRODUCTION

Production of lactate through anaerobic glycolysis in muscle is usually an indication that the oxygen demands of the exercising muscles are outstripping the rate at which oxygen supply mechanisms are delivering oxygen. Although a number of factors, from muscle enzyme activities to impaired hepatic lactate metabolism, influence lactate accumulation in blood (Jones and Ehrsam, 1982), the adequacy of oxygen supply appears to be by far the most important. It is generally assumed that lactate (La^-) and hydrogen ions (H^+) leave muscle together, plasma [La^-] increases, bicarbonate concentration falls, and carbon dioxide evolution increases. All three changes are thus assumed to be stoichiometrically equivalent—entry of 1 mol each of La^- and H^+ leads to loss of 1 mol of HCO_3^- and to evolution of 1 mol of carbon dioxide:

$$H^+ + HCO_3^- \rightarrow H_2CO_3 \rightarrow CO_2 + H_2O$$

As ventilation is controlled to keep PCO_2 fairly constant, the entry of La^- and H^+ into plasma from muscle is expected to increase carbon dioxide output from the lungs after only a short delay (the circulation time, muscle to lungs). This extra carbon dioxide is added to carbon dioxide generated by aerobic metabolism and leads to an increase in the respiratory exchange ratio (R).

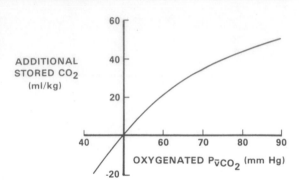

Figure 11–7. An expression of the body CO_2 storage capacity in exercise, showing the CO_2 stored as oxygenated mixed venous PCO_2 changes from a resting level of 50 mm Hg. (Modified from Jones NL, Jurkowski JE. Body carbon dioxide storage capacity in exercise. J Appl Physiol 1979;46:811–815.)

This model, which expresses the relationship between La^- production and carbon dioxide excretion, is clearly simplistic (see Chapter 2); the interaction between metabolic and ionic changes in muscle and blood is more complex. However, it does afford a method for estimating changes in blood [La^-] that has proved itself useful in a number of applications (Higgs et al., 1967; Hughes et al., 1968; Jones et al., 1971).

Various approaches have been used to estimate lactic acid accumulation from measurements of R. However, during exercise, a variable amount of carbon dioxide is accumulated in body stores and is not excreted into expired gas. Thus, more accurate estimates of lactic acid production are obtained from measurements of expired carbon dioxide and mixed venous PCO_2 by constructing a carbon dioxide balance equation that has four components.

Total CO_2 output = CO_2 produced by aerobic metabolism
$\pm$ CO_2 moving into or out of stores
$+$ CO_2 resulting from lactic acid production

$$\text{Total } \dot{V}CO_2 = \underset{1}{\text{aerobic } \dot{V}CO_2} \pm \underset{2}{\text{stored } CO_2} + \underset{3}{CO_2} \underset{4}{\text{(lactic acid)}}$$

These four components may be estimated in the following way:

1. The total $\dot{V}CO_2$ is measured for the total exercise time, or assumed constant—the total being obtained from $\dot{V}CO_2 \times$ time
2. The aerobic component is obtained by assuming an aerobic metabolic respiratory

quotient (RQ) of 0.9, or an average normal RQ for the level of exercise:

$$\text{aerobic } \dot{V}CO_2 = \dot{V}O_2 \times 0.9 \times \text{time}$$

3. Stored carbon dioxide is calculated from the change in $P\bar{v}CO_2$ from the beginning to end of the study, from values of body carbon dioxide storage capacity (Fig. 11–7):

$$\text{stored } CO_2 = \Delta\, P\bar{v}CO_2 \times \text{kg} \\ \times \text{storage capacity}$$

4. The carbon dioxide generated from La^- and H^+ is given by

$$CO_2\,(La^-) = \dot{V}CO_2 - \text{aerobic } \dot{V}CO_2 \\ \pm \text{stored } CO_2$$

This volume of carbon dioxide is converted into a molar equivalent (by dividing it by 22.26), which represents the total accumulated lactate. Theoretically, this total is distributed in total body water (0.6 × body weight), and correction for water content of blood (by division by 0.8) should yield the change in blood lactate concentration. However, when validating the method, Marie Clode found that division of the total accumulated lactate by 0.5 body weight yielded changes in blood lactate concentration that were within ± 0.5 mmol/L of the measured changes (Clode and Campbell, 1969).

INTERPRETATION OF STAGE 2 TESTS

To interpret fully stage 2 tests, one requires knowledge of the normal variation in measurements made at the given power during the steady state, including variables that depend on arterial blood analysis. Implicit in the guidelines given previously is a knowledge of the normal variations in arterial PCO_2, dead space–tidal volume ratio, and cardiac output. These are given in Chapter 12; the main purpose of this section is to indicate the logic involved in the interpretation of stage 2 tests in which the limits for these variables are explored.

Example 1

The following values were obtained in the patient whose stage 1 results were presented in Example 1, Chapter 8. After the stage 1 test, measurements were made in a steady state at 400 kpm/min and 800 kpm/min. For the sake of brevity, the results at the higher workload only will be analyzed in detail.

Patient: male, age 49 years
Height: 175 cm; Weight: 86 kg
Readings taken at 800 kpm/min were as follows:

Power output	kpm/min	800
	watts	133
f_c	b/min	140
$\dot{V}E$	L/min	48
f_b	breaths/min	20
$\dot{V}CO_2$	mL/min	2000
$\dot{V}O_2$	mL/min	2080
$PECO_2$	mm Hg	36
$PETCO_2$	mm Hg	45
$P\bar{v}CO_2$	mm Hg	75

First, we examine the relationship between oxygen uptake and power output (see Fig. 11–1); oxygen uptake is seen to lie within the normal range, indicating that the metabolic requirements are appropriate for this power output; if the values for oxygen uptake did not lie in this range, the other variables would need to be related to an equivalent oxygen uptake rather than to the power output when variables were compared with normal data (see Appendix D).

Second, the relationship between cardiac frequency and oxygen uptake is examined (see Fig. 11–1). The cardiac frequency of 140 b/min indicates an oxygen pulse of 15 mL oxygen per beat. As pointed out previously, the oxygen pulse equals the product of stroke volume and the arteriovenous oxygen content difference. Thus, the lowest value for stroke volume may be identified by a calculation that uses the widest possible arteriovenous difference, which we may take as the highest usual value recorded in athletes and patients, of 160 mL/L.

Thus

$$\dot{V}O_2/f_c = Ca - \bar{v}O_2 \times V_s \\ 15 = 160 \times V_s \\ V_s = 0.093 \text{ L}$$

This calculation indicates that stroke volume in this subject cannot be less than 93 mL, a value within the normal range for a man of this size. From stage 1 data, a stroke volume of 106 mL at maximum was estimated.

Third, we may examine the relationship between the variables involved in carbon dioxide excretion by use of the four-quadrant diagram. We may plot $PECO_2$ as a point in the upper right quadrant and $P\bar{v}CO_2$ as an isopleth in the lower left quadrant.

The two lines—a horizontal line from $P_{E}CO_2$ across into the upper left quadrant and the $P\bar{v}CO_2$ isopleth—form boundaries to establish the limits of the dead space–tidal volume ratio and the cardiac output, shown in Figure 11–8 as shaded bands. One limit represents the lowest V_D/V_T, and the other border is defined by choosing the highest possible value for cardiac output. The tidal volume is 2400 mL; the lowest value for dead space volume, including an instrumental dead space of 60 mL, is 240 mL, yielding a V_D/V_T ratio of 0.10 (Jones et al., 1966). A vertical line is dropped from the intersection of this V_D/V_T isopleth with the $P_{E}CO_2$ boundary, meeting the $PaCO_2$ abscissa at 40 mm Hg and the $P\bar{v}CO_2$ isopleth at a venoarterial carbon dioxide content difference of 13.0 mL/100 mL. At the abscissa, corrections would need to be applied for hemoglobin values above or below 15 g/100 mL and for arterial oxygen desaturation, but such corrections are not required in this example. A horizontal line from this venoarterial carbon dioxide difference meets a vertical line dropped from the $\dot{V}CO_2$ ordinate on an isopleth cardiac output of 15.4 L/min. By choosing the lowest value for V_D/V_T we have obtained the lowest value for $PaCO_2$, the highest venoarterial carbon dioxide content difference, and the lowest values for $\dot{Q}tot$ and stroke volume; thus, the lowest stroke volume is 110 mL (15,400 ÷ 140).

The diagram may be used also to obtain the highest likely values for $PaCO_2$ and V_D/V_T, by starting with the highest likely value for stroke volume and $\dot{Q}tot$. From studies of healthy subjects (Cotes et al., 1969), we estimate the highest value for stroke volume to be 2 mL/kg, or 160 mL, giving an equivalent cardiac output of 22 L/min. This point is plotted in the lower right quadrant, and a horizontal line is drawn to the $P\bar{v}CO_2$ boundary; a line extended vertically from the intersection yields a $PaCO_2$ of 48 mm Hg and V_D/V_T of 0.25; when this value is corrected for instrumental dead space of 60 mL, the V_D/V_T ratio is 0.22; this is the highest value compatible with the measurements but is still within normal limits. Using the diagram in this way, we may conclude that $PaCO_2$ lies between 40 and 48 mm Hg, V_D/V_T between 0.1 and 0.22, and $\dot{Q}tot$ between 15 and 22 L/min. This exercise in logic has allowed us to place limits on most of the variables, with an accuracy that is not much inferior to that attained by invasive techniques. Because this patient also had normal pulmonary function, we may use the end-tidal PCO_2 to obtain an estimate of $PaCO_2$; estimated $PaCO_2$ is 42 mm Hg, yielding a cardiac output of 16.7 L/min.

Finally, we may construct the carbon dioxide balance to obtain an estimate of lactate production by use of the data in the table with one additional

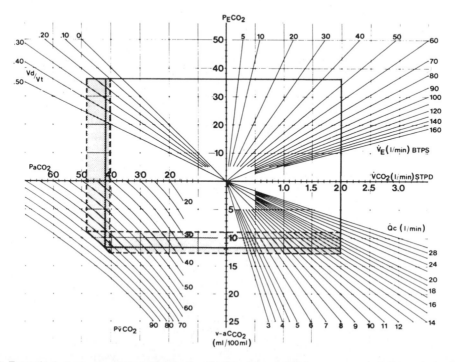

Figure 11–8. Example 1 measurements plotted on the diagram. The dotted lines represent limits to derived variables implied by the lowest V_D/V_T ratios (0.1) and highest cardiac output (22 L/min). The solid lines indicate values derived from the measured arterial PCO_2. The shaded area indicates how narrow the limits are when all the variables are normal.

measurement—$P\bar{v}CO_2$ at the start of the power output. This was 65 mm Hg, measured at the end of a preceding exercise level (400 kpm/min). We need also to know the duration of the exercise (5 minutes).

1. Total carbon dioxide output is determined:

$$\text{Total } CO_2 \text{ output} = \dot{V}CO_2 \times \text{time}$$
$$= 2000 \times 5$$
$$= 10,000 \text{ mL}$$

2. Aerobic carbon dioxide production is estimated (RQ is assumed to be 0.9.):

$$\text{Aerobic } \dot{V}CO_2 = \dot{V}O_2 \times RQ \times \text{time}$$
$$= 2080 \times 0.9 \times 5$$
$$= 9360 \text{ mL}$$

3. Stored carbon dioxide is calculated from the product of change in $P\bar{v}CO_2 \times$ slope $\times$ weight, where slope is the slope of the body stores carbon dioxide dissociation curve. The volume of carbon dioxide in milliliters per kilogram is derived from the two values of $P\bar{v}CO_2$ (beginning and end of test) by use of Figure 11–8. For the example, $P\bar{v}CO_2$ changed from 65 to 75 mm Hg. From Figure 11–8, the additional carbon dioxide stored increases from 28 to 39 mL/kg, an increase of 11 mL/kg.

Thus

$$CO_2 \text{ stored} = 11 \times 85$$
$$= 935 \text{ mL}$$

4. Carbon dioxide from lactic acid is calculated:

$$CO_2 \text{ (lactic acid)} = 10,000 - 9360 + 935$$
$$= 1575 \text{ mL}$$
$$= 71 \text{ mmol}$$

This is equivalent to 71 mmol of lactic acid, increasing lactate concentration by 71 ÷ (0.5 × 85) or 1.7 mmol/L.

Thus, from this noninvasive study, we may conclude that cardiac output and stroke volume are within normal limits, alveolar ventilation and dead space are also normal, and an oxygen intake of over 2 L/min is not accompanied by significant muscle lactate production.

Example 2

The following values were obtained in the patient whose stage 1 test results were presented in Example 2, Chapter 8. Studies were performed at two power outputs, 200 kpm/min and 400 kpm/min. The results at 400 kpm/min only are discussed here and are analyzed exactly as in the preceding example.

Patient: female, age 35 years
Height: 165 cm; Weight: 70 kg

Power output	kpm/min	400
	watts	67
f_c	b/min	168
$\dot{V}E$	L/min	51
f_b	breaths/min	30
$\dot{V}CO_2$	mL/min	1340
$\dot{V}O_2$	mL/min	1120
$PECO_2$	mm Hg	22.3
$PETCO_2$	mm Hg	31
$P\bar{v}CO_2$	mm Hg	65

Oxygen intake is appropriate to the power output (see Fig. 11–1). Cardiac frequency is high for the oxygen intake, the oxygen pulse being 6.7 mL/beat. Thus, if the arteriovenous oxygen difference is normal at 10.5 mL/100 mL, stroke volume is 62 mL, a reduced value.

Analyzing carbon dioxide transport measurements using the four-quadrant diagram (Fig. 11–9), we are unable to infer normal values for both VD/VT and $\dot{Q}tot$. Note that the bands joining the limiting values, implied by normal VD/VT and stroke volume, are wider than in the first example, and $PaCO_2$ may lie anywhere between 25 and 40 mm Hg. If we use the value for end-tidal PCO_2 as an indication of $PaCO_2$, the implied variables indicate a high VD/VT, a $\dot{Q}tot$ within the lowest normal limit, and a low stroke volume. However, in this situation, it is unwise to assume that end-tidal PCO_2 yields a reasonable estimate of $PaCO_2$ in view of the fact that the presence of an alveolar dead space may lead to an appreciable underestimation of $PaCO_2$. Thus, in this situation, blood gas measurements are needed for the unique solution to be obtained. Note, however, that because cardiac frequency is close to the maximum value expected for a subject of this age, even a normal value of cardiac output implies that the maximum cardiac output is considerably reduced. The measured $PaCO_2$ in this patient (34 mm Hg) indicated an increased VD/VT ratio (0.33), a $\dot{Q}tot$ that is within normal limits

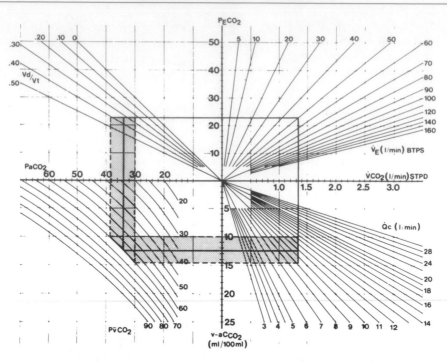

Figure 11–9. Example 2 measurements plotted on the diagram. In this case, the limiting values are much wider apart; the dotted lines have been drawn to represent the limits implied by the highest normal VD/VT (0.22) and normal cardiac output (13 L/min). It is impossible for both to be within normal limits.

(11 L/min), and a stroke volume that is reduced (65 mL). These values are discussed in more detail in Chapter 12.

The carbon dioxide balance equation may be constructed for this patient as follows:

$$1340 \times 6 = (1120 \times 0.9 \times 6) + (5 \times 70) + CO_2 \text{ (lactic acid)}$$

$$CO_2 \text{ (lactic acid)} = 8040 - 6048 + 600$$

$$= 2592 \text{ mL}$$

$$= 116 \text{ mmol}$$

Thus, the increase in blood $[La^-]$ is predicted at 3.3 mmol/L. A change of this amount is higher than normal at this oxygen intake.

The noninvasive measurements indicate a limited cardiovascular reserve, probably associated with a pulmonary gas exchange disturbance.

Example 3

The following values were obtained in the patient whose stage 1 test results were presented in Example 3, Chapter 8. Measurements were made at 150 kpm/min and 300 kpm/min; the values at 300 kpm/min only are given here.

Patient: female, age 41 years
Height: 155 cm; Weight: 51 kg

Power output	kpm/min	300
	watts	50
f_c	b/min	136
$\dot{V}E$	L/min	28.5
f_b	breaths/min	25
$\dot{V}CO_2$	mL/min	1060
$\dot{V}O_2$	mL/min	1040

$PECO_2$	mm Hg	32
$PETCO_2$	mm Hg	51
$P\bar{v}CO_2$	mm Hg	83

Oxygen intake is appropriate to the power output.

Cardiac frequency is high for the oxygen intake; oxygen pulse is 7 mL/beat, which is at the lowest limit of normal (see Fig. 11–1).

Examining the measurements with the use of the four-quadrant diagram (Fig. 11–10), we find that the cardiac output implied by the highest normal VD/VT (0.23) is only 7.3 L/min, which is low. A normal cardiac output would imply a high VD/VT. Because neither alternative leads to a normal solution, we need an estimate of $PaCO_2$ so that the unique values can be obtained. End-tidal PCO_2 was 51 mm Hg, suggesting that VD/VT is

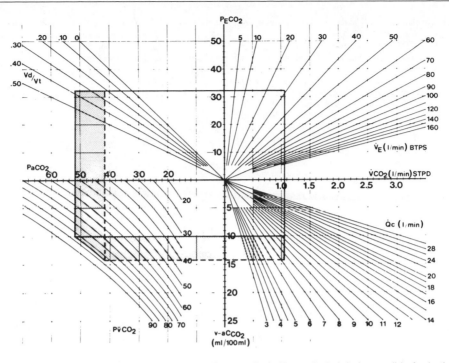

Figure 11–10. Example 3 measurements plotted on the diagram. As in Example 2, it is impossible for both VD/VT and cardiac output to be within normal limits.

high and $\dot{Q}$tot normal. However, this patient has abnormal pulmonary function, and the estimated value of PaCO₂ may be in error. The measured arterial PCO₂ (the solid line in Fig. 11–10) is consistent with alveolar underventilation, an increased VD/VT ratio (0.33), a normal cardiac output (10.3 L/min), and a stroke volume in the low-normal range.

The carbon dioxide balance equation may be constructed, as with the previous two examples; the 11 mm Hg rise in PⱽCO₂ from the end of the 150 kpm/min power output (72 mm Hg) to that at the end of the 300 kpm/min power output (83 mm Hg) implies an appreciable increase in carbon dioxide stores.

The carbon dioxide balance is as follows:

$$1060 \times 5 = (1040 \times 0.9 \times 5) + (11 \times 51) + CO_2 \text{ (lactic)}$$

$$CO_2 \text{ (lactic)} = 5300 - 4680 + 671$$

$$= 1181 \text{ mL}$$

$$= 53 \text{ mmol}$$

Thus, the estimated change in blood [La⁻] is 2 mmol/L.

In this patient, who in a stage 1 test reached a level of exercise associated with a ventilation approximately equal to ventilatory capacity, the stage 2 test results suggested that alveolar underventilation (high PETCO₂ and PⱽCO₂) was present and thus that cardiac output was not significantly impaired. The "normal" ventilation was due to a combination of increased VD/VT and reduced V̇A. Although greater than expected in normal subjects, the calculated lactate increase was small, suggesting that the cardiovascular response was not impaired.

SUMMARY

In many laboratories, arterial blood sampling is deemed necessary in the work-up of most pulmonary and cardiac patients. However, the use of a noninvasive technique may be more applicable to studies carried out in laboratories lacking the facilities and the medical help necessary for arterial catheterization. The stage 2 test offers a good compromise and, when used to explore the linkage between mechanisms with the logic outlined above, falls only a little short of the stage 3 procedure.

REFERENCES

Campbell RD, McKelvie RS, Heigenhauser GJF, Jones NL. Estimation of cardiac output by CO₂ rebreathing during incremental exercise in patients with coronary artery disease. Am J Noninvasive Cardiol 1989;3:147–153.

Clode M, Campbell EJM. The relationship between gas exchange and changes in blood lactate concentrations during exercise. Clin Sci 1969;37:263–272.

Cotes JE, Davies CTM, Edholm OG, et al. Factors relating to the aerobic capacity of 46 healthy British males and females, ages 18 to 28 years. Proc R Soc Lond B 1969;174:91–114.

Gadhoke S, Jones NL. The responses to exercise in boys aged 9 to 15. Clin Sci 1969;37:789–801.

Harris EA, Seelye ER, Whitlock RML. Gas exchange during exercise in healthy people. Clin Sci 1976;51:335–344.

Higgs BE, Clode M, McHardy GJR, et al. Changes in ventilation, gas exchange and circulation during exercise in normal subjects. Clin Sci 1967;32:329–337.

Hughes RL, Clode M, Edwards RHT, et al. Effect of inspired O2 on cardiopulmonary and metabolic responses to exercise in man. J Appl Physiol 1968;24:336–347.

Jones NL, Ehrsam RE. The anaerobic threshold. Exerc Sports Sci Rev 1982;10:49–83.

Jones NL, Jones G, Edwards RHT. Exercise tolerance in chronic airway obstruction. Am Rev Respir Dis 1971;103:477–491.

Jones NL, Jurkowski JE: Body carbon dioxide storage capacity in exercise. J Appl Physiol 1979;46:811–815.

Jones NL, McHardy GJR, Naimark A, et al. Physiological dead space and alveolar-arterial gas pressure differences during exercise. Clin Sci 1966;31:19–29.

Lands LC, Heigenhauser GJF, Jones NL. Analysis of factors limiting maximal exercise performance in cystic fibrosis. Clin Sci 1992;83:391–397.

Massey G, Becklake MR, McKenzie JM, et al. Criculatory and ventilatory response to exercise in thyrotoxicosis. N Engl J Med 1967;276:1104–1112.

McHardy GJR: Relationship between the difference in pressure and content of carbon dioxide in arterial and venous blood. Clin Sci 1967;32:299–309.

McHardy GJR, Jones NL, Campbell EJM: Graphical analysis of carbon dioxide transport during exercise. Clin Sci 1967; 32:289–298.

McKelvie RS, Heigenhauser GJF, Jones NL. Measurement of cardiac output by CO2 rebreathing in unsteady state exercise. Chest 1987;92:777–782.

McKelvie RS, Jones NL. Cardiopulmonary exercise testing. Clin Chest Med 1989;10:277–291.

Spiro SG, Hahn HL, Edwards RHT, et al: Cardiorespiratory adaptations at the start of exercise in normal subjects and in patients with chronic obstructive bronchitis. Clin Sci 1974;47:165–172.

Wicks JR, Lymburner K, Dinsdale SM, et al: The use of multistage exercise testing with wheelchair ergometry and arm cranking in subjects with spinal cord lesions. Paraplegia 1977;15:252–261.

12

Interpretation of Stage 3 Test Results: Steady State Cardiac Output and Pulmonary Gas Exchange

To some readers it must seem puzzling that in the interpretation of stage 1 and stage 2 test results, physiological juggling was needed so that limits could be placed on some of the more important mechanisms that investigators would like to assess in an exercise study. Why not measure arterial blood gases and be done with it? The answer has been hinted at in several sections of the book already. Mainly, the reasons are practical—an arterial blood study requires more time and greater technical skill, and it requires more from the patient. Such studies are best reserved for clinical situations in which the information may be important for diagnostic reasons or because the functional abnormality requires precise measurement. Valvular heart disease, cardiomyopathy, pulmonary vascular disease, and diffuse alveolitis are conditions in which the increase in information may outweigh the cost. For some research purposes, arterial blood studies may be needed for sufficient precision for calculation of cardiac output and other variables to be obtained, but many studies in healthy subjects have shown that an acceptable accuracy is obtained without blood sampling (Faulkner et al., 1977).

In addition to the measured and derived variables that are obtained in a stage 2 test, the following variables are obtained in the stage 3 test:

- Arterial PCO_2 (Pa_{CO_2})
- Arterial pH and HCO_3^- concentration ($[HCO_3^-]$)
- Arterial PO_2 (Pa_{O_2}) and oxygen saturation (Sa_{O_2})
- Alveolar ventilation ($\dot{V}A$)
- VD/VT ratio and physiological dead space (VD)
- Alveolar-arterial PO_2 difference ($PA - aO_2$)
- Venous admixture ($\dot{Q}VA/\dot{Q}tot$) ratio
- Cardiac output ($\dot{Q}tot$)
- Stroke volume (Vs)
- Plasma lactate concentration ($[La^-]$)

These variables may be examined by use of the following guidelines derived from studies in normal subjects and reviewed in Chapter 9 to obtain assessments of pulmonary gas exchange and cardiac output.

STEADY STATE PULMONARY GAS EXCHANGE

1. Arterial PCO_2 shows little change with increasing submaximal exercise, remaining within $\pm$ 2 mm Hg within a subject and between 35 and 45 mm Hg, until substantial lactate accumulation occurs; at higher power, there is a progressive fall to 25 to 35 mm Hg. If high-level exercise is continued for a long time ($>$ 15 minutes), a correction may be needed for changes in body temperature.

2. The fall of arterial $[HCO_3^-]$ with heavy exercise is approximately equimolar to the rise in $[La^-]$, leading to pH values of 7.1 to 7.3.

3. Arterial PO_2 remains within 10 mm Hg of resting values in normal subjects: changes are interpreted through changes in $PA - aO_2$ and $\dot{Q}VA/\dot{Q}tot$ (see below).

4. The VD/VT ratio normally falls from resting values of 0.25 to 0.35 to below 0.20 during exercise. For a more precise estimate of the normal expected value, the expected resting VD—approximately the product of body weight (kilograms) $\times$ 2—is calculated and the VD is increased by 100 mL for every liter of VT: this yields a value with a variance of $\pm$ 15 per cent (Jones et al., 1966).

Thus

$$VD \text{ pred} = (kg \times 2) + 0.1 \ VT$$

where VT is expressed in milliliters. A careful study by Harris and colleagues (1976) yielded a number of regression equations that enable V_D to be calculated from age, height, $\dot{V}CO_2$, $\dot{V}E$, and f_b, and that yield values slightly higher than predicted from our work (Jones et al., 1966). Harris and colleagues made the point that in normal subjects, a correction for changes in pulmonary capillary blood temperature should be made to P_aCO_2; this correction leads to an increase in calculated V_D. In most studies made in patients, this is less important because the power outputs often are relatively low, the duration of exercise is relatively short, and the error becomes less as V_D increases. A representative equation that predicts V_D for rest and exercise in men and women with a 95 per cent upper confidence limit of 81 mL is as follows (Harris et al., 1976):

$$V_D \text{ (mL)} = 0.92 \text{ age (y)} + 1.24 \text{ ht (cm)}$$
$$- 0.36 \ \dot{V}CO_2 \text{ (mL/min)}$$
$$+ 20.8 \ \dot{V}E \text{ (L/min)} - 7.8 \ f_b \text{ (breaths/min)}$$

5. The alveolar-arterial P_{O_2} difference in normal subjects shows no change or a minor decrease from resting values in moderate exercise, with a progressive increase at high power outputs ($\dot{V}O_2 > 2$ L/min). The $P_A - aO_2$ difference cannot be used by itself in assessing gas exchange efficiency, but it is used to calculate venous admixture.*

6. Venous admixture in normal subjects falls from resting values of around 6 per cent to less than 3 per cent of the total cardiac output (Jones et al., 1966; Harris et al., 1976) at moderate workloads. Harris and associates (1976) suggested that there is a small increase with heavy exercise, but 3 per cent of the cardiac output remains an upper limit.*

---

*Theoretically, the three-compartment model analysis (ideal ventilation-perfusion, dead space, and venous admixture compartments), as usually performed by assuming P_aCO_2 is equal to ideal alveolar P_{CO_2}, is not completely valid in situations in which gross venous admixture occurs, particularly if the venoarterial carbon dioxide difference is wide. This is because the venous admixture results in a P_aCO_2 that is significantly higher than the P_{CO_2} in the "ideal" compartment. Although in practice there is little to be gained by correcting for this effect, if necessary it may be performed by a second approximation procedure. This applies the calculated venous admixture to the measured P_aCO_2 so that a corrected P_aCO_2 is then used to calculate a corrected V_D/V_T ratio, $P_A - aO_2$ difference, and $\dot{Q}_{VA}/\dot{Q}_{tot}$. The procedure leads to a slightly higher V_D/V_T and slightly lower $\dot{Q}_{VA}/\dot{Q}_{tot}$ than that calculated by use of uncorrected values (Jones et al., 1966).

STEADY STATE CARDIAC OUTPUT

1. Many studies have demonstrated a linear increase of cardiac output with oxygen uptake, with a slope of 4.5 to 6.1 L/min for every liter increase in $\dot{V}O_2$. Faulkner and colleagues (1977) reviewed previous work and suggested that the intercept of the relationship was related to body weight and was, on average, 66 mL/kg/min in active men. They found that the intercept was lower in older men (49 mL/kg/min) and also concluded that too few data were available for adequate prediction equations for women to be constructed. However, a study of men and women younger and older than 40 years did not show any differences between men and women at given power outputs (Higgs et al., 1967). More recent studies have yielded very similar results in middle-aged men (Campbell et al., 1989), but a study of older men and women showed a lower intercept, averaging 2.9 L/min in both sexes (McElvaney et al., 1989). Taking all this information into account, a reasonable prediction may be obtained from the following equation:

$$\dot{Q}_{tot} = (0.06 \times \text{wt}) + 5.0 \ \dot{V}O_2 \text{ L/min}$$

where wt is in kilograms, $\dot{V}O_2$ is in L/min, and 95 per cent confidence limits are ± 2 L/min.

2. Normal standards for stroke volume during exercise are difficult to find, but taking the previously mentioned studies of cardiac output in untrained healthy men and women and children (see Chapter 2), we obtain values of 1.0 to 1.6 mL/kg in females and 1.4 to 2.0 mL/kg in males (Blimkie et al., 1980; Cunningham et al., 1984). Not surprisingly there is a good correlation between stroke volume and maximal oxygen intake: highly trained athletes may achieve stroke volumes in excess of 2.5 mL/kg (Åstrand and Rodahl, 1970).

3. Changes in plasma lactate concentration are interpreted according to standards derived for other measurements, such as maximal oxygen intake ($\dot{V}O_2$max). In healthy untrained persons, plasma $[La^-]$ increases from resting levels (1.5 $\pm$ 1 mmol/L) at 50 to 75 per cent $\dot{V}O_2$max and reaches 6 to 10 mmol/L at maximum power. In athletes,

plasma [La⁻] may not increase until 80 per cent $\dot{V}O_2$max is exceeded, and very high levels ($\leq$ 20 mmol/L) may be reached. Increases in plasma [La⁻] are used to indicate anaerobic metabolism and thus an imbalance between the rate of muscle glycolysis and the supply of oxygen. However, too literal an interpretation is to be avoided in view of other factors that may influence La⁻ accumulation, such as the blood acid-base status (Jones et al., 1977; Jones and Ehrsam, 1982).

Results of stage 3 measurements are supplied for the patients discussed in the examples in Chapters 8 and 11, for the interpretation and evaluation of the additional information obtained from arterial blood studies. Complete stage 2 and stage 3 measurements are presented together for all the studies.

INTERPRETATION OF STAGE 4 DATA

Although theoretically the placement of a catheter in the pulmonary artery allows measurement of cardiac output by the direct Fick oxygen, dye dilution, or thermodilution methods, such measurements may not be easy if a very small-bore catheter has been floated in place. Of more importance is the measurement of pulmonary arterial pressures, especially in the investigation of pulmonary vascular obstructive disorders (Weber et al., 1984); measurement of left atrial pressures during exercise may also be helpful in assessing the reserve of the left ventricle in mitral and aortic valvar disease or cardiomyopathy.

Pulmonary vascular pressures need to be interpreted in relation to the subject's age and the intensity of the exercise as reflected in $\dot{V}O_2$. Normal standards for pressures are available from the reports of Tartulier and associates (1972) and Ehrsam and colleagues (1983). Tartulier and his colleagues provided the following prediction equations that are similar to those of Ehrsam and co-workers:

$$PAP(syst) = 0.138\dot{Q} + 0.035A\dot{Q} - 0.008A + 11.7$$

$$PAP(diast) = 0.107\dot{Q} + 0.015A\dot{Q} + 0.033A + 1.6$$

$$PcapP(mean) = 0.025A\dot{Q} - 0.487\dot{Q} + 3.4$$

where PAP refers to pulmonary artery pressure, PcapP refers to mean pulmonary capillary wedge pressure, $\dot{Q}$ is cardiac output in L/min, A is age in years, and pressures are in mm Hg. (See also Figure 2–12.)

Example 1

Patient: male, age 49 years
Height: 175 cm; Weight: 86 kg
Referred for: possible coronary artery disease

MEASUREMENTS

Stage 2

W	kpm/min	0	400	800
$\dot{V}O_2$	mL/min	280	1240	2080
$\dot{V}CO_2$	mL/min	230	1120	2000
R		0.82	0.90	0.96
f_c	b/min	68	110	140
$\dot{V}E$	L/min	7	28	48
f_b	breaths/min	10	16	20
V_T	mL	700	1780	2400
$PECO_2$	mm Hg	28.5	34	36
$PETCO_2$	mm Hg	41	43	45
$P\bar{v}CO_2$	mm Hg	52	67	70

Stage 3

$PaCO_2$	mm Hg	42.5	42.0	42.5
PaO_2	mm Hg	86	93	92.0
pH	units	7.37	7.36	7.33
Lactate	mmol/L	1.2	1.8	3.8

DERIVED VARIABLES FOR STAGE 3

VD/VT		0.24	0.16	0.13
$\dot{Q}tot$	L/min	6.8	12.0	17.0
V_s	mL	100	110	120
$PA-aO_2$	mm Hg	10	8	12
SaO_2	%	96	97	97
$\dot{Q}VA/\dot{Q}tot$	%	5	2	2
HCO_3^-	mmol/L	23.5	23.0	21.2

Stage 2 measurements are not commented on further (see page 173).

If the stage 3 results are examined by use of the guidelines previously presented, all will be found to be within normal limits. Arterial PCO_2, PO_2, and pH change very little with exercise, the VD/VT ratio is normal at rest and falls normally with exercise, and cardiac output and stroke volume are normal. Plasma $[La^-]$ shows a small increase, and there is a comparable fall in $[HCO_3^-]$, but at this oxygen intake, these changes do not indicate a serious degree of anaerobic metabolism. In this subject, the stage 1 test results (see page 142) allowed us to state that cardiovascular and respiratory function in exercise were normal and that stroke volume and pulmonary gas exchange must lie within the expected normal range. Considering the clinical condition of this patient, there would be little point in going on to perform stage 2 and stage 3 tests, even though more precise information regarding the variables may be obtained. Similarly, the stage 2 results allowed limits to be placed on the VD/VT ratio and cardiac output that were sufficiently narrow to imply that arterial blood gas measurements would add little to the precision of the interpretation, as may be appreciated from the stage 3 measurements given.

Example 2

Patient: female, age 35 years
Height: 165 cm; Weight: 70 kg
Referred for: investigation of dyspnea

MEASUREMENTS

Stage 2

W	kpm/min	0	200	400
$\dot{V}O_2$	mL/min	210	760	1120
$\dot{V}CO_2$	mL/min	185	745	1340
R		0.89	0.90	1.19
f_c	b/min	84	130	168
$\dot{V}E$	L/min	6.7	28	51
f_b	breaths/min	10	24	30
V_T	mL	640	1165	1700
$PECO_2$	mm Hg	24	23	22.5
$PETCO_2$	mm Hg	34	32	31
$P\bar{v}CO_2$	mm Hg	47	50	65

Stage 3

$PaCO_2$	mm Hg	37	35	34
PaO_2	mm Hg	90	87	85
pH	units	7.40	7.38	7.32
Lactate	mmol/L	1.6	3.1	6.1

DERIVED VARIABLES FOR STAGE 3

VD/VT		0.27	0.28	0.31
$\dot{Q}tot$	L/min	4.8	7.8	10.7
V_s	mL	57	60	64
$PA - aO_2$	mm Hg	16	25	34
SaO_2	%	0.963	0.956	0.946
$\dot{Q}VA/\dot{Q}tot$	%	7	5	7
HCO_3^-	mmol/L	22	20	17

The stage 2 measurements (see page 175) indicated a limited cardiac response to exercise and a probable pulmonary gas exchange disturbance. Arterial PCO_2, PO_2, and pH all showed small progressive falls with increasing exercise. The VD/VT ratio, although within normal limits at rest, increases with exercise: taken with the $PaCO_2$ to $PETCO_2$ difference, this finding implies an increase in alveolar dead space owing to ventilation of poorly perfused areas of the lung. Although arterial PO_2 shows only a small fall, the $PA - aO_2$ difference increases during exercise through an increase in alveolar PO_2. However, when expressed in terms of the venous admixture ratio ($\dot{Q}VA/\dot{Q}tot$), little change is seen with exercise: the $\dot{Q}VA/\dot{Q}tot$ ratio is high, indicating perfusion of some poorly ventilated areas of the lung or a minor degree of right-to-left shunt. The cardiac output is within the lower part of the normal range, but stroke volume is low and fixed, this means that the maximum cardiac output is limited. Blood $[La^-]$ is high in relation to oxygen intake, indicating appreciable anaerobic metabolism.

Pulmonary artery catheterization was performed for pulmonary angiography. Pulmonary artery pressures were elevated at rest (60/30 mm Hg) and increased during exercise (oxygen intake 1 L/min) to 85/50 mm Hg. Normal pulmonary artery pressures at age 41 and cardiac output of 10 L/min are 28/10 mm Hg (Tartulier et al., 1972).

This patient underwent the full range of tests, from stage 1 (see page 144) through stage 3, and finally stage 4 measurements were made. A diagnosis of severe pulmonary thromboembolic hypertension was made, and angiography revealed obstruction of several major pulmonary arteries. Although stage 1 results demonstrated a severe limitation with abnormal ventilatory and heart rate responses, a stage 3 test was needed for quantification of pulmonary gas exchange and cardiac output. In addition to yielding clinical diagnostic information, the stage 3 test elucidated the factors contributing to hyperventilation. Note that ventilation in this patient exceeded the ventilation of the patient in Example 1 during exercise of twice the power (800 kpm/min). This dramatic difference was due to the combination of increased carbon dioxide output (owing to anaerobic metabolism), high alveolar ventilation (low arterial P_{CO_2}), and an increase in dead space ventilation (high V_D/V_T ratio).

Example 3

Patient: female, age 41 years
Height: 155 cm; Weight: 51 kg
Referred for: dyspnea after mitral valvulotomy, and chronic airway obstruction

MEASUREMENTS

Stage 2

W	kpm/min	0	150	300
$\dot{V}O_2$	mL/min	185	680	1040
$\dot{V}CO_2$	mL/min	160	645	1060
R		0.87	0.95	1.02
f_c	b/min	88	104	136
$\dot{V}E$	L/min	5.0	18.0	28.5
f_b	breaths/min	11	17	25
V_T	mL	420	1050	1140
P_{ECO_2}	mm Hg	28	31	32
P_{ETCO_2}	mm Hg	45	49.5	51
$P\bar{v}CO_2$	mm Hg	58	72	83

Stage 3

$PaCO_2$	mm Hg	47	51	52
PaO_2	mm Hg	61	66	71
pH	units	7.38	7.35	7.32
Lactate	mmol/L	1.7	2.2	3.8

DERIVED VARIABLES FOR STAGE 3

V_D/V_T		0.31	0.33	0.33
$\dot{Q}tot$	L/min	4.0	7.8	10.3
V_s	mL	45	75	76
$P_A - aO_2$	mm Hg	33	28	26
SaO_2	%	0.895	0.904	0.910
$\dot{Q}VA/\dot{Q}tot$	%	30	13	9
HCO_3^-	mmol/L	27.0	27.5	26.0

During the stage 1 test (see page 146) the maximum power output was 500 kpm/min; steady state measurements were made at rest, at 150 kpm/min, and at 300 kpm/min.

Arterial PCO_2 is high at rest and increases with exercise in association with a fall in pH. Arterial PO_2 is low at rest but increases with exercise. Although the $P_A - aO_2$ difference is large at rest, it becomes smaller with exercise and the $\dot{Q}VA/\dot{Q}tot$ ratio falls from 30 per cent to 10 per cent of the cardiac output. This suggests that poorly ventilated, well-perfused alveoli at rest become better ventilated during exercise, owing to the increase in V_T. The V_D/V_T is high and does not fall in exercise, also indicating that the increased V_T has led to ventilation of poorly perfused areas. Cardiac output is normal, and stroke volume is low-normal. Plasma lactate concentration increases a small amount, suggesting that some anaerobic metabolism occurs. The stage 3 results show that $P_A - aO_2$ and $\dot{Q}VA/\dot{Q}tot$ improve with exercise despite overall alveolar underventilation (high $PaCO_2$) and that the cardiac output response is adequate. Note that the "normal" value for ventilation is due to a combination of increased dead space and reduced alveolar ventilation.

In most patients assessed for chronic air flow obstruction, there is usually little point in going farther than a stage 1 test, particularly if arterial oxygen saturation is measured by ear oximetry during the test. Stage 2 and stage 3 test results may help in differentiating a cardiac from a pulmonary problem, as in the present example, and in assessing pulmonary gas exchange in detail in some patients. The finding of a progressive diminution in the $P_A - a_{O_2}$ difference in this patient may be taken as evidence against significant alveolar destruction by emphysema.

REFERENCES

Åstrand P-O, Rodahl K. Textbook of Work Physiology. New York: McGraw-Hill Book Co.; 1970.

Blimkie CJR, Cunningham DA, Nichol PM. Gas transport capacity and echocardiographically determined cardiac size in children. J Appl Physiol 1980;49:994–999.

Campbell RD, McKelvie RS, Heigenhauser GJF, Jones NL. Estimation of cardiac output by CO2 rebreathing during incremental exercise in patients with coronary artery disease. Am J Noninvas Cardiol 1989;3:147–153.

Cunningham DA, Paterson DH, Blimkie CJR, Donner AP. Development of cardiorespiratory function in circumpubertal boys: A longitudinal study. J Appl Physiol 1984;56:302–307.

Ehrsam RE, Perruchoud A, Oberholzer M, et al. Influence of age on pulmonary haemodynamics at rest and during supine exercise. Clin Sci 1983;65:653–660.

Faulkner JA, Heigenhauser GF, Shork A. The cardiac output–oxygen uptake relationship of men during graded bicycle ergometry. Med Sci Sports 1977;9:143–147.

Harris EA, Seelye ER, Whitlock RML. Gas exchange during exercise in healthy people. Clin Sci 1976;51:335–344.

Higgs BE, Clode M, McHardy GJR, et al. Changes in ventilation, gas exchange and circulation during exercise in normal subjects. Clin Sci 1967;32:329–337.

Jones NL. Hydrogen ion balance during exercise. Clin Sci 1980;59:85–91.

Jones NL, Ehrsam RE. The anaerobic threshold. Exerc Sports Sci Rev 1982;10:49–83.

Jones NL, McHardy GJR, Naimark A, Campbell EJM. Physiological dead space and alveolar-arterial gas pressure differences during exercise. Clin Sci 1966;31:19–29.

Jones NL, Sutton JR, Taylor R, et al. Effect of pH on cardiorespiratory and metabolic responses to exercise. J Appl Physiol 1977;43:959–964.

McElvaney GN, Blackie SP, Morrison NJ, et al. Cardiac output at rest and in exercise in elderly subjects. Med Sci Sports Exerc 1989;21:293–298.

Tartulier M, Bourret M, Deyrieux F. Pulmonary arterial pressures in normal subjects: Effects of age and exercise. Bull Physiopathol Respir 1972;8:1295–1321.

Weber KT, Wilson JR, Janicki JS, Likoff MJ. Exercise testing in the evaluation of the patient with chronic cardiac failure. Am Rev Respir Dis 1984;129:S60–S62.

13

Interpretation—Further Examples

This chapter allows the reader to interpret data obtained in several examples, which serve also to emphasize the type of information obtained from exercise tests. For each example, I suggest that data from each test (stage 1, stage 2, and stage 3) be analyzed separately; in this way, the additional information gained from more complex data can be readily appreciated. The reader may prefer to construct graphs from the data, similar to those used in the preceding chapters. Some normal standards are given in Appendix D. A brief interpretation follows each set of data, with comments regarding points of interest. Most of the examples appeared in previous editions of the book; with changes in the approach and some of the normal predictive standards, some minor discrepancies may appear, and some irrelevant data have been omitted.

I have avoided writing a section entitled "Patterns of Response" and presenting a series of responses "typical" for each of the diagnoses. I did not wish to give the impression that interpretation of test results mainly involves a search for a diagnostic pattern. The first need is to describe the physiological changes and obtain a picture of the responses in the patient under study. Any diagnostic information is a bonus and may be appreciated in the physiological context. The examples that follow are actual case studies and consist of reasonably straightforward considerations. The diagnosis for each is given after the interpretation; the examples typify the changes usually found. As will be appreciated, some physiological changes are common to several diagnoses, so that their use in indicating a diagnostic response pattern is limited.

Example 1

Stage 1 Measurements

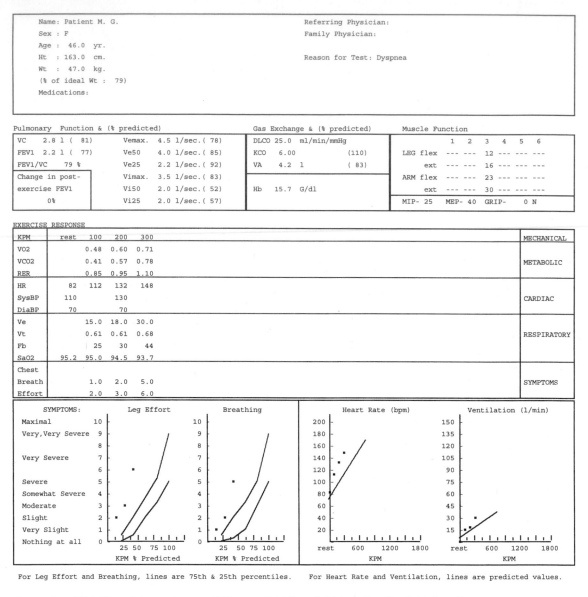

```
Name: Patient M. G.                    Referring Physician:
Sex : F                                Family Physician:
Age : 46.0 yr.
Ht  : 163.0 cm.                        Reason for Test: Dyspnea
Wt  : 47.0 kg.
(% of ideal Wt : 79)
Medications:
```

Pulmonary Function & (% predicted)

VC	2.8 1 (81)	Vemax.	4.5 1/sec. (78)
FEV1	2.2 1 (77)	Ve50	4.0 1/sec. (85)
FEV1/VC	79 %	Ve25	2.2 1/sec. (92)
Change in post-		Vimax.	3.5 1/sec. (83)
exercise FEV1		Vi50	2.0 1/sec. (52)
0%		Vi25	2.0 1/sec. (57)

Gas Exchange & (% predicted)

DLCO	25.0 ml/min/mmHg	
KCO	6.00	(110)
VA	4.2 1	(83)
Hb	15.7 G/dl	

Muscle Function

	1	2	3	4	5	6
LEG flex	---	---	12	---	---	---
ext	---	---	16	---	---	---
ARM flex	---	---	23	---	---	---
ext	---	---	30	---	---	---

MIP- 25   MEP- 40   GRIP-   0 N

EXERCISE RESPONSE

KPM	rest	100	200	300	MECHANICAL
VO2		0.48	0.60	0.71	
VCO2		0.41	0.57	0.78	METABOLIC
RER		0.85	0.95	1.10	
HR	82	112	132	148	
SysBP	110		130		CARDIAC
DiaBP	70		70		
Ve		15.0	18.0	30.0	
Vt		0.61	0.61	0.68	
Fb		25	30	44	RESPIRATORY
SaO2	95.2	95.0	94.5	93.7	
Chest					
Breath		1.0	2.0	5.0	SYMPTOMS
Effort		2.0	3.0	6.0	

For Leg Effort and Breathing, lines are 75th & 25th percentiles.   For Heart Rate and Ventilation, lines are predicted values.

Max. work: 300 (40% pred) kpm   Max. ventilation: 30 (30% pred) l/min   Max. HR 148 (87% pred)

Spirometry shows values that are just below the normal limits for the patient's stature, and flow-volume measurements show a reduction in maximum inspiratory flow; note that she is underweight (79 per cent of ideal weight), suggesting that lean body mass is reduced. Carbon monoxide uptake (KCO) is in the high-normal range, and single-breath lung volume (VA) is in the low-normal range. Respiratory muscle strength is reduced, and skeletal muscle strength is also low.

Stage 1 results show a severe reduction in maximum power output to 40 per cent of that predicted. This is due in part to the low lean body mass, but even if this is taken into account, the maximum power output is less than 50 per cent of that expected, and $\dot{V}O_2$max also is less than 50 per cent of that predicted. The $\dot{V}O_2$ is appropriate at all power outputs, but $\dot{V}CO_2$ shows a relative increase with increasing power, with the RER rising to above 1.0, suggesting that plasma lactate concentration has increased. The cardiac frequency is elevated at all power outputs, and although the value during maximal exercise is not at the

Stage 2 Measurements

		0	200
W	kpm/min	0	200
$\dot{V}O_2$	mL/min	203	605
$\dot{V}CO_2$	mL/min	160	557
R		0.79	0.92
f_c	b/min	90	135
$\dot{V}E$	L/min	9.4	24.0
f_b	breaths/min	27	38
VT	mL	351	630
$PECO_2$	mm Hg	15	21
$PETCO_2$	mm Hg	31	29
$P\bar{v}CO_2$	mm Hg	44	52
min			6

Stage 3 Measurements

		0	200
W	kpm/min	0	200
$PaCO_2$	mm Hg		33
VD/VT	ratio	0.30	0.23
$\dot{Q}tot$	L/min	2.9	5.5
V_s	mL	32	41
PaO_2	mm Hg	90	99
$PA - aO_2$	mm Hg	16	14
SaO_2		0.96	0.97
$\dot{Q}VA/\dot{Q}tot$	%	2.6	1.4
pH		7.34	7.31
HCO_3^-	mmol/L	17.5	15.0
Lactate	mmol/L	0.64	3.0

maximal level predicted for the patient's age (87 per cent of predicted), extrapolation of the submaximal values shows that had she accomplished a further workload, a maximal cardiac frequency would have been reached. Thus, she is close to a maximum cardiac output. Maximum estimated cardiac output is 6.5 L/min, implying a low cardiac stroke volume of 44 mL. Blood pressure is in the low-expected range. There were no electrocardiographic changes with exercise. Ventilation is in the high-normal range when related to power output, but a disproportionate increase in $\dot{V}E$ occurs at the highest power output, owing partly to an increase in $\dot{V}CO_2$. Although $\dot{V}E$ is high, there is still plenty of ventilation reserve in that the ventilation at the maximum power output is only 40 per cent of the predicted maximal voluntary ventilation (77 L/min); however, the pattern of breathing shows a high frequency and a low VT. Ratings of symptoms showed that both leg effort and dyspnea were much greater than expected for the power outputs relative to predicted maximum power, with leg effort being rated slightly greater. Factors identified as contributing to leg muscle fatigue are muscle weakness as well as lactate production secondary to reduced stroke volume and poor muscle perfusion. Factors contributing to dyspnea are increased $\dot{V}E$ secondary to high $\dot{V}CO_2$, hyperventilation and low VT, respiratory muscle weakness, and small lungs.

The stage 2 results show a high cardiac frequency, increased ventilation, high frequency of breathing, and low tidal volume. The mixed venous PCO_2 is low, so alveolar hyperventilation must have been present. However, it is impossible to fit normal values for cardiac output to the data; assuming the highest value for VD/VT compatible with airway dead space alone (0.3; high owing to the low VT), arterial PCO_2 is 30 mm Hg, cardiac output is 5 L/min, and stroke volume is only 38 mL. This solution would be compatible with the low end-tidal PCO_2. The carbon dioxide output is high, and a carbon dioxide balance indicates an increase in lactate of 2 mmol/L.

The stage 3 results confirm the low arterial PCO_2, the normal VD/VT ratio, and the reduced cardiac output (5.5 L/min) and stroke volume (41 mL). Although pulmonary gas exchange is normal (normal VD/VT, $PA - aO_2$, and $\dot{Q}VA/\dot{Q}tot$), lactate accumulation has occurred, indicating an abnormal degree of anaerobic metabolism for this metabolic demand; this finding is consistent with a cardiovascular impairment with inadequate oxygen delivery.

Comments

This patient was referred for assessment of dyspnea of gradually increasing severity since mitral valvotomy 5 years previously. Stage 1 results suggested a cardiovascular limitation with low stroke volume and anaerobic metabolism (Holmgren and Ström, 1959), with severe disability and handicap due to several factors (Holmgren et al., 1958). The stage 2 results suggested that cardiac output was very low and that lactate was being produced at a low work rate. The stage 3 results added the measurement of a low cardiac output and stroke volume. Some other points are pertinent in this patient: it is important to take body size into account when analyzing exercise data; it is an advantage to relate some variables, such as cardiac output and heart rate, to $\dot{V}O_2$ and $\dot{V}E$ to $\dot{V}CO_2$ rather than to power output; hyperventilation and a low tidal volume are commonly seen in patients with left-sided cardiac and pulmonary vascular disease (Gazetopoulos et al., 1966; Gallagher and Younes, 1986).

Example 2

Stage 1 Measurements

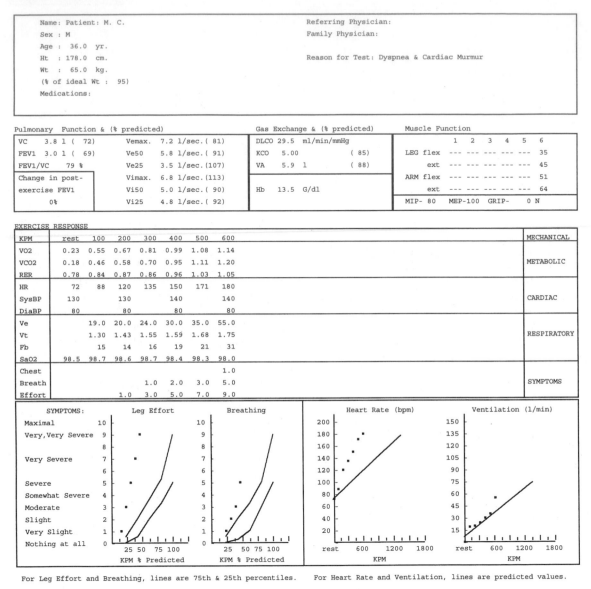

```
Name: Patient: M. C.                      Referring Physician:
Sex : M                                   Family Physician:
Age : 36.0 yr.
Ht : 178.0 cm.                            Reason for Test: Dyspnea & Cardiac Murmur
Wt : 65.0 kg.
(% of ideal Wt : 95)
Medications:
```

Pulmonary Function & (% predicted)		Gas Exchange & (% predicted)		Muscle Function	
VC 3.8 l (72)	Vemax. 7.2 1/sec. (81)	DLCO 29.5 ml/min/mmHg			1 2 3 4 5 6
FEV1 3.0 l (69)	Ve50 5.8 1/sec. (91)	KCO 5.00 (85)		LEG flex --- --- --- --- --- 35
FEV1/VC 79 %	Ve25 3.5 1/sec. (107)	VA 5.9 1 (88)		ext --- --- --- --- --- 45
Change in post-	Vimax. 6.8 1/sec. (113)			ARM flex --- --- --- --- --- 51
exercise FEV1	Vi50 5.0 1/sec. (90)	Hb 13.5 G/dl		ext --- --- --- --- --- 64
0%	Vi25 4.8 1/sec. (92)			MIP- 80 MEP-100 GRIP- 0 N

EXERCISE RESPONSE

KPM	rest	100	200	300	400	500	600		MECHANICAL
VO2	0.23	0.55	0.67	0.81	0.99	1.08	1.14		
VCO2	0.18	0.46	0.58	0.70	0.95	1.11	1.20		METABOLIC
RER	0.78	0.84	0.87	0.86	0.96	1.03	1.05		
HR	72	88	120	135	150	171	180		
SysBP	130		130		140		140		CARDIAC
DiaBP	80		80		80		80		
Ve		19.0	20.0	24.0	30.0	35.0	55.0		
Vt		1.30	1.43	1.55	1.59	1.68	1.75		RESPIRATORY
Fb		15	14	16	19	21	31		
SaO2	98.5	98.7	98.6	98.7	98.4	98.3	98.0		
Chest						1.0			
Breath			1.0	2.0	3.0	5.0			SYMPTOMS
Effort		1.0	3.0	5.0	7.0	9.0			

For Leg Effort and Breathing, lines are 75th & 25th percentiles.   For Heart Rate and Ventilation, lines are predicted values.

Max. work: 600 (44% pred) kpm   Max. ventilation: 55 (36% pred) l/min   Max. HR 180 (102% pred)

This 36-year-old man is slightly underweight (95 per cent of ideal). Spirometry values are just below normal limits, with normal flow rates and a lung volume that is in the low-normal range. Carbon monoxide uptake is normal, respiratory muscle strength is normal, and leg muscle strength is in the low-normal range.

The stage 1 test shows reduced maximal power output (44 per cent of that predicted). The patient experienced very severe leg muscle effort and severe dyspnea; he experienced "very, very

severe" effort at a power output normally described as "very slight." Peak $\dot{V}O_2$ was 1.14 L/min. The cardiac frequency is high at all levels and reaches the maximal heart rate predicted for the patient's age. At the peak $\dot{V}O_2$, a cardiac output of 8 to 12 L/min is expected, suggesting a reduced cardiac stroke volume of 45 to 60 mL (oxygen pulse is only 6 mL/beat). Ventilation is normal at all workloads but increases disproportionately at the highest levels: this is associated with a relative increase in $\dot{V}CO_2$ and

Stage 2 Measurements

W	kpm/min	0	200	400
$\dot{V}_{O_2}$	mL/min	220	725	992
$\dot{V}_{CO_2}$	mL/min	190	710	1080
R		0.88	0.98	1.09
f_c	b/min	76	130	168
$\dot{V}_E$	L/min	8.6	26	42
f_b	breaths/min	14	18	25
V_T	mL	600	1450	1700
P_{ECO_2}	mm Hg	20	24	22
P_{ETCO_2}	mm Hg	34	43	40
$P_{\bar{v}CO_2}$	mm Hg	56.0	67.0	80.5
min			6	5

Stage 3 Measurements

W	kpm/min	0	200	400
Pa_{CO_2}	mm Hg	40	40	38
V_D/V_T ratio		0.4	0.35	0.38
$\dot{Q}_{tot}$	L/min	3.2	6.3	7.7
V_s	mL	42	48	46
Pa_{O_2}	mm Hg	80	90	85
$P_A - a_{O_2}$	mm Hg	22	17	28
Sa_{O_2}		0.95	0.95	0.94
$\dot{Q}_{VA}/\dot{Q}_{tot}$	%	3	1	1
pH		7.38	7.32	7.27
HCO_3^-	mmol/L	22	20	17
Lactate	mmol/L	0.8	2.0	4.5

suggests that blood lactate concentration has increased. The pattern of breathing is normal, and the maximal voluntary ventilation (105 L/min) is not reached.

Arterial oxygen saturation is maintained within the normal range. These results suggest a dominant cardiac limitation, with very reduced maximum cardiac output and cardiac stroke volume, and poor muscle blood flow with lactate production accounting for the severe leg muscle fatigue and contributing also to dyspnea through an increase in $\dot{V}_{CO_2}$.

The stage 2 results confirm the increased cardiac frequency for a given oxygen intake and the increased ventilation. The mixed expired P_{CO_2} is low, and the gross elevation in mixed venous P_{CO_2} suggests that the low P_{ECO_2} cannot be due to alveolar overventilation alone. It is impossible to give normal values for either the V_D/V_T ratio or the cardiac output in order to fit the results; at the highest normal level for V_D/V_T (0.22), arterial P_{CO_2} is 31 mm Hg; the calculated venoarterial content difference is nearly 20 mL/100 mL, which, when converted to oxygen content, exceeds the blood oxygen capacity (1.3 × Hb = 17.5). Thus, the V_D/V_T ratio must be increased in addition to cardiac output's being low. The carbon dioxide balance shows an increase in lactate concentration of 1.3 mmol/L during the first stage and 2 mmol/L during the second stage of the study; both are greater than expected for the low power output.

The stage 3 results show that the V_D/V_T ratio is increased, and cardiac output is low, with a very low stroke volume. The arterial P_{O_2} is normal; although the alveolar-arterial P_{O_2} difference is increased (28 mm Hg), this is accounted for by a high alveolar P_{O_2} and a wide arteriovenous oxygen content difference; venous admixture is normal (1 per cent of total pulmonary blood flow). There is a fall in arterial pH, which is due to the increase in lactate concentration.

Comments

In this patient, who was investigated because of dyspnea and a systolic cardiac murmur, the stage 1 results identified a reduced maximum power output owing to a grossly reduced cardiac reserve and a low stroke volume, as well as evidence of lactate production. The main symptom was leg muscle fatigue, probably related to poor muscle blood flow and muscle lactate accumulation; increased dyspnea was related to an increase in $\dot{V}_{CO_2}$ and a reduction in ventilatory capacity (nonobstructive, suggesting increased elastance). Stage 2 results supplemented our information by demonstrating that in addition to cardiac output's being low, the V_D/V_T ratio was high. The stage 3 results quantified these abnormalities. Another point brought up in the analysis concerns the effect of a wide arteriovenous oxygen difference on the interpretation of the alveolar-arterial P_{O_2} difference. Subsequent cardiac catheterization confirmed a low cardiac output with severe mitral incompetence (Holmgren et al., 1958).

Example 3

Stage 1 Measurements

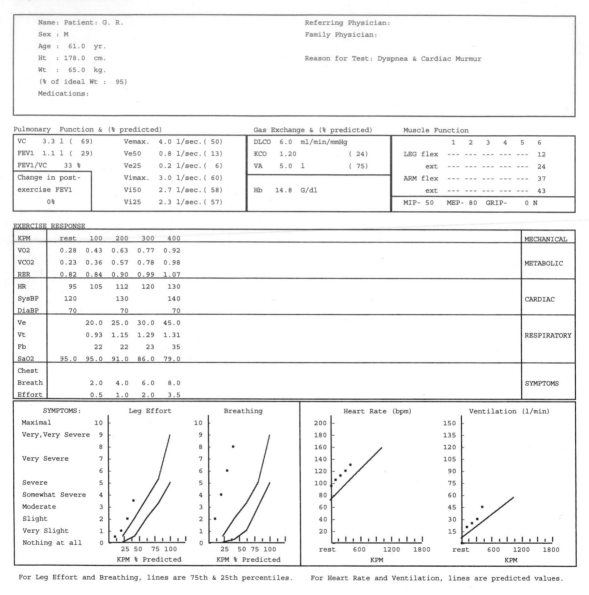

```
Name: Patient: G. R.              Referring Physician:
Sex : M                           Family Physician:
Age : 61.0 yr.
Ht  : 178.0 cm.                   Reason for Test: Dyspnea & Cardiac Murmur
Wt  : 65.0 kg.
(% of ideal Wt :  95)
Medications:
```

Pulmonary Function & (% predicted)		Gas Exchange & (% predicted)	Muscle Function	
VC 3.3 l (69)	Vemax. 4.0 l/sec.(50)	DLCO 6.0 ml/min/mmHg		1 2 3 4 5 6
FEV1 1.1 l (29)	Ve50 0.8 l/sec.(13)	KCO 1.20 (24)	LEG flex --- --- --- --- --- 12
FEV1/VC 33 %	Ve25 0.2 l/sec.(6)	VA 5.0 l (75)	ext --- --- --- --- --- 24
Change in post-	Vimax. 3.0 l/sec.(60)		ARM flex --- --- --- --- --- 37
exercise FEV1	Vi50 2.7 l/sec.(58)	Hb 14.8 G/dl	ext --- --- --- --- --- 43
0%	Vi25 2.3 l/sec.(57)		MIP- 50 MEP- 80 GRIP- 0 N

EXERCISE RESPONSE

KPM	rest	100	200	300	400		MECHANICAL
VO2	0.28	0.43	0.63	0.77	0.92		METABOLIC
VCO2	0.23	0.36	0.57	0.78	0.98		
RER	0.82	0.84	0.90	0.99	1.07		
HR	95	105	112	120	130		CARDIAC
SysBP	120		130		140		
DiaBP	70		70		70		
Ve		20.0	25.0	30.0	45.0		RESPIRATORY
Vt		0.93	1.15	1.29	1.31		
Fb		22	22	23	35		
SaO2	95.0	95.0	91.0	86.0	79.0		
Chest							SYMPTOMS
Breath		2.0	4.0	6.0	8.0		
Effort		0.5	1.0	2.0	3.5		

For Leg Effort and Breathing, lines are 75th & 25th percentiles.   For Heart Rate and Ventilation, lines are predicted values.

Max. work: 400 (38% pred) kpm   Max. ventilation: 45 (34% pred) l/min   Max. HR 130 (82% pred)

Spirometry shows severe airway obstruction, with low flow rates in both expiration and inspiration, and also a reduced lung volume; these results indicate a severe reduction in ventilatory capacity (FEV$_1$ × 35 = 38 L/min). Also DLCO is severely reduced (24 per cent of that predicted) when it is corrected for alveolar volume, indicating marked impairment of pulmonary gas exchange that is consistent with emphysema. Respiratory muscle strength is normal, but leg muscle strength is in the low-expected range.

The stage 1 results show a severe reduction in the maximal power output to 38 per cent of predicted. The ventilatory response is slightly higher than normal and reaches a level at which further increases are limited by the reduced ventilatory capacity. The estimated maximal voluntary ventilation of 38 L/min is exceeded, probably because inspiratory flow is less reduced than is expiratory flow. The frequency of breathing is low at the lower power outputs, and the tidal volume is well maintained, considering the reduction in FEV$_1$, although there is a sharp increase in the frequency of breathing at the highest load. Although cardiac frequency is above the average normal value, it does not reach a level close to the maximum predicted for his age. Arterial oxygen saturation (measured by ear

Stage 2 Measurements				Stage 3 Measurements			
W	kpm/min	0	250	W	kpm/min	0	250
$\dot{V}O_2$	mL/min	290	855	$PaCO_2$	mm Hg	32	41.5
$\dot{V}CO_2$	mL/min	288	830	VD/VT		0.43	0.48
R		1.0	0.97	$\dot{Q}tot$	L/min	5.3	11.0
f_c	b/min	95	120	V_s	mL	56	92
$\dot{V}E$	L/min	15.5	40.1	PaO_2	mm Hg	83	47.5
f_b	breaths/min	20	29	$PA - aO_2$	mm Hg	35.5	62.0
VT	mL	80	1370	SaO_2		0.96	0.82
$PECO_2$	mm Hg	16	18	$\dot{Q}VA/\dot{Q}tot$	%	14	15
$PETCO_2$	mm Hg	34	43	pH		7.4	7.38
$P\bar{v}CO_2$	mm Hg	44	58	HCO_3^-	mmol/L	25	23
min			5	Lactate	mmol/L	1.0	2.5

oximeter) showed a marked fall with increasing exercise, indicating a severe pulmonary gas exchange defect, with a 16 per cent fall associated with less than 1 L/min increase in $\dot{V}O_2$. It is possible that the increase in cardiac frequency represents an adaptive increase in cardiac output secondary to hypoxemia. Dyspnea was the dominant limiting symptom and was related to the increase in ventilation and reduction in ventilatory capacity. Leg muscle effort was also increased for the relative workload and was probably related to some muscle weakness and also lactate production, in turn related to hypoxemia. The results suggest that the patient's severe limitation is due to the combined effects of severe air flow obstruction and a gas exchange defect typical of severe emphysema.

The stage 2 results yield similar quantitative information to that of the stage 1 test. The cardiac frequency is high for the level of oxygen uptake but is within the normal range. Ventilation is high for the carbon dioxide output, as shown by the reduced PCO_2. The mixed venous PCO_2 is normal. Testing the data with the four-quadrant diagram (see Fig. 11–6) shows that the results are not compatible with a normal VD/VT ratio and cardiac output. Because the cardiac frequency is within normal limits and the ventilatory capacity limited the maximum power output in the stage 1 test, it is likely that cardiac output is normal and thus that the VD/VT ratio is elevated. $PaCO_2$ may be normal or high, although a normal value is suggested by the normal end-tidal PCO_2. The respiratory exchange ratio is high, indicating a high carbon dioxide output for this level of oxygen uptake; however, because mixed venous PCO_2 has increased, we may conclude that the high $\dot{V}CO_2$ is not due to the washing out of carbon dioxide from body stores. A carbon dioxide balance calculation shows a change in plasma lactate concentration of 2 mmol/L, which is higher than would normally be expected at this level of oxygen intake.

The stage 3 results show that the arterial PCO_2 is low at rest and normal during exercise; the VD/VT ratio is high, but cardiac output and stroke volume are normal. The arterial PO_2 is low at rest and falls markedly during exercise, with an increase in the alveolar-arterial PO_2 difference and a fall in arterial oxygen saturation. The venous admixture ratio increases. The blood lactate concentration shows an increase similar to that predicted from the stage 2 results and appears to be secondary to arterial hypoxemia.

Note that a correction must be applied to the venoarterial content difference derived from the PCO_2 difference because of arterial oxygen saturation, which is not detected in the bloodless (stage 2) test. However, this correction amounts to only 0.8 mL/100 mL, which does not affect the qualitative stage 2 interpretation.

Comments

The stage 1 results demonstrated the severity of the functional impairment and identified the limiting factor as reduced ventilatory capacity, which was compromised by hyperventilation and associated with hypoxemia. The stage 2 results showed that cardiac output was probably normal. The severity of the pulmonary gas exchange abnormality, with a gross oxygen transfer defect (Dantzker and D'Alonzo, 1986), was confirmed by the stage 3 results, which also confirmed that the cardiac response was normal (Light et al., 1984). This patient had long-standing chronic airway obstruction. The results of other pulmonary function tests were compatible with the diagnosis of severe pulmonary emphysema. A severe gas exchange disturbance (Wagner, 1991) was associated with an increase in the ventilation, which encroached on the reduced ventilatory capacity and resulted in a severe reduction in effort tolerance (Gallagher, 1990).

Example 4

Stage 1 Measurements

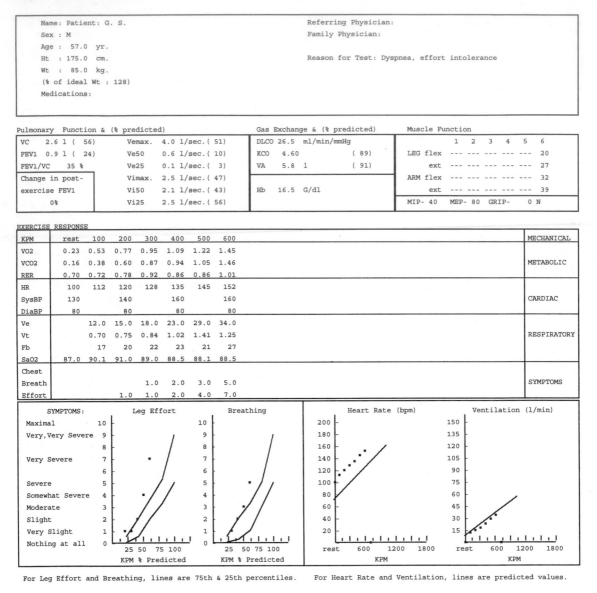

```
Name: Patient: G. S.               Referring Physician:
Sex : M                            Family Physician:
Age : 57.0 yr.
Ht  : 175.0 cm.                    Reason for Test: Dyspnea, effort intolerance
Wt  : 85.0 kg.
(% of ideal Wt : 128)
Medications :
```

Pulmonary Function & (% predicted)

VC	2.6 l	(56)	Vemax.	4.0 l/sec.	(51)
FEV1	0.9 l	(24)	Ve50	0.6 l/sec.	(10)
FEV1/VC	35 %		Ve25	0.1 l/sec.	(3)
Change in post-			Vimax.	2.5 l/sec.	(47)
exercise FEV1			Vi50	2.1 l/sec.	(43)
0%			Vi25	2.5 l/sec.	(56)

Gas Exchange & (% predicted)

DLCO	26.5	ml/min/mmHg	
KCO	4.60		(89)
VA	5.8 l		(91)
Hb	16.5	G/dl	

Muscle Function

	1	2	3	4	5	6
LEG flex	---	---	---	---	---	20
ext	---	---	---	---	---	27
ARM flex	---	---	---	---	---	32
ext	---	---	---	---	---	39
MIP- 40	MEP- 80		GRIP-		0 N	

EXERCISE RESPONSE

KPM	rest	100	200	300	400	500	600		MECHANICAL
VO2	0.23	0.53	0.77	0.95	1.09	1.22	1.45		
VCO2	0.16	0.38	0.60	0.87	0.94	1.05	1.46		METABOLIC
RER	0.70	0.72	0.78	0.92	0.86	0.86	1.01		
HR	100	112	120	128	135	145	152		
SysBP	130		140		160		160		CARDIAC
DiaBP	80		80		80		80		
Ve		12.0	15.0	18.0	23.0	29.0	34.0		
Vt		0.70	0.75	0.84	1.02	1.41	1.25		RESPIRATORY
Fb		17	20	22	23	21	27		
SaO2	87.0	90.1	91.0	89.0	88.5	88.1	88.5		
Chest									
Breath			1.0	2.0	3.0	5.0			SYMPTOMS
Effort		1.0	1.0	2.0	4.0	7.0			

For Leg Effort and Breathing, lines are 75th & 25th percentiles.   For Heart Rate and Ventilation, lines are predicted values.

Max. work: 600 (58% pred) kpm   Max. ventilation: 34 (26% pred) l/min   Max. HR 152 (94% pred)

This 57-year-old man is overweight, and spirometry shows severe airway obstruction, together with some reduction in vital capacity (56 per cent of that predicted). Flow rates were low in both inspiration and expiration. However, DLCO was normal, and other pulmonary function test results showed that total lung capacity was normal and residual volume increased. Respiratory muscle strength is in the low-normal range, and skeletal muscle strength also low-normal for this age. Hemoglobin is raised at 16.5 g/dL.

The stage 1 results reveal a moderately reduced exercise performance (58 per cent of predicted). The patient was limited mainly by leg muscle discomfort, although intensity of dyspnea was also increased. Metabolic measurements show an excess of carbon dioxide output at the highest load only, representing some lactate accumulation. Cardiac frequency is high at all power outputs and at the maximal power output is close (94 per cent) to the maximal heart rate predicted from age. At the measured peak V̇O₂, cardiac output is predicted

Stage 2 Measurements

W	kpm/min	0	200	400
$\dot{V}_{O_2}$	mL/min	254	1080	1350
$\dot{V}_{CO_2}$	mL/min	216	900	1430
R		0.85	0.87	1.05
f_c	b/min	85	130	150
$\dot{V}_E$	L/min	7.8	23	31
f_b	breaths/min	18	19.5	19.5
V_T	mL	430	1170	1580
P_{ECO_2}	mm Hg	24	34	40
P_{ETCO_2}	mm Hg	48	53	58
$P_{\bar{v}CO_2}$	mm Hg	66	86	97
min			6	7

Stage 3 Measurements

W	kpm/min	0	200	400
Pa_{CO_2}	mm Hg	58	60.5	63
V_DV_T	ratio	0.42	0.39	0.33
$\dot{Q}tot$	L/min	8.4	11	14
V_s	mL	100	77	93
Pa_{O_2}	mm Hg	58	62	64
$P_A - a_{O_2}$	mm Hg	22	16	24
Sa_{O_2}		0.86	0.87	0.87
$\dot{Q}_{VA}/\dot{Q}tot$	%	20	12	14
pH		7.36	7.32	7.28
HCO_3^-	mmol/L	31	30	29
Lactate	mmol/L	0.7	1.4	2.4

to be 11 to 13 L/min, suggesting a stroke volume of 70 to 85 mL, within the low-normal range. Ventilation is low at all levels of power output and reaches a value close to the predicted maximal voluntary ventilation (32 L/min). The pattern of breathing shows a normal frequency and a V_T that exceeds the FEV_1, although it shows a fall at the highest load. Arterial oxygen saturation is low at rest but shows a small increase in exercise, suggesting improved $\dot{V}_A/\dot{Q}_C$ distribution during exercise. Because of the severe air flow limitation, the slightly low ventilatory response may indicate hypoventilation during exercise.

The stage 2 results confirm that cardiac frequency is high at both 200 and 400 kpm/min, partly because of the high $\dot{V}_{O_2}$ at both levels, but even when this is allowed for, cardiac frequency is at the upper limit of normal. Ventilation is low for the $\dot{V}_{CO_2}$, and P_{ECO_2} is elevated to 40 mm Hg; the mixed venous P_{CO_2} is also very high. These results indicate that Pa_{CO_2} must be high: if $\dot{Q}tot$ were normal, Pa_{CO_2} would be at least 58 mm Hg at 400 kpm/min. The increased carbon dioxide output together with the increased mixed venous P_{CO_2} at the higher workload indicates lactate accumulation, and a carbon dioxide balance shows an increase of 1.7 mmol/L during this workload.

The stage 3 results confirm the high arterial P_{CO_2} both at rest and during exercise, with increased V_D/V_T ratio and normal cardiac output and stroke volume. Arterial P_{O_2} is low at rest but increases during exercise, with little change in the alveolar-arterial P_{O_2} difference. The calculated venous admixture falls with exercise. The fall in arterial pH is due partly to the increase in P_{CO_2} and partly to a small increase in lactate concentration.

Comments

The stage 1 results demonstrated a relatively well-maintained exercise tolerance, underventilation, and limitation owing to reduced ventilatory capacity. The stage 2 results suggested that severe underventilation occurred during exercise. The stage 3 results confirmed this quantitatively and also demonstrated a normal cardiac output. Although a severe pulmonary gas exchange abnormality was present, this improved with exercise, presumably owing to better distribution of ventilation-perfusion relationships (Jones, 1966; Wagner, 1991).

This patient had severe chronic bronchitis with long-standing airway obstruction and abnormal gas exchange. Underventilation in this patient allowed a relatively high power output to be achieved before a ventilatory limit was reached, and the increase in arterial P_{O_2} with exercise allowed oxygen delivery to be maintained.

Example 5

Stage 1 Measurements

```
Name: Patient P. H.                    Referring Physician:
Sex : M                                Family Physician:
Age :  71.0  yr.
Ht  : 168.0  cm.                       Reason for Test: Fitness programme
Wt  :  71.0  kg.
(% of ideal Wt : 114)
Medications: VENTOLIN QID  BECLOVENT QID  THEODUR BID
```

Pulmonary Function & (% predicted)		Gas Exchange & (% predicted)		Muscle Function	
VC 2.3 l (58)	Vemax. 4.0 l/sec.(59)	DLCO 12.3 ml/min/mmHg		1 2 3 4 5 6	
FEV1 1.2 l (39)	Ve50 0.6 l/sec.(11)	KCO 2.56 (55)		LEG flex --- --- --- --- --- 21	
FEV1/VC 52 %	Ve25 0.1 l/sec.(4)	VA 4.8 l (83)		ext --- --- --- --- --- 23	
Change in post-	Vimax. 4.7 l/sec.(94)			ARM flex --- --- --- --- --- 34	
exercise FEV1	Vi50 4.3 l/sec.(93)	Hb 15.5 G/dl		ext --- --- --- --- --- 40	
0%	Vi25 2.9 l/sec.(67)			MIP- 70 MEP-110 GRIP- 0 N	

EXERCISE RESPONSE

KPM	rest	100	200	300	400	500	600	700	800		MECHANICAL
VO2	0.35	0.49	0.67	0.79	0.91	1.08	1.22	1.42	1.57		
VCO2	0.29	0.37	0.50	0.60	0.76	0.97	1.15	1.42	1.65		METABOLIC
RER	0.82	0.75	0.74	0.76	0.83	0.89	0.95	1.00	1.05		
HR	93	102	104	106	109	116	122	131	142		
SysBP	120		155		150		180		185		CARDIAC
DiaBP	85		85		85		85		85		
Ve	12.3	14.2	18.4	21.0	26.5	32.0	37.0	45.0	53.8		
Vt	1.00	1.02	1.10	1.27	1.35	1.50	1.61	1.66	1.68		RESPIRATORY
Fb	12	14	17	17	20	21	23	28	32		
SaO2	94.9	95.3	94.9	95.3	95.5	95.2	94.5	93.5	93.4		
Chest											
Breath		0.5	1.0	2.0	2.5	3.0	3.0	5.0			SYMPTOMS
Effort			0.5	1.0	1.5	2.0	2.0				

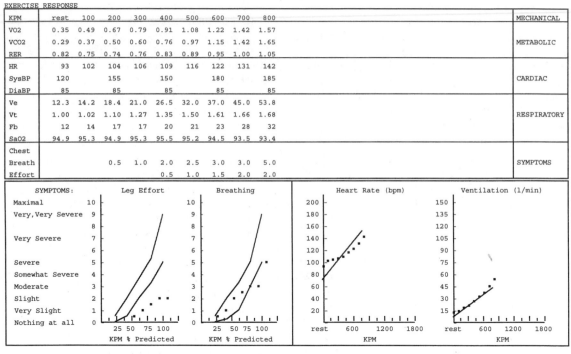

For Leg Effort and Breathing, lines are 75th & 25th percentiles.   For Heart Rate and Ventilation, lines are predicted values.

Max. work: 800 (103% pred) kpm   Max. ventilation: 54 (50% pred) l/min   Max. HR 142 (94% pred)

The patient is of average weight (114 per cent of ideal). Spirometry shows a severe expiratory flow limitation, suggesting a ventilatory capacity of only 39 per cent of that predicted. However, the flow-volume loop shows excellent inspiratory flow, suggesting that ventilatory capacity might actually exceed 100 L/min. Carbon monoxide uptake is severely reduced to 55 per cent of predicted when it is corrected for lung volume, suggesting emphysema. Both respiratory and skeletal muscle

strength are in the normal range for the patient's age (71 years).

In the stage 1 study, the patient achieves a normal maximum exercise capacity (103 per cent of predicted). He is limited by dyspnea, but the intensity is appropriate to the relative workload. Oxygen intake is appropriate, and excess carbon dioxide output is seen at the highest two workloads, suggesting a normal lactate accumulation. Heart rate and blood pressure increase in the normal range, and the electrocardiogram shows no changes. Ventilation is appropriate to the metabolic demands, and the tidal volume at maximal exercise (1.68 L) exceeds the rest FEV_1 (1.2 L). FEV_1 value following exercise is identical to the pre-exercise value.

Comments

It may appear surprising that this patient achieved a normal exercise capacity, in view of the severe impairment of both FEV_1 and DLCO, illustrating the fallacy of predicting disability on the basis of these measurements made at rest. The explanation lies in good skeletal and respiratory muscle strength, good inspiratory air flow, and presumably good $\dot{V}A/\dot{Q}C$ matching during exercise. The patient was a very active individual; the low rating for dyspnea was presumably due to normal exercise ventilation, good inspiratory flow, strong respiratory muscles, and the sensory adaptation associated with long-standing airway obstruction. Inspiratory flow capacity is very variable among patients with severe expiratory air flow obstruction (Stubbing et al., 1980) and is one factor accounting for variability in dyspnea during exercise (Leblanc et al., 1986).

Example 6A

Stage 1 Measurements

```
Name: Patient J. K.                    Referring Physician:
Sex : M                                Family Physician:
Age :  18.0  yr.
Ht  : 175.0  cm.                       Reason for Test: Evaluation, alveolitis
Wt  :  72.0  kg.
(% of ideal Wt : 109)
Medications:
```

Pulmonary Function & (% predicted)

			Gas Exchange & (% predicted)	Muscle Function						
VC 3.3 l (60)	Vemax. 7.5 l/sec.(95)		DLCO 14.0 ml/min/mmHg			1	2	3	4	5 6
FEV1 2.8 l (60)	Ve50 6.2 l/sec.(114)		KCO 3.10 (48)	LEG flex	--- --- --- --- ---	32
FEV1/VC 85 %	Ve25 4.1 l/sec.(130)		VA 4.5 l (69)	ext	--- --- --- --- ---	57
Change in post-	Vimax. 6.5 l/sec.(108)			ARM flex	--- --- --- --- ---	48
exercise FEV1	Vi50 5.5 l/sec.(100)		Hb 16.9 G/dl	ext	--- --- --- --- ---	55
0%	Vi25 5.2 l/sec.(100)			MIP-120 MEP-150 GRIP- 0 N		

EXERCISE RESPONSE

KPM	rest	100	200	300	400	500	600	700	800		MECHANICAL
VO2	0.35	0.49	0.67	0.79	0.91	1.03	1.25	1.42	1.58		
VCO2	0.29	0.37	0.55	0.68	0.85	0.98	1.32	1.65	1.95		METABOLIC
RER	0.83	0.76	0.82	0.86	0.93	0.95	1.06	1.16	1.23		
HR	110	125	138	145	152	162	176	182	191		
SysBP	120		125		135		150		170		CARDIAC
DiaBP	80		80		80		80		80		
Ve		22.0	27.0	31.0	35.0	47.0	79.0	93.0	99.0		
Vt		0.61	0.65	0.73	0.93	1.11	1.33	1.60	1.51		RESPIRATORY
Fb		36	42	43	38	42	59	58	66		
SaO2	95.1	94.5	93.0	91.5	91.1	90.5	87.6	83.1	79.5		
Chest											
Breath			1.0	1.0	2.0	4.0	6.0	8.0			SYMPTOMS
Effort				1.0	1.0	3.0	5.0	8.0			

For Leg Effort and Breathing, lines are 75th & 25th percentiles.   For Heart Rate and Ventilation, lines are predicted values.

Max. work: 800 (56% pred) kpm   Max. ventilation: 99 (61% pred) l/min   Max. HR 191 (101% pred)

This 18-year-old man has a normal weight. Spirometry shows a moderate reduction in the ventilatory capacity of nonobstructive type, with VC and single-breath VA being 60 and 69 per cent of predicted, respectively. DLCO is very reduced, at 48 per cent of that predicted, indicating a severe gas exchange impairment. Respiratory muscle strength and skeletal muscle strength are normal.

The stage 1 results show that the maximum power output is reduced to 56 per cent of predicted for the patient's age and height. Oxygen uptake is appropriate to the power output, but there is a progressive increase in $\dot{V}CO_2$, suggesting marked lactate accumulation. Cardiac frequency is increased at all levels and reaches the maximum predicted for the patient's age. Ventilation is also increased at the higher power outputs and at the highest level is close to the maximal voluntary ventilation (96 L/min). Tidal volume is reduced at all levels. Arterial oxygen saturation is normal at rest but falls progressively with increasing exercise, with a maximum fall of 15 to 16 per

Stage 2 Measurements

Stage 3 Measurements

W	kpm/min	0	300	500
$\dot{V}_{O_2}$	mL/min	252	816	1240
$\dot{V}_{CO_2}$	mL/min	190	160	180
R		0.76	1.05	1.05
f_c	b/min	120	160	180
$\dot{V}_E$	L/min	9	34	74
f_b	breaths/min	24	31	56
V_T	mL	370	1090	1320
P_{ECO_2}	mm Hg	18	21	15
P_{ETCO_2}	mm Hg	31	29	24
$P_{\bar{v}CO_2}$	mm Hg	46	55	61
min			5	6

W	kpm/min	0	300	500
Pa_{CO_2}	mm Hg	32	30	26
V_D/V_T	ratio	0.26	0.23	0.36
$\dot{Q}_{tot}$	L/min	2.7	7.2	8.4
V_s	mL	23	45	47
Pa_{O_2}	mm Hg	76	70	61
$P_A - a_{O_2}$	mm Hg	32	48	62
Sa_{O_2}		0.95	0.94	0.91
$\dot{Q}_{VA}/\dot{Q}_{tot}$	%	7	8	10
pH		7.39	7.38	7.37
HCO_3^-	mmol/L	18.8	17.5	14.6
Lactate	mmol/L	0.8	2.2	4.8

cent. Thus, although a cardiovascular abnormality is suggested by the high cardiac frequency, it is also possible that it represents a high cardiac output in response to hypoxemia. Thus, the stage 1 results show a severe reduction in capacity, limitation due to both dyspnea and leg muscle fatigue, progressive hypoxemia, evidence of lactate formation, and much-increased ventilatory and cardiac responses.

The stage 2 results show a gross increase in ventilation with a very low P_{ECO_2} (15 mm Hg at the higher load). The pattern of breathing was that of a high frequency with a low tidal volume. The mixed venous P_{CO_2} was normal. It is impossible to fit normal values for V_D/V_T ratio and cardiac output to the data; the low end-tidal P_{CO_2} suggests that there was marked alveolar hyperventilation, implying a low cardiac output in addition to an increased V_D/V_T, and a carbon dioxide balance indicates an increase in lactate concentration of about 2 mmol/L at each of the two workloads.

The stage 3 results reveal a marked alveolar hyperventilation, an increased V_D/V_T ratio, and low cardiac output and stroke volume. In addition, the arterial P_{O_2} is low at rest and falls with exercise, with a very large alveolar-arterial P_{O_2} difference and increasing venous admixture. There is a decrease in bicarbonate and pH, which coincides with the increase in blood lactate concentration.

This patient shows a gross increase in the alveolar-arterial P_{O_2} difference and thus provides an opportunity to examine the calculations made using the "three-compartment lung model"

approach, in which arterial P_{CO_2} is assumed to be equal to the ideal alveolar P_{CO_2} in the calculation of alveolar P_{O_2}. Arterial P_{CO_2} is 26 mm Hg at 500 kpm/min; using the calculated value for venous admixture (10 per cent) and the measured mixed venous P_{O_2}, we may calculate the extent to which the arterial P_{CO_2} is higher than the ideal alveolar P_{CO_2} (Riley et al., 1951):

$$0.9 \text{ (ideal } Pa_{CO_2}) + 0.1 (61) = 26$$

$$\text{Ideal } Pa_{CO_2} = 22.2 \text{ mm Hg}$$

Using this value instead of Pa_{CO_2}, V_D/V_T is 0.28 (compared with 0.36), Pa_{O_2} is 127 mm Hg (instead of 123 mm Hg), and alveolar-arterial P_{O_2} is 66 mm Hg (instead of 62 mm Hg). The differences between these figures are not great and do not lead to important errors of interpretation. However, in a patient with such a severe gas exchange disturbance, the use of the rebreathing method for measurement of cardiac output must be questioned. During the higher workload, there was a progressive hyperventilation and reduction in Pa_{CO_2}, and it is quite likely that equilibration of carbon dioxide stores was not complete; this would lead to a falsely high $P_{\bar{v}CO_2}$ in relation to Pa_{CO_2} and would lead to an erroneous underestimate of cardiac output.

Two months later, clinical features of alveolitis had cleared, and the patient was free of symptoms. Clinical and laboratory examination revealed the following results in a stage 1 test (see Example 6B).

Example 6B

Stage 1 Measurements

```
Name: Patient J. K.                    Referring Physician:
Sex : M                                Family Physician:
Age : 18.0  yr.
Ht  : 175.0  cm.                       Reason for Test: Post Rx allergic alveolitis
Wt  : 80.0  kg.
(% of ideal Wt : 121)
Medications: PREDNISONE
```

Pulmonary Function & (% predicted)			Gas Exchange & (% predicted)		Muscle Function	
VC 4.8 l (87)	Vemax. 0.0 l/sec.(0)		DLCO 24.5 ml/min/mmHg		1 2 3 4 5 6	
FEV1 4.3 l (93)	Ve50 0.0 l/sec.(0)		KCO 4.20 (65)		LEG flex --- --- --- --- --- 41	
FEV1/VC 90 %	Ve25 0.0 l/sec.(0)		VA 5.9 l (90)		ext --- --- --- --- --- 67	
Change in post-	Vimax. 0.0 l/sec.(0)				ARM flex --- --- --- --- --- 57	
exercise FEV1	Vi50 0.0 l/sec.(0)		Hb 15.5 G/dl		ext --- --- --- --- --- 64	
0%	Vi25 0.0 l/sec.(0)				MIP-110 MEP-150 GRIP- 0 N	

EXERCISE RESPONSE

KPM	rest	100	200	300	400	500	600	700	800	900	1000	1100	1200	1300		MECHANICAL
VO2	0.29	0.51	0.65	0.89	1.02	1.20	1.36	1.59	1.81	2.04	2.20	2.37	2.56	2.73		
VCO2	0.24	0.42	0.55	0.72	0.79	0.91	1.02	1.22	1.39	1.58	1.71	1.98	2.57	2.85		METABOLIC
RER	0.83	0.82	0.85	0.81	0.77	0.76	0.75	0.77	0.77	0.78	0.78	0.84	1.00	1.04		
HR	95	96	100	102	110	118	128	138	145	156	159	174	180	191		
SysBP	110			130				150			170					CARDIAC
DiaBP	70			70				75			70					
Ve	12.0	15.0	19.0	23.0	27.0	32.0	36.0	38.0	48.0	51.0	52.0	70.0	87.0	101.0		
Vt	1.20	1.25	1.36	1.43	1.42	1.60	1.71	1.90	2.18	2.13	2.70	2.50	3.00	2.90		RESPIRATORY
Fb	10	12	14	16	19	20	21	20	22	24	19	28	29	35		
SaO2	98.1	98.7	98.1	97.9	97.5	97.3	96.8	96.2	96.1	95.8	95.5	94.1	93.2	91.8		
Chest																
Breath						1.0	1.0	1.0	2.0	3.0	5.0	6.0	7.0			SYMPTOMS
Effort					1.0	2.0	2.0	3.0	4.0	5.0	6.0	7.0	8.0			

For Leg Effort and Breathing, lines are 75th & 25th percentiles.   For Heart Rate and Ventilation, lines are predicted values.

Max. work: 1300 (92% pred) kpm   Max. ventilation: 101 (62% pred) l/min   Max. HR 191 (101% pred)

Resting measurements show an improvement in spirometry values to within the low-normal range; carbon monoxide uptake remains impaired at 65 per cent of predicted, when corrected for lung volume. In comparison to the first study, the repeat stage 1 study shows an increase in maximal power output from 56 per cent of predicted to 92 per cent. Symptom intensity is less, and the patient is limited mainly by severe leg muscle effort, which now exceeds the intensity of breathing effort at all loads. Oxygen uptake and carbon dioxide output are appropriate to the power output, and the respiratory exchange ratio does not exceed unity until 1200 kpm/min (previously 600 kpm/min) is reached, indicating that lactate is not accumulating until a much higher load than in the previous test. Heart rate increases normally and is 40 to 50 b/min lower. The ventilation response is also normal, and the pattern of breathing shows a higher VT at any given ventilation—for example,

Stage 2 Measurements

W	kpm/min	0	400	800
$\dot{V}O_2$	mL/min	260	1270	2130
$\dot{V}CO_2$	mL/min	210	1080	2120
R		0.8	0.85	0.99
f_c	b/min	100	135	174
$\dot{V}E$	L/min	8.8	32.6	59.0
f_b	breaths/min	15	22	26
V_T	mL	590	1440	2270
$PECO_2$	mm Hg	21	30	31
$PETCO_2$	mm Hg	34	39	37
$P\bar{v}CO_2$	mm Hg	43	57	67
min			5.5	6

Stage 3 Measurements

W	kpm/min	0	400	800
$PaCO_2$	mm Hg	36	38	36
VD/VT	ratio	0.31	0.17	0.11
$\dot{Q}tot$	L/min	7	12.4	17.7
V_s	mL	70	92	101
PaO_2	mm Hg	80	88	84
$PA - aO_2$	mm Hg	15	13	26
SaO_2		0.96	0.96	0.96
$\dot{Q}VA/\dot{Q}tot$	%	7	2	3
pH		7.40	7.38	7.35
HCO_3^-	mmol/L	24	22	19
Lactate	mmol/L	0.6	1.5	4.2

at a $\dot{V}E$ of 100 L/min, V_T is now 2.9 L, compared with 1.5 L. Oximetry shows that SaO_2 is maintained at close to rest values until the highest loads, when there is a small 4 per cent decrease.

The stage 2 test shows a normal relationship of ventilation to carbon dioxide output with a higher $PECO_2$ and $PETCO_2$ and little change in $P\bar{v}CO_2$—the results being compatible with normal cardiac output and VD/VT ratio.

The results of the stage 3 test confirm these conclusions in showing a normal cardiac output and stroke volume, a normal VD/VT ratio and venous admixture, and maintained arterial PO_2.

Comments

In this patient with allergic alveolitis, the severe gas exchange disturbance and hypoxemia and the associated cardiovascular and ventilatory changes were shown in the stage 1 test. The stage 3 test quantified the cardiac and gas exchange impairments. Comparison of the results on the two occasions shows the importance of retesting. Also, the data obtained from the stage 1 test were adequate to indicate the degree of improvement. A final point of interest is that the pathological condition was not only impairing pulmonary gas exchange but also embarrassing the circulation, both through the strain of adapting to the hypoxemia and presumably by causing pulmonary hypertension. The patient was finally tested 6 months after the second study; at this point, spirometry and carbon monoxide uptake were in the high-normal range, and maximum power had increased further to 1600 kpm/min (110 per cent of predicted), consistent with a very active lifestyle but also indicating that the reduction in capacity at the time of the first test was probably greater than indicated by the reduction expressed as per cent of predicted.

Example 7

Stage 1 Measurements

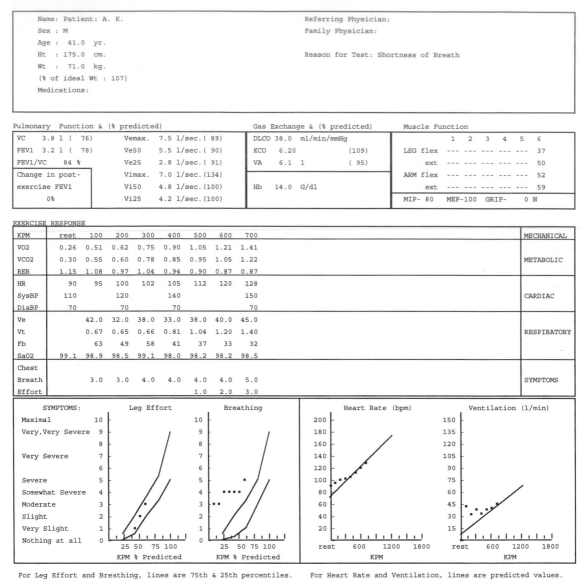

```
Name: Patient: A. K.                    Referring Physician:
Sex : M                                 Family Physician:
Age : 41.0 yr.
Ht  : 175.0 cm.                         Reason for Test: Shortness of Breath
Wt  : 71.0 kg.
(% of ideal Wt : 107)
Medications:
```

Pulmonary Function & (% predicted)

VC 3.8 l (76)	Vemax. 7.5 l/sec.(89)
FEV1 3.2 l (78)	Ve50 5.5 l/sec.(90)
FEV1/VC 84 %	Ve25 2.8 l/sec.(91)
Change in post-	Vimax. 7.0 l/sec.(134)
exercise FEV1	Vi50 4.8 l/sec.(100)
0%	Vi25 4.2 l/sec.(100)

Gas Exchange & (% predicted)

DLCO 38.0 ml/min/mmHg	
KCO 6.20	(109)
VA 6.1 l	(95)
Hb 14.0 G/dl	

Muscle Function

	1	2	3	4	5	6
LEG flex	---	---	---	---	---	37
ext	---	---	---	---	---	50
ARM flex	---	---	---	---	---	52
ext	---	---	---	---	---	59
MIP- 80	MEP-100	GRIP-	0 N			

EXERCISE RESPONSE

KPM	rest	100	200	300	400	500	600	700		
VO2	0.26	0.51	0.62	0.75	0.90	1.05	1.21	1.41		MECHANICAL
VCO2	0.30	0.55	0.60	0.78	0.85	0.95	1.05	1.22		METABOLIC
RER	1.15	1.08	0.97	1.04	0.94	0.90	0.87	0.87		
HR	90	95	100	102	105	112	120	128		
SysBP	110		120		140			150		CARDIAC
DiaBP	70		70		70			70		
Ve		42.0	32.0	38.0	33.0	38.0	40.0	45.0		
Vt		0.67	0.65	0.66	0.81	1.04	1.20	1.40		RESPIRATORY
Fb		63	49	58	41	37	33	32		
SaO2	99.1	98.9	98.5	99.1	98.0	98.2	98.2	98.5		
Chest										
Breath		3.0	3.0	4.0	4.0	4.0	4.0	5.0		SYMPTOMS
Effort						1.0	2.0	3.0		

For Leg Effort and Breathing, lines are 75th & 25th percentiles.   For Heart Rate and Ventilation, lines are predicted values.

Max. work: 700 (57% pred) kpm   Max. ventilation: 45 (31% pred) l/min   Max. HR 128 (74% pred)

This patient's weight is close to ideal; spirometry is normal, and flow is normal at all lung volumes in inspiration and expiration; carbon monoxide uptake is normal. Respiratory and skeletal muscle strength are normal.

In the stage 1 test, the patient achieved a maximum power that was only 57 per cent of predicted. He was limited by shortness of breath, but the intensity of dyspnea was very high at low workloads and became relatively less with increases in work. Oxygen uptake is appropriate to the loads, but carbon dioxide output is high at low workloads, with a high respiratory exchange ratio, which becomes less with increasing power, suggesting that lactate has not accumulated. Apart from mild tachycardia at low work, the heart rate response is normal, as is the blood pressure; there is no abnormality in the electrocardiogram at rest and exercise. Ventilation is very high and variable at low levels of exercise, with a high frequency of breathing, in spite of encouragement to breathe more slowly; however, at higher work, ventilation is normal. Oxygen saturation is normal throughout. Neither the cardiac frequency nor the ventilation reaches values considered to be limiting. Blood lactate concentration, measured shortly after the cessation of exercise, was only 2.5 mmol/L.

Because of apparent apprehension, the test was repeated a week later, with almost identical results being obtained.

Comments

This pattern of response is typical of psychogenic dyspnea associated with hyperventilation, which confirmed the clinical impression: the patient showed clinical evidence of an anxiety reaction, together with episodes of dizziness and tingling that generally occurred at times of stress. The exercise test results excluded pulmonary hypertension and significant cardiac or pulmonary disease, allowing the physician to reassure the patient and pursue an expectant course of management. Stage 2 and stage 3 tests were not required, because there was no indication of a cardiac, respiratory, or metabolic abnormality. This clinical problem is not uncommon and deserves to be diagnosed promptly, before undue attention reinforces the patient's anxiety (Burns and Howell, 1969).

Example 8

Stage 1 Measurements

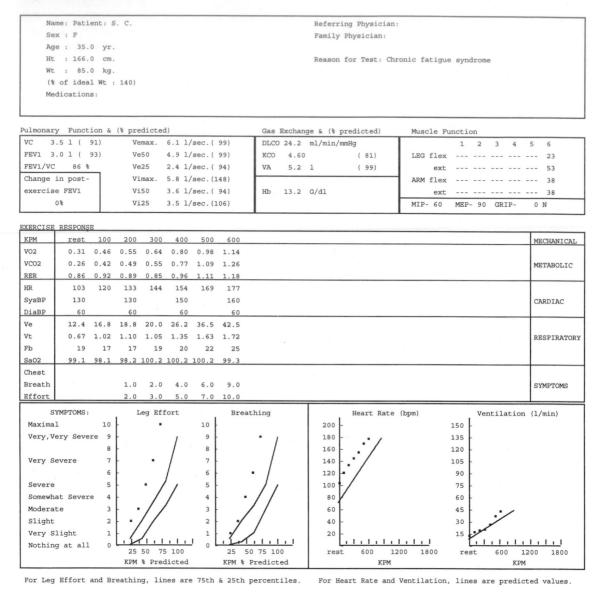

```
Name: Patient: S. C.                    Referring Physician:
Sex : F                                 Family Physician:
Age : 35.0  yr.
Ht  : 166.0 cm.                         Reason for Test: Chronic fatigue syndrome
Wt  : 85.0  kg.
(% of ideal Wt : 140)
Medications:
```

Pulmonary Function & (% predicted)

VC	3.5 l (91)	Vemax.	6.1 l/sec. (99)
FEV1	3.0 l (93)	Ve50	4.9 l/sec. (99)
FEV1/VC	86 %	Ve25	2.4 l/sec. (94)
Change in post-		Vimax.	5.8 l/sec.(148)
exercise FEV1		Vi50	3.6 l/sec. (94)
0%		Vi25	3.5 l/sec.(106)

Gas Exchange & (% predicted)

DLCO	24.2 ml/min/mmHg	
KCO	4.60	(81)
VA	5.2 l	(99)
Hb	13.2 G/dl	

Muscle Function

	1	2	3	4	5	6
LEG flex	---	---	---	---	---	23
ext	---	---	---	---	---	53
ARM flex	---	---	---	---	---	38
ext	---	---	---	---	---	38
MIP- 60	MEP- 90	GRIP-	0 N

EXERCISE RESPONSE

KPM	rest	100	200	300	400	500	600	
VO2	0.31	0.46	0.55	0.64	0.80	0.98	1.14	MECHANICAL
VCO2	0.26	0.42	0.49	0.55	0.77	1.09	1.26	METABOLIC
RER	0.86	0.92	0.89	0.85	0.96	1.11	1.18	
HR	103	120	133	144	154	169	177	
SysBP	130		130		150		160	CARDIAC
DiaBP	60		60		60		60	
Ve	12.4	16.8	18.8	20.0	26.2	36.5	42.5	
Vt	0.67	1.02	1.10	1.05	1.35	1.63	1.72	RESPIRATORY
Fb	19	17	17	19	20	22	25	
SaO2	99.1	98.1	98.2	100.2	100.2	100.2	99.3	
Chest								
Breath			1.0	2.0	4.0	6.0	9.0	SYMPTOMS
Effort			2.0	3.0	5.0	7.0	10.0	

For Leg Effort and Breathing, lines are 75th & 25th percentiles.   For Heart Rate and Ventilation, lines are predicted values.

Max. work: 600 (69% pred) kpm   Max. ventilation: 43 (37% pred) l/min   Max. HR 177 (100% pred)

This patient is overweight (140 per cent of ideal). Spirometry values are in the low-normal range, and flow rates are normal in inspiration and expiration. Carbon monoxide uptake is normal. Respiratory and skeletal muscle strength are normal.

In the stage 1 study the patient achieves a power output that is moderately reduced (69 per cent of predicted), and exercise capacity is limited by severe leg muscle discomfort. The Borg ratings for both dyspnea and leg effort are markedly increased at all power outputs. Oxygen uptake is appropriate, but carbon dioxide output is increased at the higher loads, with R exceeding 1.0 at 500 kpm/min, suggesting that blood lactate concentration has increased. Heart rate is elevated at all power outputs and reaches 100 per cent of the predicted maximum. Blood pressure increases in the low-expected range. The electrocardiographic results are normal at rest and exercise. Ventilation and the pattern of breathing are normal, and oximetry shows no change in Sao2.

Stage 2 Measurements

W	kpm/min	0	300
$\dot{V}O_2$	mL/min	250	940
$\dot{V}CO_2$	mL/min	214	920
R		0.86	0.98
f_c	b/min	90	159
$\dot{V}E$	L/min	7.6	24.6
f_b	breaths/min	14	27
V_T	mL	541	910
$PECO_2$	mm Hg	24.3	30.2
$PETCO_2$	mm Hg	38	38
$P\bar{v}CO_2$	mm Hg	46	55
min			5

Stage 3 Measurements

W	kpm/min	0	300
$PaCO_2$	mm Hg	37	38
VD/VT	ratio	0.22	0.14
$\dot{Q}tot$	L/min	4.9	12.5
V_s	mL	56	79
PaO_2	mm Hg	92	97
$PA-aO_2$	mm Hg	12	11
SaO_2		0.96	0.97
$\dot{Q}VA/\dot{Q}tot$	%	4	2
pH		7.38	7.33
HCO_3^-	mmol/L	21.6	20.3
Lactate	mmol/L	1.0	2.6

Low maximum power output, high heart rate, evidence of lactate formation, and severe muscle effort and dyspnea conventionally suggest a cardiac limitation with impaired cardiac stroke volume, but in a patient with no clinical evidence of heart disease, these findings may be explained by poor peripheral vascular control, with increased cardiac output but poor distribution to the active muscle.

Stage 2 results are all normal, apart from a high cardiac frequency, and are compatible with a high cardiac output and VD/VT ratio and normal lactate production.

Stage 3 results confirm that cardiac output is high; at an oxygen intake of 0.94 L/min, cardiac output is expected to be about 9.5 L/min but is 12.5 L/min. Pulmonary gas exchange variables are normal. A small increase in lactate concentration is seen.

Comments

In this patient, who was referred for investigation of severe effort intolerance associated with fatigue, the stage 1 results suggested a low cardiac stroke volume, but the stage 2 and 3 results were compatible with a high cardiac output and normal VD/VT ratio and were helpful in excluding an occult problem, such as pulmonary vascular disease. Stage 1 results provided a quantitative picture of her disability and handicap; at an exercise intensity equal to 50 per cent of the predicted maximum, she experienced an intensity of leg effort and dyspnea that were three to four times that expected in a healthy individual. Bearing in mind that the demands of daily activities involving weight bearing are higher than for someone who is less heavy, symptom intensity is a serious limitation to an active occupation.

The results, together with the clinical assessment, were compatible with the diagnosis of vasoregulatory asthenia (Holmgren et al., 1957), one of the syndromes included in the chronic fatigue syndrome. Although the etiology remains controversial, the combination of increased effort representing an increase in central motor command, poor circulatory control, and lactate formation is a common pathophysiological feature of this condition.

Example 9

Stage 1 Measurements

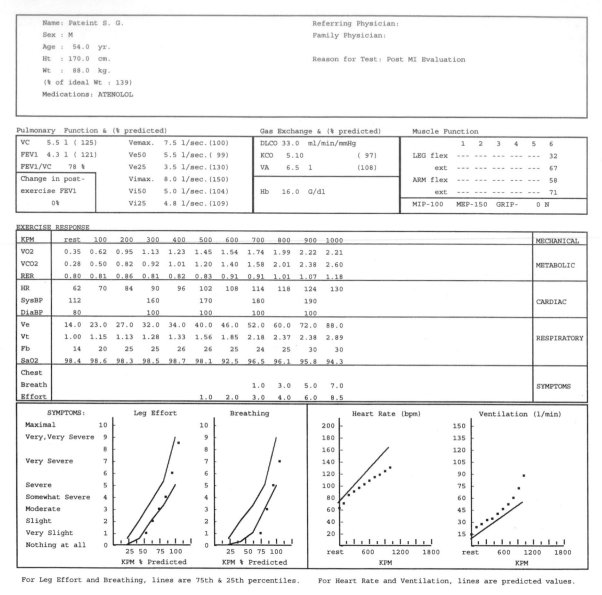

Name: Pateint S. G.
Sex : M
Age : 54.0 yr.
Ht : 170.0 cm.
Wt : 88.0 kg.
(% of ideal Wt : 139)
Medications: ATENOLOL

Referring Physician:
Family Physician:

Reason for Test: Post MI Evaluation

Pulmonary Function & (% predicted)

VC	5.5 l (125)	Vemax.	7.5 l/sec.(100)	
FEV1	4.3 l (121)	Ve50	5.5 l/sec.(99)	
FEV1/VC	78 %	Ve25	3.5 l/sec.(130)	
Change in post-		Vimax.	8.0 l/sec.(150)	
exercise FEV1		Vi50	5.0 l/sec.(104)	
0%		Vi25	4.8 l/sec.(109)	

Gas Exchange & (% predicted)

DLCO 33.0 ml/min/mmHg		
KCO	5.10	(97)
VA	6.5 l	(108)
Hb	16.0 G/dl	

Muscle Function

	1	2	3	4	5	6
LEG flex	---	---	---	---	---	32
ext	---	---	---	---	---	67
ARM flex	---	---	---	---	---	58
ext	---	---	---	---	---	71

MIP-100   MEP-150   GRIP-   0 N

EXERCISE RESPONSE

KPM	rest	100	200	300	400	500	600	700	800	900	1000	
VO2	0.35	0.62	0.95	1.13	1.23	1.45	1.54	1.74	1.99	2.22	2.21	MECHANICAL
VCO2	0.28	0.50	0.82	0.92	1.01	1.20	1.40	1.58	2.01	2.38	2.60	METABOLIC
RER	0.80	0.81	0.86	0.81	0.82	0.83	0.91	0.91	1.01	1.07	1.18	
HR	62	70	84	90	96	102	108	114	118	124	130	
SysBP	112		160		170		180		190			CARDIAC
DiaBP	80		100		100		100		100			
Ve	14.0	23.0	27.0	32.0	34.0	40.0	46.0	52.0	60.0	72.0	88.0	
Vt	1.00	1.15	1.13	1.28	1.33	1.56	1.85	2.18	2.37	2.38	2.89	RESPIRATORY
Fb	14	20	25	25	26	26	25	24	25	30	30	
SaO2	98.4	98.6	98.3	98.5	98.7	98.1	92.5	96.5	96.1	95.8	94.3	
Chest												
Breath						1.0	3.0	5.0	7.0			SYMPTOMS
Effort					1.0	2.0	3.0	4.0	6.0	8.5		

SYMPTOMS:

Leg Effort / Breathing	
Maximal	10
Very,Very Severe	9
	8
Very Severe	7
	6
Severe	5
Somewhat Severe	4
Moderate	3
Slight	2
Very Slight	1
Nothing at all	0

KPM % Predicted

Heart Rate (bpm)   Ventilation (l/min)

For Leg Effort and Breathing, lines are 75th & 25th percentiles.   For Heart Rate and Ventilation, lines are predicted values.

Max. work: 1000 (101% pred) kpm   Max. ventilation: 88 (71% pred) l/min   Max. HR 130 (79% pred)

This man is moderately overweight. Spirometry and flow values are in the high-normal range; carbon monoxide uptake is normal. Respiratory and skeletal muscle strength are normal. In the stage 1 test, the maximum power output of 1000 kpm/min was 101 per cent of predicted, and the patient stopped because of leg fatigue and dyspnea, with these symptoms remaining within the range of intensity expected in a healthy individual. Oxygen intake is high at all power outputs, probably related to the patient's weight, and he reached a "plateau," with a maximum oxygen intake of 2220 mL/min, or 25.2 mL/kg, in the lower-normal range. Carbon dioxide output shows a relative increase at the highest three loads, suggesting that lactic acid production occurred, a conclusion confirmed by the blood lactate measurement during the second minute of recovery, which was 6.5 mmol/L. The cardiac frequency is low at all power outputs and at maximum is 79 per cent of the maximum predicted for the patient's age (175 b/min). Ventilation is normal at the lower power outputs but high at the submaximal levels, related to increasing carbon dioxide output and lactic acidosis; however, the ventilation at maximum is well below the predicted maximum ventilatory capacity.

The resting electrocardiogram shows changes compatible with an old anterior infarction, but no ST segment changes occur during or after exercise.

In view of the low cardiac frequency, itself compatible with moderate beta blockade, stroke volume must be normal. A maximal oxygen intake of 2.22 L/min suggests a cardiac output of at least 16 L/min and thus a stroke volume of 123 mL. The inability of cardiac frequency to increase further may be a factor limiting maximal exercise.

Comments

This patient, who had suffered a myocardial infarction a year previously, was referred for exercise testing before enrollment in an activity program. From the results of the test, a training level was chosen that was equivalent to an oxygen intake of 1.8 L/min or 6 mets (multiples of resting oxygen intake) and at which cardiac frequency was 110 to 120 b/min. Further studies were not required.

Example 10

Stage 1 Measurements

```
Name: Patient: J. B.                    Referring Physician:
Sex : M                                 Family Physician:
Age : 52.0 yr.
Ht  : 169.0 cm.                         Reason for Test: Shy-Drager Syndrome
Wt  : 75.0 kg.
(% of ideal Wt : 120)
Medications:
```

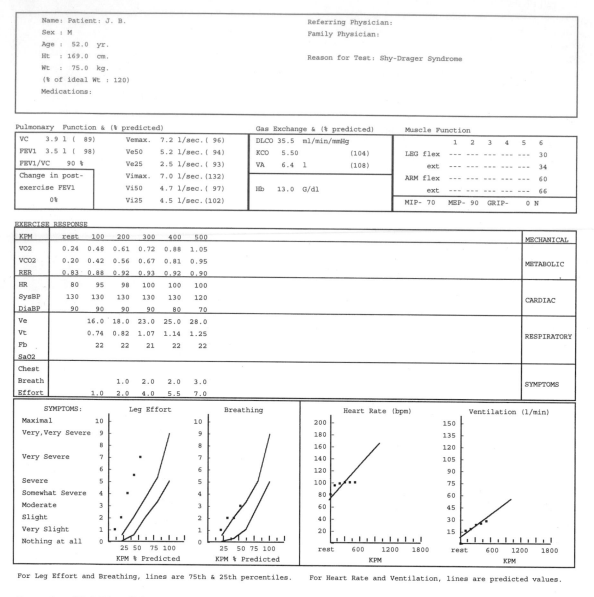

Pulmonary Function & (% predicted)

VC	3.9 l	(89)	Vemax.	7.2 l/sec.	(96)
FEV1	3.5 l	(98)	Ve50	5.2 l/sec.	(94)
FEV1/VC	90 %		Ve25	2.5 l/sec.	(93)
Change in post-			Vimax.	7.0 l/sec.	(132)
exercise FEV1			Vi50	4.7 l/sec.	(97)
0%			Vi25	4.5 l/sec.	(102)

Gas Exchange & (% predicted)

DLCO	35.5 ml/min/mmHg	
KCO	5.50	(104)
VA	6.4 l	(108)
Hb	13.0 G/dl	

Muscle Function

	1	2	3	4	5	6
LEG flex	---	---	---	---	---	30
ext	---	---	---	---	---	34
ARM flex	---	---	---	---	---	60
ext	---	---	---	---	---	66
MIP- 70	MEP- 90	GRIP-	0 N			

EXERCISE RESPONSE

KPM	rest	100	200	300	400	500		MECHANICAL
VO2	0.24	0.48	0.61	0.72	0.88	1.05		
VCO2	0.20	0.42	0.56	0.67	0.81	0.95		METABOLIC
RER	0.83	0.88	0.92	0.93	0.92	0.90		
HR	80	95	98	100	100	100		
SysBP	130	130	130	130	130	120		CARDIAC
DiaBP	90	90	90	90	80	70		
Ve		16.0	18.0	23.0	25.0	28.0		
Vt		0.74	0.82	1.07	1.14	1.25		RESPIRATORY
Fb		22	22	21	22	22		
SaO2								
Chest								
Breath			1.0	2.0	2.0	3.0		SYMPTOMS
Effort		1.0	2.0	4.0	5.5	7.0		

For Leg Effort and Breathing, lines are 75th & 25th percentiles.   For Heart Rate and Ventilation, lines are predicted values.

Max. work: 500 (50% pred) kpm   Max. ventilation: 28 (22% pred) l/min   Max. HR 100 (60% pred)

This patient is a little overweight (120 per cent of ideal). Spirometry is normal, and carbon monoxide uptake is normal. Respiratory muscle strength is normal, arm strength is normal, and leg muscle strength is in the low-normal range.

In the stage 1 test, maximum power output is reduced to 50 per cent of that expected for age and size. The patient is limited by very severe leg muscle discomfort, and rating of effort is much higher than expected at all loads. Oxygen intake and carbon dioxide output are appropriate to the

workloads, with no evidence of lactate production. The heart rate response to exercise is abnormal, with an initial increase and then a flat response. Blood pressure is also flat, with a decrease at the highest load, and also shows a decrease with change in position at rest. Ventilation and breathing pattern are normal. The electrocardiogram is normal.

The stage 2 study shows a metabolic rate ($\dot{V}O_2$ and $\dot{V}CO_2$) that is in the high-normal range for the power output. Although ventilation is high for the

Stage 2 Measurements

W	kpm/min	0	200	400
$\dot{V}_{O_2}$	mL/min	260	900	1540
$\dot{V}_{CO_2}$	mL/min	196	690	141
R		0.75	0.76	0.90
f_c	b/min	80	104	108
$\dot{V}_E$	L/min	7	22	46
f_b	breaths/min	12	24	33
V_T	mL	580	940	1410
P_{ECO_2}	mm Hg	25	28	27
P_{ETCO_2}	mm Hg	40	39	36
$P_{\bar{v}CO_2}$	mm Hg	50	59	69
min			6	5

power output, the increase is accounted for mainly by the increase in $\dot{V}_{CO_2}$, and the P_{ECO_2} is within the expected range. If the end-tidal P_{CO_2} is used to estimate arterial P_{CO_2}, values for Pa_{CO_2} of 40 and 35 mm Hg, respectively, are obtained at 200 and 400 kpm/min; the estimated cardiac output is 8.9 and 10.3 L/min. At the levels of $\dot{V}_{O_2}$ measured in the studies, the expected cardiac outputs are 10.0 and 13.2 L/min. We may interpret these values as representing a reduced cardiac output response to exercise, owing to a low heart rate without a compensating increase in stroke volume. Note, in addition, that values for $\dot{V}_E$ and heart rate in the stage 1 test are much lower than the steady state values at the same power output, suggesting that the rate of adaptation of these variables is also impaired. This means that muscle blood flow does not increase in parallel with the power output, leading to accumulation of lactate and carbon dioxide in muscle, which in turn contributes to muscle fatigue.

Comments

The clinical diagnosis in this patient was Shy-Drager syndrome. The abnormal blood pressure and heart rate response to positional change and exercise were accounted for by the autonomic nervous system paralysis found in this condition. It is likely that this also led to a slow adaptation to exercise and to reduced myocardial contractility.

Example 11A

Stage 1 Measurements

```
Name: Patient O. G.              Referring Physician:
Sex : M                          Family Physician:
Age :  26.0  yr.
Ht  : 173.0  cm.                 Reason for Test: Effort intolerance, dyspnea
Wt  : 140.0  kg.
(% of ideal Wt : 216)
Medications:
```

Pulmonary Function & (% predicted)

VC	5.0 l (96)	Vemax.	6.5 l/sec.(74)
FEV1	3.4 l (78)	Ve50	3.1 l/sec.(50)
FEV1/VC	68 %	Ve25	1.8 l/sec.(57)
Change in post-		Vimax.	5.5 l/sec.(91)
exercise FEV1		Vi50	4.3 l/sec.(78)
0%		Vi25	4.1 l/sec.(78)

Gas Exchange & (% predicted)

DLCO	31.2 ml/min/mmHg	
KCO	5.20	(84)
VA	6.0 l	(95)
Hb	15.4 G/dl	

Muscle Function

	1	2	3	4	5	6
LEG flex	---	---	---	---	---	31
ext	---	---	---	---	---	57
ARM flex	---	---	---	---	---	78
ext	---	---	---	---	---	86
MIP- 80	MEP-130	GRIP-			0 N	

EXERCISE RESPONSE

KPM	rest	100	200	300	400	500	600	700	800	900		
VO2	0.52	0.78	0.84	0.98	1.10	1.22	1.58	1.80	1.89	2.08		MECHANICAL
VCO2	0.46	0.64	0.71	0.84	0.90	1.06	1.50	1.89	2.02	2.39		METABOLIC
RER	0.88	0.82	0.85	0.86	0.82	0.87	0.95	1.05	1.07	1.15		
HR	75	110	120	132	141	150	161	173	179	182		
SysBP	150		160		175		190		215			CARDIAC
DiaBP	90		90		90		90		90			
Ve	15.0	20.0	26.0	32.0	45.0	57.0	62.0	83.0	95.0	110.0		
Vt	1.10	1.18	1.23	1.30	1.41	1.52	1.62	1.79	2.16	2.30		RESPIRATORY
Fb	14	17	21	25	32	38	39	46	44	48		
SaO2	98.2	98.1	98.2	97.5	97.8	97.5	97.8	98.2	98.0	97.7		
Chest												
Breath			1.0	1.0	2.0	2.0	4.0	5.0	7.0			SYMPTOMS
Effort				1.0	3.0	3.0	4.0	6.0				

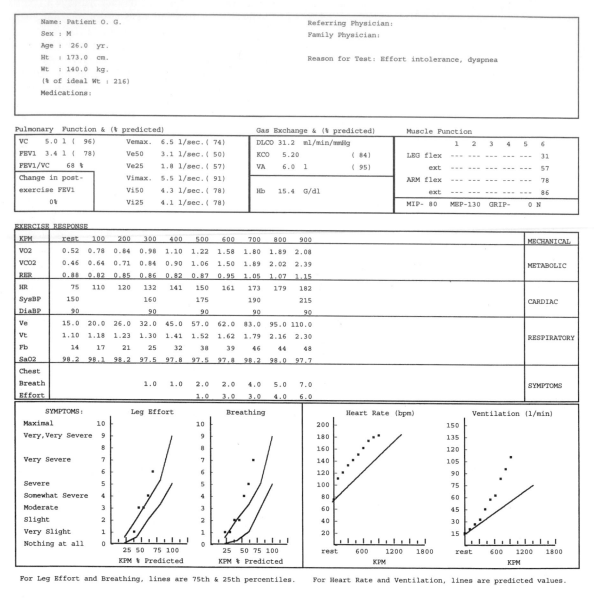

For Leg Effort and Breathing, lines are 75th & 25th percentiles.   For Heart Rate and Ventilation, lines are predicted values.

Max. work: 900 (66% pred) kpm   Max. ventilation: 110 (72% pred) l/min   Max. HR 182 (99% pred)

The anthropometric results show a severe degree of obesity (216 per cent of ideal weight), body fat being at least 50 per cent of body weight. Spirometry showed reductions in vital capacity, FEV$_1$ and FEV$_1$/VC ratio, and also in maximal flow rates at all lung volumes, indicating air flow limitation. The stage 1 results show that the maximal power output is moderately reduced to 66 per cent of predicted. Symptom ratings indicated increased effort in leg muscles and breathing, with dyspnea being the dominant symptomatic limitation. Oxygen uptake is high at all workloads, consistent with severe obesity, and there is evidence of excess carbon dioxide output at higher power outputs, indicating lactate accumulation. Cardiac frequency is above normal at all workloads and reaches a value close to the maximum heart rate predicted by age. The increase in heart rate is in part related to the high $\dot{V}O_2$; maximum cardiac output is estimated at 15

Stage 2 Measurements

W	kpm/min	0	300	600
$\dot{V}O_2$	mL/min	310	1159	1850
$\dot{V}CO_2$	mL/min	250	1031	1585
R		0.80	0.85	0.86
f_c	b/min	72	135	162
$\dot{V}E$	L/min	10.8	33	56
f_b	breaths/min	15	25	38
V_T	mL	720	1350	1460
$PECO_2$	mm Hg	20	27	25
$PETCO_2$	mm Hg	30	32	29
$P\bar{v}CO_2$	mm Hg	42	52	54
min		6	6	

Stage 3 Measurements

W	kpm/min	0	300	600
$PaCO_2$	mm Hg	34	34	32
VD/VT	ratio	0.33	0.17	0.19
$\dot{Q}tot$	L/min	7.0	12.8	15.7
V_s	mL	100	95	97
PaO_2	mm Hg	80	83	85
$PA - aO_2$	mm Hg	25	20	25
SaO_2		0.95	0.95	0.96
$\dot{Q}VA/\dot{Q}tot$	%	13	3	3
pH		7.40	7.38	7.34
HCO_3^-	mmol/L	20	19	17
Lactate	mmol/L	0.8	1.2	2.8

L/min, and stroke volume, 82 mL. Ventilation is high at all power outputs and reaches a value close to the maximal voluntary ventilation (120 L/min); the pattern of breathing is normal, but a maximum frequency of 48 is reached. Thus, both the ventilatory and the cardiovascular systems appear to be reaching maximal adaptation, combining to limit performance. Contributing to severe dyspnea are the high ventilation, high frequency of breathing, reduced lung volume, and flow limitation. Although exercise capacity is only moderately reduced compared with the value predicted on the basis of his height, when the patient's weight is taken into account, this translates into considerable handicap in daily activities associated with weight bearing; the calculated oxygen demands for such activities as stair climbing are huge. Maximal oxygen intake is less than 15 mL/min/kg, which suggests that the demands for any active occupation cannot be sustained.

The stage 2 results reveal a cardiac frequency that is high for the oxygen intake. Ventilation is also increased, shown by the low values for $PECO_2$. The mixed venous PCO_2 is also low, indicating that the increase in ventilation is partly due to an increase in alveolar ventilation. The mixed venous to mixed expired PCO_2 difference is consistent with normal values for cardiac output and VD/VT ratio. A carbon dioxide balance suggests that only a small lactate accumulation occurred at the work rates studied.

The stage 3 results confirm alveolar hyperventilation with low $PaCO_2$ and normal VD/VT ratio, cardiac output, and stroke volume (approximately 100 mL). The arterial PO_2 is slightly reduced, with a widened alveolar-arterial PO_2 difference; this improves during exercise when the venous admixture ratio falls to normal values. The blood lactate concentration has increased to an extent that is normal for the oxygen intake.

Comments

The stage 1 results indicated a reduction in exercise capacity and suggested considerable handicap in activities of daily living. Dyspnea was the limiting symptom, and several contributing factors could be identified. The excess oxygen costs of exercise were shown; the cardiovascular responses were virtually normal once the increased metabolic demands were allowed for. The stage 2 and stage 3 results mainly confirmed these findings and, although documenting the changes more precisely, added little to the assessment. Cardiac output was shown to be in the high-normal range, suggesting a poor blood flow distribution. The carbon dioxide balance technique underestimated lactate accumulation; reasons for this may be the utilization of free fatty acids as a fuel source, with a lower value for the muscle respiratory quotient than that assumed for the purposes of the calculation and possibly an overestimate of the distribution volume relative to total body weight. All the changes may be explained by the patient's obesity, although the contributing factors are quite complex, involving increased metabolic demands, increased impedance to breathing, and poor cardiovascular control. The patient successfully undertook a weight reduction and exercise regimen and was retested 6 months after these tests (see Example 11B).

Example 11B

Stage 1 Measurements

Name: Patient O. G.

Sex : M

Age : 26.0 yr.

Ht : 173.0 cm.

Wt : 108.0 kg.

(% of ideal Wt : 166)

Medications:

Referring Physician:

Family Physician:

Reason for Test: Re-Evaluation

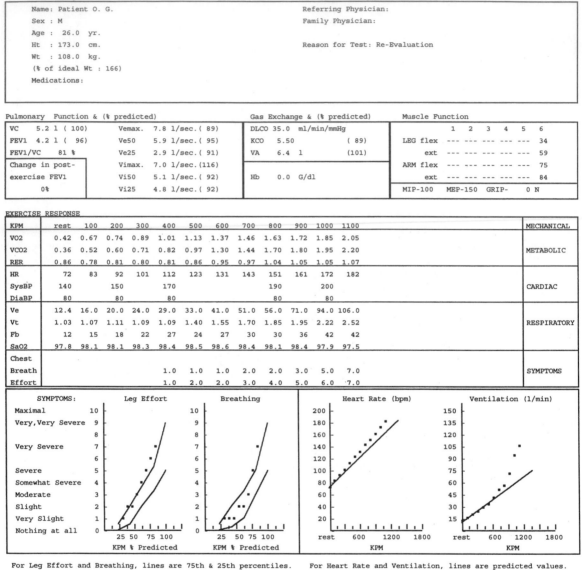

Pulmonary Function & (% predicted)				Gas Exchange & (% predicted)			Muscle Function							
VC 5.2 l (100)	Vemax.	7.8 l/sec.(89)		DLCO 35.0 ml/min/mmHg				1	2	3	4	5	6	
FEV1 4.2 l (96)	Ve50	5.9 l/sec.(95)		KCO 5.50	(89)		LEG flex	---	---	---	---	---	34	
FEV1/VC 81 %	Ve25	2.9 l/sec.(91)		VA 6.4 l	(101)		ext	---	---	---	---	---	59	
Change in post-	Vimax.	7.0 l/sec.(116)					ARM flex	---	---	---	---	---	75	
exercise FEV1	Vi50	5.1 l/sec.(92)		Hb 0.0 G/dl			ext	---	---	---	---	---	84	
0%	Vi25	4.8 l/sec.(92)					MIP-100 MEP-150 GRIP- 0 N							

EXERCISE RESPONSE

KPM	rest	100	200	300	400	500	600	700	800	900	1000	1100	MECHANICAL
VO2	0.42	0.67	0.74	0.89	1.01	1.13	1.37	1.46	1.63	1.72	1.85	2.05	
VCO2	0.36	0.52	0.60	0.71	0.82	0.97	1.30	1.44	1.70	1.80	1.95	2.20	METABOLIC
RER	0.86	0.78	0.81	0.80	0.81	0.86	0.95	0.97	1.04	1.05	1.05	1.07	
HR	72	83	92	101	112	123	131	143	151	161	172	182	
SysBP	140		150		170			190		200			CARDIAC
DiaBP	80		80		80			80		80			
Ve	12.4	16.0	20.0	24.0	29.0	33.0	41.0	51.0	56.0	71.0	94.0	106.0	
Vt	1.03	1.07	1.11	1.09	1.09	1.40	1.55	1.70	1.85	1.95	2.22	2.52	RESPIRATORY
Fb	12	15	18	22	27	24	27	30	30	36	42	42	
SaO2	97.8	98.1	98.1	98.3	98.4	98.5	98.6	98.4	98.1	98.4	97.9	97.5	
Chest													
Breath				1.0	1.0	1.0	2.0	2.0	3.0	5.0	7.0		SYMPTOMS
Effort				1.0	2.0	2.0	3.0	4.0	5.0	6.0	7.0		

SYMPTOMS:

Maximal	10
Very,Very Severe	9
	8
Very Severe	7
	6
Severe	5
Somewhat Severe	4
Moderate	3
Slight	2
Very Slight	1
Nothing at all	0

For Leg Effort and Breathing, lines are 75th & 25th percentiles.   For Heart Rate and Ventilation, lines are predicted values.

Max. work: 1100 (80% pred) kpm   Max. ventilation: 106 (69% pred) l/min   Max. HR 182 (99% pred)

The stage 1 test was repeated after 6 months, at which time the patient's weight had fallen by 32 kg to 108 kg (166 per cent of ideal weight), and his exercise symptoms had improved considerably. Improvements occurred in the spirometric and flow-volume measurements, reflecting increased ventilatory capacity, and in the maximum power output. The metabolic demands, in terms of $\dot{V}O_2$ and $\dot{V}CO_2$, were less, reflecting the loss of weight and more efficient energy expenditure. Cardiac frequency and ventilation were less at all power outputs, approximately parallel to the reductions in $\dot{V}O_2$ and $\dot{V}CO_2$, and at maximum power output, the cardiac frequency and $\dot{V}E$ were similar to the values recorded in the previous test at a lower power. Ventilation, although close to the previous maximal value, was now only 73 per cent of the predicted maximal voluntary ventilation (145 L/

min). The pattern of breathing had also improved, as shown by the increase in tidal volume at any given $\dot{V}E$. The "ventilatory anaerobic threshold" was shifted to a higher power, indicating less lactate formation and improved balance between glycolytic flux and aerobic metabolism. Maximal $\dot{V}O_2$ when expressed per kilogram of weight increased to 19 mL/min/kg; although there has been an improvement, it is likely that the patient will continue to experience handicap in an active occupation.

Example 12

Stage 1 Measurements

Name: Patient H. B.
Sex : M
Age : 58.0 yr.
Ht : 177.0 cm.
Wt : 95.5 kg.
(% of ideal Wt : 142)
Medications:

Referring Physician:
Family Physician:

Reason for Test: Discomfort in left arm

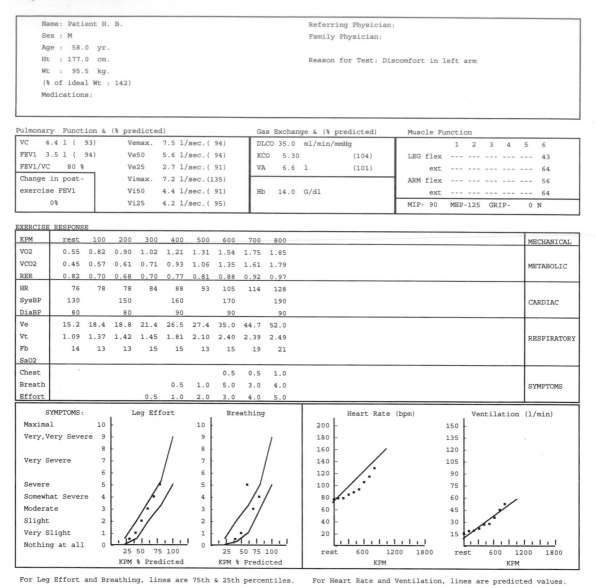

Pulmonary Function & (% predicted)				Gas Exchange & (% predicted)			Muscle Function						
VC 4.4 l (93)	Vemax. 7.5 l/sec.(94)			DLCO 35.0 ml/min/mmHg				1	2	3	4	5	6
FEV1 3.5 l (94)	Ve50 5.6 l/sec.(94)			KCO 5.30 (104)			LEG flex	---	---	---	---	---	43
FEV1/VC 80 %	Ve25 2.7 l/sec.(91)			VA 6.6 l (101)			ext	---	---	---	---	---	64
Change in post-	Vimax. 7.2 l/sec.(135)						ARM flex	---	---	---	---	---	56
exercise FEV1	Vi50 4.4 l/sec.(91)			Hb 14.0 G/dl			ext	---	---	---	---	---	64
0%	Vi25 4.2 l/sec.(95)						MIP- 90 MEP-125 GRIP- 0 N						

EXERCISE RESPONSE

KPM	rest	100	200	300	400	500	600	700	800		
VO2	0.55	0.82	0.90	1.02	1.21	1.31	1.54	1.75	1.85		MECHANICAL
VCO2	0.45	0.57	0.61	0.71	0.93	1.06	1.35	1.61	1.79		METABOLIC
RER	0.82	0.70	0.68	0.70	0.77	0.81	0.88	0.92	0.97		
HR	76	78	78	84	88	93	105	114	128		
SysBP	130		150		160		170		190		CARDIAC
DiaBP	80		80		90		90		90		
Ve	15.2	18.4	18.8	21.4	26.5	27.4	35.0	44.7	52.0		
Vt	1.09	1.37	1.42	1.45	1.81	2.10	2.40	2.39	2.49		RESPIRATORY
Fb	14	13	13	15	15	13	15	19	21		
SaO2											
Chest						0.5	0.5	1.0			
Breath				0.5	1.0	5.0	3.0	4.0			SYMPTOMS
Effort				0.5	1.0	2.0	3.0	4.0	5.0		

For Leg Effort and Breathing, lines are 75th & 25th percentiles.   For Heart Rate and Ventilation, lines are predicted values.

Max. work: 800 (76% pred) kpm   Max. ventilation: 52 (39% pred) l/min   Max. HR 128 (79% pred)

The patient was overweight by about 18 kg (142 per cent of ideal weight). Spirometry and flow rates were normal; carbon monoxide uptake was normal. Respiratory and skeletal muscle strength were normal. Stage 1 testing showed maximum power and $\dot{V}O_2$ to be 76 and 75 per cent of that predicted, respectively, with leg effort being the most prominent symptom; both leg effort and dyspnea were appropriate for the relative workload, but slight chest discomfort was also present. Carbon dioxide output showed a small increase relative to $\dot{V}O_2$ at the two highest loads, suggesting a normal lactate accumulation. Heart rate and blood pressure increased normally, and at maximum exercise, the heart rate of 128 was only 79 per cent of the expected maximum heart rate. The electrocardiogram showed ST depression in lead V_5 that was first noticed at 600 kpm/min and increased to 2.2 mm at maximum exercise (R-wave amplitude, 1.5 mm). The respiratory responses to exercise were appropriate to the carbon dioxide output, and the pattern of breathing was also normal.

The patient was referred for evaluation of a constricting discomfort in the neck radiating to the left arm, often but variably related to effort and usually subsiding with rest. Nitroglycerin was not always effective in relieving the discomfort, and the patient considered alkali to be at least as effective. The referring cardiologist considered this to be atypical angina. The abnormalities in this test consisted of a maximum power just below the lowest limit of normal, chest discomfort, and electrocardiographic changes. ST depression of 2.2 mm occurred at 80 per cent of maximum predicted power and at a heart rate appropriate to that power; ST depression corrected for the reduced power was 2.75 mm (2.2/0.8). These changes may be interpreted with the guidelines given in Figure 7–10. The prevalence of coronary artery narrowing in a man aged 58 years is 10 per cent; the likelihood ratio for atypical angina is 20, and estimated pretest probability is thus 70 per cent; the likelihood ratio for ST depression of more than 2.5 mm is 39, leading to a calculated post-test probability of more than 95 per cent. Narrowing of the left anterior descending coronary artery was shown by angiography.

Example 13

Stage 1 Measurements

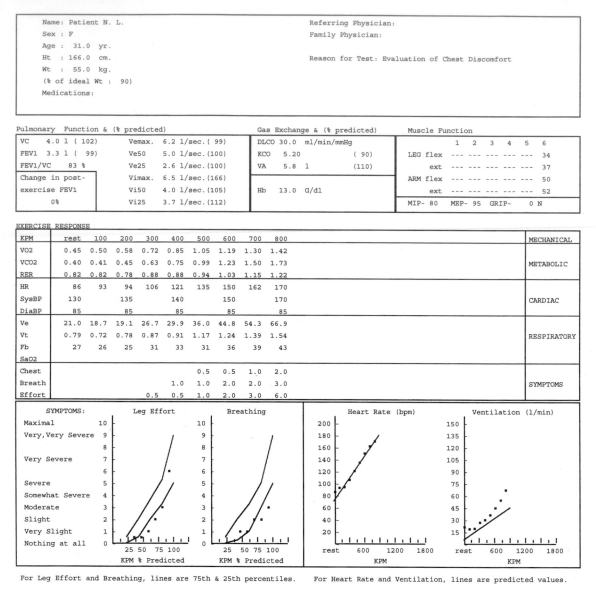

```
Name: Patient N. L.                    Referring Physician:
Sex : F                                Family Physician:
Age : 31.0  yr.
Ht  : 166.0  cm.                       Reason for Test: Evaluation of Chest Discomfort
Wt  : 55.0  kg.
(% of ideal Wt :  90)
Medications:
```

Pulmonary Function & (% predicted)

VC 4.0 l (102)	Vemax. 6.2 l/sec.(99)	
FEV1 3.3 l (99)	Ve50 5.0 l/sec.(100)	
FEV1/VC 83 %	Ve25 2.6 l/sec.(100)	
Change in post-	Vimax. 6.5 l/sec.(166)	
exercise FEV1	Vi50 4.0 l/sec.(105)	
0%	Vi25 3.7 l/sec.(112)	

Gas Exchange & (% predicted)

DLCO 30.0 ml/min/mmHg		
KCO 5.20	(90)	
VA 5.8 l	(110)	
Hb 13.0 G/dl		

Muscle Function

	1	2	3	4	5	6
LEG flex	---	---	---	---	---	34
ext	---	---	---	---	---	37
ARM flex	---	---	---	---	---	50
ext	---	---	---	---	---	52
MIP- 80	MEP- 95	GRIP-	0 N			

EXERCISE RESPONSE

KPM	rest	100	200	300	400	500	600	700	800		
VO2	0.45	0.50	0.58	0.72	0.85	1.05	1.19	1.30	1.42		MECHANICAL
VCO2	0.40	0.41	0.45	0.63	0.75	0.99	1.23	1.50	1.73		METABOLIC
RER	0.82	0.82	0.78	0.88	0.88	0.94	1.03	1.15	1.22		
HR	86	93	94	106	121	135	150	162	170		
SysBP	130		135		140		150		170		CARDIAC
DiaBP	85		85		85		85		85		
Ve	21.0	18.7	19.1	26.7	29.9	36.0	44.8	54.3	66.9		
Vt	0.79	0.72	0.78	0.87	0.91	1.17	1.24	1.39	1.54		RESPIRATORY
Fb	27	26	25	31	33	31	36	39	43		
SaO2											
Chest					0.5	0.5	1.0	2.0			
Breath				1.0	1.0	2.0	2.0	3.0			SYMPTOMS
Effort			0.5	0.5	1.0	2.0	3.0	6.0			

```
SYMPTOMS:            Leg Effort      Breathing          Heart Rate (bpm)      Ventilation (l/min)
Maximal        10        10              10
Very,Very Severe 9        9               9
               8         8               8
Very Severe    7         7               7
               6         6               6
Severe         5         5               5
Somewhat Severe 4        4               4
Moderate       3         3               3
Slight         2         2               2
Very Slight    1         1               1
Nothing at all 0         0               0
                    25 50  75 100     25  50  75 100    rest    600   1200  1800   rest    600   1200  1800
                    KPM % Predicted    KPM % Predicted      KPM                      KPM
```

For Leg Effort and Breathing, lines are 75th & 25th percentiles.   For Heart Rate and Ventilation, lines are predicted values.

Max. work: 800 (89% pred) kpm   Max. ventilation: 67 (57% pred) l/min   Max. HR 170 (94% pred)

The patient is underweight (90 per cent of ideal weight). Spirometric results are normal, with normal air flow, and carbon monoxide uptake is normal. Respiratory and skeletal muscle strength are normal. The cardiovascular system is clinically normal apart from resting tachycardia; the electrocardiogram is normal at rest. There is a considerable degree of hyperventilation at rest.

During exercise, the patient reaches a power output and maximal $\dot{V}O_2$ close to the values predicted for age and height (900 kpm/min and 1.78 L/min) and in the low-normal range (89 per cent of predicted); this is to be expected in someone of low body weight because it implies a reduction in lean body mass. The main limiting symptom is leg fatigue, of appropriate intensity, but chest discomfort also occurred. Oxygen uptake is appropriate, and carbon dioxide output exceeds oxygen intake at power outputs above 500 kpm/min, indicating lactate production, which is associated with an increase in ventilation. The breathing pattern is one of lower-than-average tidal volume and is of relatively high frequency (1.54 L and 43 breaths/min at maximum). Heart rate increases in the normal range, and blood pressure also increases normally. The electrocardiogram shows 1 mm of ST segment depression at maximum exercise. The ST segment depression may be evaluated in terms of the prevalence of coronary artery disease in a female of this age (< 0.5 per cent) in the presence of atypical chest pain (likelihood ratio, 20), giving a pretest probability of 10 per cent at the most. The 1-mm ST depression carries a likelihood ratio of 1:2; post-test probability is thus 10 to 20 per cent. In this situation, a thallium study may be helpful; in this patient, the scan was normal, with a likelihood ratio of 0.18, and the final probability of significant coronary artery disease is less than 5 per cent.

Comments

This patient was referred for evaluation of precordial chest discomfort occurring at rest and exercise, associated with dyspnea, but taking up to an hour to fade if she stopped exercising; the referring cardiologist judged it atypical chest pain. The stage 1 test showed normal cardiorespiratory responses, apart from anxiety-related hyperventilation and tachycardia at rest and low workloads, and the additional information of the stage 2 and stage 3 tests was not needed. The minor ST segment depression did not represent a significant increase in the likelihood of coronary artery disease.

Example 14

Stage 1 Measurements

Name: Patient: H. R.	Referring Physician:
Sex : M	Family Physician:
Age : 60.0 yr.	
Ht : 162.0 cm.	Reason for Test: Scleroderma evaluation
Wt : 60.0 kg.	
(% of ideal Wt : 102)	
Medications: PENICILLAMINE CISAPRIDE OMEPRAZOLE	

Pulmonary Function & (% predicted)

VC	3.1 l (81)	Vemax.	5.7 l/sec.(87)
FEV1	2.7 l (88)	Ve50	3.5 l/sec.(71)
FEV1/VC	87 %	Ve25	1.5 l/sec.(66)
Change in post-		Vimax.	4.2 l/sec.(79)
exercise FEV1		Vi50	3.9 l/sec.(81)
98%		Vi25	2.3 l/sec.(52)

Gas Exchange & (% predicted)

DLCO	8.3 ml/min/mmHg	
KCO	1.80	(36)
VA	4.6 l	(86)
Hb	12.4 G/dl	

Muscle Function

	1	2	3	4	5	6
LEG flex	---	---	14	---	---	---
ext	---	---	26	---	---	---
ARM flex	---	---	---	12	---	---
ext	---	---	---	7	---	---
MIP- 60	MEP- 60	GRIP-	0 N			

EXERCISE RESPONSE

KPM	rest	100	200	300	400	MECHANICAL
VO2	0.34	0.43	0.54	0.66	0.72	
VCO2	0.27	0.36	0.49	0.66	0.66	METABOLIC
RER	0.80	0.83	0.91	1.00	1.12	
HR	78	97	116	135	150	
SysBP	140		160		190	CARDIAC
DiaBP	90		90		90	
Ve	15.7	18.6	23.7	33.6	47.0	
Vt	0.90	1.05	1.38	1.49	1.46	RESPIRATORY
Fb	17	18	17	23	32	
SaO2	94.2	94.1	92.3	91.3	89.5	
Chest						
Breath				1.0	5.0	SYMPTOMS
Effort				1.0	4.0	

For Leg Effort and Breathing, lines are 75th & 25th percentiles.   For Heart Rate and Ventilation, lines are predicted values.

Max. work: 400 (49% pred) kpm   Max. ventilation: 47 (43% pred) l/min   Max. HR 150 (94% pred)

This 60-year old man is of normal weight and has spirometric and flow-volume loop measurements in the low-normal range. Carbon monoxide uptake is severely reduced to 36 per cent of predicted when it is corrected for lung volume. Respiratory muscle strength is normal. Skeletal muscle strength is reduced. Stage 1 results show a low exercise capacity (49 per cent of predicted). The patient is limited by shortness of breath, and the intensity of both dyspnea and leg effort is increased relative to power output.

Oxygen uptake is appropriate to power, but there is excess carbon dioxide output, suggesting an increase in plasma lactate concentration. The cardiovascular responses are abnormal, with a high heart rate reaching the predicted maximal rate. At the highest $\dot{V}O_2$, cardiac output is expected to be 9 L/min, suggesting a low cardiac stroke volume (60 mL). Blood pressure increase is normal; no electrocardiographic changes are seen. In the pulmonary responses, ventilation is high; in relation to both $\dot{V}O_2$ and $\dot{V}CO_2$, there is a high frequency of breathing. In spite of the high $\dot{V}_E$, there is a progressive decrease in arterial oxygen saturation of 5 per cent.

Comments

This patient had been diagnosed as having scleroderma and was referred for evaluation of dyspnea that was out of proportion to spirometric impairment. The results suggested multisystem involvement, with severe impairment of pulmonary gas exchange, impaired cardiac stroke volume, and weak muscles with lactate production at low power. Dyspnea is accounted for by an increase in ventilation, due to excess carbon dioxide output and poor pulmonary gas exchange, with mild increase in elastance and the concomitant increase in breathing frequency. Although the high heart rate might be due in part to hypoxemia, the increase is greater than expected for the mild degree of hypoxemia, suggesting a low stroke volume due to the effects of scleroderma on the myocardium (Follansbee et al., 1984).

REFERENCES

Burns BH, Howell JBL. Disproportionately severe breathlessness in chronic bronchitis. Q J Med 1969;38:277–294.

Dantzker DR, D'Alonzo GE. The effect of exercise on pulmonary gas exchange in patients with severe chronic obstructive pulmonary disease. Am Rev Respir Dis 1986;134:1135–1139.

Follansbee WP, Curtiss EI, Medsger TA Jr, et al. Myocardial function and perfusion in the CREST syndrome variant of progressive systemic sclerosis: Exercise radionuclide evaluation and comparison with diffuse scleroderma. Am J Med 1984;77:489–496.

Gallagher CG. Exercise and chronic obstructive pulmonary disease. Med Clin North Am 1990;74:619–641.

Gallagher CG, Younes MK. Breathing pattern during and following exercise in patients with chronic obstructive lung disease, interstitial lung disease and cardiac disease and in normal subjects. Am Rev Respir Dis 1986;133:581–586.

Gazetopoulos N, Davies H, Oliver C, Deuchar D. Ventilation and haemodynamics in heart disease. Br Heart J 1966;28:1–15.

Holmgren A, Jonsson B, Levander M, et al. Low physical working capacity in suspected heart cases due to inadequate adjustment of peripheral blood flow (vasoregulatory asthenia). Acta Med Scand 1957;158:413–436.

Holmgren A, Jonsson B, Linderholm H, et al. Physical working capacity in cases of mitral valvular disease in relation to heart volume, total amount of hemoglobin and stroke volume. Acta Med Scand 1958;162:99–121.

Holmgren A, Ström G. Blood lactate concentration in relation to absolute and relative work load in normal men, and in mitral stenosis, atrial septal defect and vasoregulatory asthenia. Acta Med Scand 1959;163:185–193.

Jones NL. Pulmonary gas exchange during exercise in patients with chronic airflow obstruction. Clin Sci 1966;31:39–50.

Leblanc P, Bowie DM, Summers E, et al. Breathlessness and exercise in patients with cardiorespiratory disease. Am Rev Respir Dis 1986;133:21–25.

Light RW, Mintz HM, Linden GS, et al. Hemodynamics of patients with severe chronic obstructive pulmonary disease during progressive upright exercise. Am Rev Respir Dis 1984;130:391–395.

Riley RL, Cournand A, Donald KW. Analysis of factors affecting partial pressure of oxygen and carbon dioxide in gas and blood of lungs: Methods. J Appl Physiol 1951;4:102–120.

Stubbing DG, Pengelly LD, Morse JLC, Jones NL. Pulmonary mechanics during exercise in subjects with chronic airflow obstruction. J Appl Physiol 1980;49:511–515.

Wagner PD. Effects of COPD on gas exchange. In: Cherniack NS, editor. Chronic Obstructive Pulmonary Disease. Philadelphia: WB Saunders Co.; 1991, pp. 73–79.

14

Equipment

This chapter is intended for the reader who wants to know what equipment should be used for exercise testing. It is not an exhaustive review, but is limited to general observations because the range of some items of equipment is now so large that I cannot provide a "consumer's guide" of instruments from all sources.

The question of cost is often difficult to resolve for several reasons. First, there is usually a wide range of equipment that performs a given function. Although superior specifications may suggest a costly alternative, this may not be justified if only basic measurements are required. A rugged and simple instrument is often preferable to a complex one with higher capability. Second, the hidden costs involved in the maintenance of equipment should be estimated. Finally, the technical skill required for running the machine must be taken into account.

Before choosing any equipment, decisions have to be made regarding the type of tests to be performed, the measurements to be made, and the number of patients to be studied. In general, it is best to start with simple techniques and develop more complex facilities when experience has been gained.

The reader should be aware that the costs given in the following discussion are meant as a rough guide. There is great variation among models of differing specification and among manufacturers, and in general, the price of all equipment has been increasing at well over 10 per cent per year.

In previous editions, many details were provided in order to enable readers to assemble their own exercise testing systems, usually based on an electrically braked ergometer, a gas meter, rapid gas analyzers for oxygen and carbon dioxide sampling from a chamber that mixed expired gas, an electrocardiograph, and a multichannel chart recorder. The calculations were performed by hand or by computer, and the results were displayed on a report form by hand or by computer. Now, it seems likely that anyone investing time and other resources into a busy clinical exercise testing laboratory would find the funds to buy a commercially available system that does all of this automatically (Wilmore et al., 1976). Many systems are available, and superficially, all make the measurements, do the ap-

propriate calculations, present the results on a monitor, and after the test provide a report in a customized format together with enough graphs to please the most demanding of respiratory physiologists. Some systems allow measurements to be made on a breath-by-breath basis, and a few have incorporated the rebreathing carbon dioxide cardiac output method. Although I cannot survey all the available devices, I can provide some guidelines to help in the choice of system, bearing in mind that $50,000 to $100,000 is at stake.

SCOPE OF THE SYSTEM

The first task is to decide exactly what capabilities one wants now and in the next few years, bearing in mind that an expensive system should continue to work well for longer than 10 years. This includes the projected patient load and the expected reasons for referral, for a clinical laboratory; whether breath-by-breath measurements or rebreathing is needed; the degree of sophistication of the electrocardiograph; the generation of an acceptable report and the capability to store data; and special needs related to research aims.

THE COMPONENTS

Although the general requirements of the parts that make up automatic exercise testing systems are provided later in the chapter, the following section deals briefly with each, in the context of the system specifications provided by manufacturers.

Ergometer

Several systems incorporate excellent cycle ergometers, for which the main requirements are stability, precision, ease of calibration, comfort, and compactness (see below). Electrically braked ergometers provide an electrical resistance to pedaling that is automatically controlled so that power output is constant despite variations in pedaling frequency. An electrical signal proportional to power should be displayed or made available for recording. It should be possible to calibrate the ergometer through a full range of loads and pedaling frequencies in order to establish that the presented power is within 2 per cent. Systems that provide a physical calibration device are worth any extra cost because such devices are not easy to engineer in-house. In terms of comfort, it should be possible to adjust the saddle height through a full range, and several saddles should be available, to suit children, competitive cyclists, and subjects who may be as much as three times their ideal weight. Handlebars should be adjustable from a dropped racing position to a "sit up and beg" position. The pedal shank length can be adjusted in some models, which is a great advantage if children are to be studied. Finally, the general design should allow the ergometer to fit into the laboratory and be easily moved.

Respiratory Circuitry

Tubing needs to be kept as short as possible and have an internal diameter of 4 to 5 cm so that resistance is kept to a minimum, and the resistance of valves and taps should also be kept low (< 1 cm H_2O/L/sec). This may not be easy to achieve without sacrificing a low dead space (between the inspiratory and the expiratory valves); the dead space should be kept below 100 mL and should be measurable. Electrically actuated valves are helpful, particularly if rebreathing is required. If analysis of expired gas is from a mixing chamber, the washout volume and adequacy of mixing must be documented. A mixing chamber inevitably leads to a delay between volume measurement and gas analysis that can be corrected for.

Flow and Ventilation

Although volume is accurately measured by gas meters and Tissot spirometer, in all modern systems, the signals from flowmeters are used, mainly pneumotachographs and turbines (Yeh et al., 1987), but also Pitot tubes (Porszasz et al., 1994). Capable of very accurate measurement, they do require calibration over a range of flows and volumes; a calibration routine that is easy to perform and provides on-line verification is an essential component of an automated system. Some systems provide a calibrated syringe for delivery of a constant volume at several flow rates, with on-screen presentation of the flows and the derived volume, which should be within 2 per cent of the syringe volume. The flowmeter should be capable of measuring volume to within 2 per cent, at flow rates up to 10 L/sec. Temperature, density, and humidity (Liese et al., 1974) changes should not influence performance or should be corrected by adequate software.

Gas Analysis

Mainly fuel cell (zirconium), paramagnetic, and polarographic analyzers are used for oxygen, and infrared analyzers are used for carbon dioxide. Most are rapid-response analyzers, with a 95 per cent response within 100 milliseconds. Although specifications for linearity, response, and delay times are always provided by manufacturers, sometimes it is difficult to obtain the data on which these specifications are based. Furthermore, calibration for each of these functions should be built into the routine operation of the system. If rebreathing of carbon dioxide is required, linearity to 15 per cent carbon dioxide and the absence of a pressure-broadening effect from high oxygen need to be demonstrated. Even with mass spectrometry, interference between gases is sometimes difficult to identify and thus needs to be excluded on an occasional basis. Analyzers should be accurate to within 0.03 per cent within the range required (usually, 15 to 21 per cent for oxygen, zero to 8 per cent for carbon dioxide, but up to 15 per cent for carbon dioxide if rebreathing measurements are made). The system should ideally use a two-point calibration within the measurement range. Because water vapor (Liese et al., 1974) may interfere with analysis, there should be correction for the effect or adequate sample drying. Any possible effects of temperature variations should also be addressed.

Most systems are capable of providing data ($\dot{V}E$, $\dot{V}O_2$, $\dot{V}CO_2$, $PETCO_2$) on a breath-by-breath basis (Beaver et al., 1973). Although $\dot{V}E$ and $PETCO_2$ measurements are usually reliable, the measurement of breath-by-breath $\dot{V}O_2$ and $\dot{V}CO_2$ is extremely difficult, requiring a matching of flow and gas analysis signals that is almost too close to achieve. It is essential that the way in which these measurements are derived is clearly presented and detailed, rather than being the output from a "black box." It is preferable that measurements for each breath be provided, rather than a running average; the average may always be obtained later if necessary. Often, large variability between breaths can be obscured by such averaging. Although the variability is often explained as being the result of true biological variability between breaths, it has been our experience that it is more often due to inherent instability in the method used to generate the measurements. Data that verify the accuracy of these measurements through the full range of exercise intensity in healthy subjects and patients, who may breathe at high frequencies and small tidal volumes, should be provided. A mechanical system that can test the accuracy on a week-by-week basis (Huszczuk et al., 1990) is a worthwhile investment.

Electrocardiograph

For most systems, the electrocardiograph is provided by a separate machine, whose specifications and cost vary according to the laboratory requirements. It is probably preferable to obtain the instrument from the same manufacturer as that of the gas analysis system, so that compatibility is ensured. There is a complete range of instruments, from one that provides a signal for heart rate and monitors the electrocardiogram for safety to one that provides periodic 12-lead information with electronic signal conditioning, averaging, and presentation of ST segment depression and other related variables. The requirements are detailed in a recent report of the American Heart Association (Bailey et al., 1990). At least, a heart rate signal should be provided to the central processor, and a hard copy of the electrocardiogram should be available on command. Obviously, if there are many referrals from cardiologists, a system that provides a sophisticated output and enables copies of the electrocardiograms to be provided with the report form is a great advantage.

Computer

Central to exercise testing systems is a computer; because the cost of computers has fallen, there is no point in economizing by choosing one that merely does the job. Most manufacturers offer several options; it is worth investing in the one with the greatest capacity, speed, and display characteristics. Because specifications are changing on almost a monthly basis, any recommendations will be out of date by publication time; however, the following guidelines are suggested: processor, Pentium 120, with 1.6-gigabyte hard drive, 16 megabytes of RAM; super VGA monitor; 1.44MB, 3.5-inch diskette drive; and a color inkjet or laser printer. As far as possible, the software used for various functions needs to be understood and be capable of modification. It should be possible to enter data, such as blood pressure and Borg ratings, via the keyboard while the test is going on. External inputs, such as pulse oximetry and heart rate, should be available. Other functions include control of cycle ergometer or treadmill according to one of a number of selected protocols; calculation of $\dot{V}O_2$, $\dot{V}CO_2$, and other related variables; quality control procedures for gas analysis and flow calibration and for indication of malfunction; presentation of results on-screen and in a printout, both in real time and after the end of the study as a report, which should be modifiable to suit requirements; interpretation of results; and storage of data and provision of statistics for management and research purposes. If a busy clinical service is planned, the system's computer should be capable of generating an attractive report form with minimal fuss that can be included in hospital and clinic records and to store the data for utilization statistics and research. Thus, the choice requires considerable thought because some functions, such as data storage, that do not appear very important at the time the equipment is obtained may become very desirable a few years later.

Available Systems

It is not possible to provide a critical evaluation, or even a comprehensive list, of all the available systems. However, manufacturers that supply systems appearing to meet the specifications outlined above include COSMED S.r.I., Warren E Collins, Inc., Erich Jaeger GmbH, Medical Graphics Corp., P.K. Morgan Ltd., Quinton Instrument Company, SensorMedics Corp., and Vacumed. Addresses are provided in Appendix F.

Apart from the specifications outlined above, some variations are worth indicating. Nearly all systems provide breath-by-breath and mixing chamber modes, and in our view, any that allow only breath-by-breath measurements have to be evaluated very critically, for the reasons given above. Only one of the systems is portable (Cosmed K4) (Crandall et al., 1994). Several allow the rebreathing carbon dioxide cardiac output to be measured, and some provide a fully automated system for this method (Jaeger, Medical Graphics, Morgan, SensorMedics). Some provide automatic identification of the anaerobic threshold by the V-slope method (Jaeger, Medical Graphics, Quinton, Vacumed). One has a built-in electrocardiograph (SensorMedics). One can provide a flow-volume loop during exercise (Jaeger). Two provide a mechanical pump and gas mixing system (Huszczuk et al., 1990) to validate gas exchange measurements (Medical Graphics, SensorMedics).

Most manufacturers also provide ergometers and treadmills, as well as electrocardiographs that may be interfaced to the exercise gas exchange system.

Many laboratories may wish to put their own system together to suit their particular needs; the following is offered as a guide to the specifications of the components.

ERGOMETERS (see also Kane, 1983)

Cycles

Requirements

Requirements for clinical use are as follows:

1. Constant and known power output at a given setting
2. Adjustable height of handlebars and saddle and length of pedal stroke to accommodate patients of widely differing size
3. Power output relatively independent of pedaling frequency

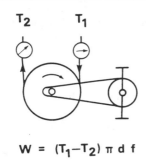

$$W = (T_1 - T_2) \pi \, d \, f$$

where d = diameter of wheel
f = frequency of rotation
$T_1 - T_2$ = braking force

Figure 14–1. Calculation of power output—mechanically braked cycle ergometer.

4. Enough inertia to maintain a cycling action in those patients unaccustomed to cycling

Types Available

MECHANICAL. In the simplest ergometers, either one wheel of a modified bicycle is braked by a strap, or a flywheel is braked in a similar way (Fig. 14–1). The power output is calculated from the difference in tension between the two ends of the strap, the circumference of the wheel, and the pedaling rate. Cycle ergometers braked by a pad are virtually useless because accurate calibration is impossible; also, the absence of a flywheel effect makes them uncomfortable.

In the most widely used machine (Monark), both ends of the strap that brakes the flywheel are attached to a weighted physical balance (von Dobeln, 1954) (Fig. 14–2). This allows the tension to be adjusted simply and to be read directly on a scale. Pedaling rate influences power output and should be controlled by use of a metronome. Friction in the bearings and other moving parts leads to a power output 8 to 10 per cent higher than calculated as above. Cost: $800 U.S.

ELECTROMECHANICAL. In electrically braked and stabilized ergometers, work is performed against an electrically produced resistance (Fig. 14–3). Specifications vary widely, and a flywheel may or may not be used. Usually, variations in pedaling frequency of between 50 and 70 per minute do not significantly affect the power output. Calibration is more difficult than with mechanical ergometers, but it is extremely important if an accurately known and constant power output is required. Biological calibration (measurement of oxygen intake and heart rate in a subject whose performance

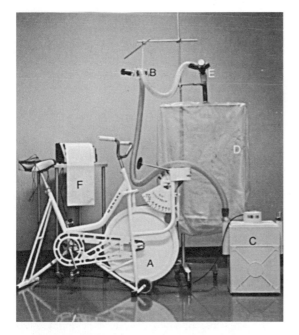

Figure 14–2. Simple system suitable for exercise testing: *A,* mechanically braked cycle ergometer; *B,* Otis-McKerrow valve; *C,* dry gas meter measuring inspired volume and fitted with potentiometer; *D,* Douglas bag collecting expired gas; *E,* stop-watch for accurate timing of expired gas collections; *F,* recorder for electrocardiographic and potentiometer signals.

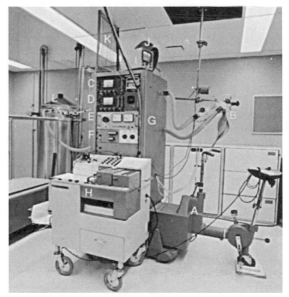

Figure 14–3. System for stage 2 and stage 3 exercise tests: *A,* electrically braked ergometer; *B,* mouthpiece assembly with rebreathing bag on adjustable rig; *C,* CO_2 analyzer; *D,* O_2 analyzer; *E,* ergometer control; *F,* solenoid controls; *G,* cabinet containing analyzers, dry gas meter, mixing chamber *(not seen),* and control panels; *H,* recorder; *I,* oscilloscope; *J,* fan; *K,* calibration gas inlets; *L,* Tissot spirometer.

has been previously established) is a method that can be used periodically. However, calibration is required at least once a year with a physical balance over the full range of work and pedaling frequencies. Cost: $4000 to $6000 U.S.

RECOMMENDED. For clinical studies an electromechanical ergometer is recommended because precise regulation of pedaling rate is unnecessary. In addition, small increases in resistance may be made more accurately than with a mechanical ergometer. However, for field studies and epidemiological work, a mechanical ergometer is adequate and has the advantages of being portable, free from the need of an electrical supply, and less expensive. Mechanical ergometers are easily adapted for arm work, if such is required in patients who are unable to perform leg exercise because of orthopedic or vascular problems or paraplegia. Suitable calibrating machines may be purchased (Vacumed) or made in a laboratory workshop (Cumming and Alexander, 1968).

Treadmills

Requirements

Requirements are as follows:

1. Easily adjustable grade from zero to 25 per cent and speed from 1 to 25 mph (40 km/h) if high power outputs are to be studied. However, for most clinical purposes, zero to 14 per cent grade and 1 to 10 mph are sufficient (Fig. 14–4).
2. Accurate timing of belt velocity
3. A main platform of at least 150 by 75 cm in area
4. Sturdy construction with handrails, side platforms, and a safety mechanism to stop the treadmill instantly in an emergency
5. Quiet operation

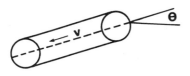

W = Wt × v × sine Θ

where v = speed

Θ = angle of elevation

Figure 14–4. Calculation of power output—treadmill.

There is a wide range in the specifications and cost of treadmills. The less powerful motors of cheaper machines are less reliable than those of more expensive machines, and it is therefore advisable to obtain a treadmill having high specifications. Most treadmills are bulky and require 220-V electric supply and are therefore not suitable for field work. Cost: $6000 to $20,000 U.S.

Steps

Requirements

1. One or two steps, adjustable in height between 2 and 12 in (5 to 30 cm)
2. Stable and covered with a nonslip surface
3. Attached handrail

A set of steps to these specifications is easily constructed. A convenient portable unit is described by Sharrock and associates (1972). An electrically controlled stair treadmill (StairMaster) has proved useful for training purposes, but it has not been used for exercise testing (Fedde and Pieschl, 1995).

MEASUREMENT OF VENTILATION

General Requirements

1. Accuracy over large ranges of volume and flow rates
2. Low resistance and inertia
3. Facility for electrical output suitable for a direct wiring recorder

Types of Equipment

Rotating Vane Flowmeters

The Wright anemometer (Wright, 1958) can be used for measurement of ventilation in simple exercise tests but is unreliable at high flow rates, when some gas may not be registered. It is inconvenient to read and may be damaged by high flow rates and by water vapor and should be used on the inspired side of a respiratory valve. Cost: $900 U.S.

Jewel-mounted turbine flowmeters are available that incorporate electro-optical detectors and electronic circuitry to correct for inertia and the effects of varying expired flow profiles, enabling ventilation to be measured with great accuracy (Jones, 1984). The cost of such a system is about $4000 U.S.

Dry Gas Meter

Models are available that have low resistance and sufficient accuracy through a full range of flow rates (see Fig. 14–2). Some contain bellows, which tend to deteriorate, so they should be calibrated regularly. Although the volume registered by a full revolution is accurate, some nonlinearity may be present within a single revolution; these characteristics need to be studied for each meter. A potentiometer may be fitted in order to obtain an electrical output, or a photoelectric device may be used to correct for nonlinearity (Reynolds, 1968). They may be damaged by the moisture of expired air, and they have a large washout volume. For these reasons, they are better used for measuring inspired rather than expired flow. The addition of bellows between the subject and the meter improves the accuracy of measurement of total ventilation by damping wide fluctuations in flow through the meter (Cotes, 1965). Cost: $1500 U.S.

Tissot Spirometer

Tissot spirometers are of 50- to 600-L capacity (see Fig. 14–3). Volume is recorded by measuring the vertical movement of the bell on a scale, from a kymograph, or from a potentiometer attached to one of the suspension pulleys. If expired gas is collected, the requisite flushing leads to unavoidable interruptions in the ventilation record; nowadays, they are rarely used for routine exercise testing, but their accuracy makes them useful for quality control. They are expensive; cost: $6000 to $8000 U.S.

Pneumotachograph

Until recently, methods for integrating flow to obtain volume were insufficiently stable for accurate measurement during exercise, but now signal conditioning electronics adjust for electrical drift and reset the signal after each breath. The output is affected by temperature changes and by the accumulation of water on the pneumotachograph screen. The head of the pneumotachograph is heated if expired flow is measured: this is a source of error that may be countered by a good heating control system. If the device is used for inspired flow, heating is not required because the temperature of the gas passing through is constant. Calibration needs to be dynamic, using a motor-driven syringe, because nonlinearity may be present at low and very high flows. For these reasons, this method is relatively unsuitable for routine exercise testing unless breath-by-breath measurements are required. With adequate signal processing, two pneumotachographs may be used to separately obtain inspired and expired flow and volume. The volume signal can be automatically processed with the output from gas analyzers to obtain breath-by-breath oxygen intake and carbon dioxide output (Wasserman et al., 1967). A suitable system has been detailed by Davies and associates (1974). Cost of pneumotachograph plus signal conditioning: about $4000 U.S.

MIXING AND COLLECTION OF EXPIRED GAS FOR ANALYSIS

Ideally, the system used to mix expired gas for continuous analysis and storage should have the following characteristics:

1. Gas is mixed rapidly and completely.
2. Stored gas is maintained at constant composition (i.e., the system does not leak and is impermeable to diffusion).
3. Resistance to flow is low.
4. If storage is needed, the spirometer or the bag should accommodate at least 100 L, preferably 200 L.

Mixing Chambers

Mixing chambers of about 5 to 15 L in volume contain either a number of baffles or a fan for mixing expired gas. Expired gas composition is measured distal to the chamber and should not show tidal fluctuations. Size of the chamber is chosen with regard to the type of study to be performed: a large volume ensures good mixing but takes time to wash out; a small volume does not mix gases completely when the tidal volume is high. A fan enables a small-volume chamber to be used, but care is needed to ensure that it does not pull gas through respiratory valves. An excellent cone-shaped mixing chamber is described by Davies and associates (1974).

Douglas Bags

Bags of 50- to 200-L capacity are suitable for the collection of expired gas (see Fig. 14–2). Polyvinyl and Mylar bags are less permeable to carbon dioxide than the older canvas and rubber types, which usually deteriorate with time. Regular checks should be made in order to detect leakage and changes in gas concentration. Volume is measured after collection by either gas meter or Tissot spirometer. Cost: about $150 U.S.

Before a gas collection, bags should be evacuated by a vacuum pump or washed out by expired gas. They should be hung vertically to diminish resistance. If volume is to be measured, accuracy is increased by the use of a stopwatch actuated by opening and closing the inlet tap (Åstrand and Rodahl, 1970). A bag-in-box system may be used to collect gas and record ventilation at the same time (Donald and Christie, 1949); it can be adapted inexpensively to provide multiple gas collections and automatic fill-empty cycles.

Tissot Spirometer

Expired gas may be collected and stored for analysis, but because the spirometer has a large washout volume, repeated flushing with expired gas is necessary, and a fan is required for adequate mixing.

TUBING, VALVES, AND TAPS

The main requirement for the respiratory circuit, including gas meters and spirometers, is a low resistance. The total resistance to inspiration or expiration should be less than 6 cm H_2O at flows up to 300 L/min (that is, approximately 1 cm $H_2O/L/sec$). Although the most reliable method of connecting the subject to the circuit is by a flanged silicon rubber or plastic mouthpiece, some patients find this very uncomfortable, and some may even gag. For this reason and for some other applications, a closely fitting face mask may be used.

Tubing

Tubing should be smooth internally and should have an internal diameter of 4 to 5 cm so that resistance is low. The total length of tubing used in a circuit should be as small as possible in order to minimize the total resistance, but angles, constrictions, and junctions are more resistive than a straight length of tubing. It is better to permit longer tubing than to clutter the space around the subject. Tubing should be gas sterilized periodically to prevent bacterial or fungal growth.

Valves

There is a wide selection of respiratory valves. The choice is dictated by a balance between dead space volume and resistance. The smallest valves generally have the highest resistance. Valves with very low resistance, such as the Otis-McKerrow valve (McKerrow and Otis, 1956), are required if maximal exercise is studied, but the dead space volume is often high, variable, and not amenable to accurate measurement. A low dead space volume is required for accurate measurement of V_D/V_T ratio and in children, in whom a large dead space may compromise alveolar ventilation.

A plastic flap valve of the Lloyd type (Cunningham et al., 1965) achieves a good compromise between volume (46 mL) and resistance (< 0.1 cm/L/sec) and is ideal for clinical testing. Daily cleaning is required in order to keep the valve working well. Cost: $400 U.S.

The Koegel valve (Lenox and Koegel, 1974) is also small, but the silicone rubber flaps have a tendency to leak. Cost: $400 U.S. An innovative valve (the Mijnhardt or Radiax valve) that allows axial flow with little turbulence and has a very small dead space (20 mL) is incorporated into the Jaeger Oxycon exercise system.

A wide variety of precision-engineered valves and taps is available from Hans Rudolph, Inc. (See Appendix F.)

Taps

Respiratory taps should be of similar bore to the valves and tubing, should avoid excessive turbulence owing to angulation, and should be easy to operate. The most widely used taps are made of cast aluminum and have a 2- to 3-cm bore. Three-way taps having a 60-degree angle are preferable to those with a 90-degree angle. If the circuit is to be controlled remotely, large-bore solenoid valves may be used. However, because they close forcibly, we use instead taps consisting of a piston moved by air pressure controlled remotely by small solenoids. For rebreathing, a tap is placed between the mouthpiece and the respiratory valve; the volume of this assembly is kept low by use of a sliding tap (Fig. 14–5) or a rotary four-channel tap (Lloyd and Wright, 1956). An alternative method to the pistons in the pneumatic taps described above is to use inflatable rubber balloons, which act in a similar way (Ellis and Lampman, 1980). A valve and rebreathing tap assembly similar to that shown in Figure 14–5 is commercially available (Hans Rudolph, Inc.). Cost: $1200 U.S.

ANALYSIS OF EXPIRED GAS

If large numbers of exercise tests are being performed, physical gas analyzers permit many analyses to be carried out with a considerable saving of time. The basis of their accuracy, however, is accurate analysis of the calibrating gases, performed with a Lloyd-Haldane apparatus or the Scholander microanalyzer. There are many types of physical analyzers, and the choice depends on several factors: the required response time, the availability of service and repair facilities, the type of output required (meter, null point, analogue, or digital readout), and the cost.

Carbon Dioxide

The measurement of carbon dioxide at the mouth during tidal breathing and during rebreathing requires a rapid analyzer. There are two main methods.

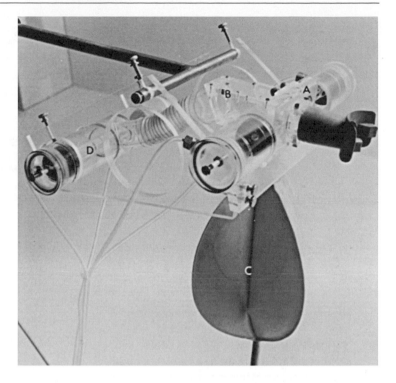

Figure 14–5. Respiratory valve and tap assembly showing sliding tap for rebreathing *(A)*, two-way flap valve *(B)*, rebreathing bag *(C)*, and two-way tap *(D)*.

Mass Spectrometer

The mass spectrometer is expensive to install but has several advantages: extremely fast response, low sampling flow, linear output, and freedom from interference by other gases (Scheid, 1983). Some difficulty may be experienced with water vapor, which travels through the sampling system at a lower rate than other gases. The mass spectrometer may also be used to measure a wide range of physiologically important gases. However, most laboratories are unable to justify the cost, which is in excess of $30,000 U.S.

Infrared Carbon Dioxide Meter

Infrared carbon dioxide meters are less expensive, and the response time is a little slower but still fast enough to enable the rapid changes in gas concentration during breathing to be followed accurately. Because the infrared analyzer is not specific for carbon dioxide, some foreign gases, such as nitrous oxide, interfere with its measurement. The oxygen concentration of the background gas has a small effect on the carbon dioxide concentration reading (Severinghaus, 1960), but this is overcome by calibrating with mixtures of carbon dioxide in concentrations of oxygen close to those in the gases to be analyzed. With careful calibration, carbon dioxide can be analyzed with an accuracy of $\pm$ 0.05 per cent. Infrared meters with adequate specifications are obtainable from several manufac-

turers, and the only major differences between models lie in the linearity of the electrical output and the response characteristics.

Although most carbon dioxide meters are linear to 6 per cent carbon dioxide, in some, the output becomes progressively less with higher concentrations. This is a serious drawback in carbon dioxide rebreathing, when concentrations of 12 per cent carbon dioxide or greater have to be accurately analyzed. The response characteristics are important if rapid changes in carbon dioxide are being measured, such as end-tidal P_{CO_2}, for which a 90 per cent response to a step input of carbon dioxide of 0.5 second or less is recommended (Jones et al., 1979). Solid-state analyzers with these specifications cost $5000 to $10,000 U.S.

Oxygen

For most purposes in exercise testing, there is no need for oxygen analysis to be rapid, but a high degree of accuracy is required. A paramagnetic oxygen meter is capable of analyzing oxygen with an accuracy of $\pm$ 0.03 per cent. Although the meter is not significantly affected by other respired gases, water vapor dilutes the sample. If dry calibration gases are used, humid samples should be passed over silica gel before analysis. Unless the analyzer has an electrical output, it should use the null balance reading principle to provide the necessary accuracy. Cost: $2000 to $6000 U.S.

Electrochemical analyzers use discs of zirconium or palladium oxides heated to high temperatures, when the potential difference across the disc is proportional to the oxygen pressure difference across the membrane. They are sensitive and fast responding; although early models were fragile and short lived, these analyzers are now much more robust. Their specifications are close to those of the mass spectrometer, but they cost less ($6000 U.S.).

EQUIPMENT FOR MEASUREMENT OF MIXED VENOUS Pco_2 BY REBREATHING

A 5-L anesthetic bag connected to the mouth-piece tap (see Fig. 14–5) is filled with a known volume and concentration of carbon dioxide in oxygen obtained by use of one of the methods to be described. The choice depends on the availability of engineering resources.

1. A series of mixtures of carbon dioxide in oxygen in 2 per cent steps between 7 and 15 per cent can be stored in gas cylinders and used to fill the rebreathing bag by opening the appropriate cylinder valve by hand. This method is convenient but may ultimately be expensive, owing to wastage of gas.
2. A system consisting of a 5-L plastic piston attached to a cylinder of 7 per cent carbon dioxide in 93 per cent oxygen and a 100-mL plastic syringe attached to a cylinder of 100 per cent carbon dioxide enables any concentration of carbon dioxide in oxygen to be mixed in the required volume (Fig. 14–6). Although minor engineering may be required, this method is simple to use and cheap to run because commercially available carbon dioxide is used.

3. Gas pressure from cylinders of 7 per cent carbon dioxide in oxygen and 100 per cent carbon dioxide is regulated by high-performance reducing valves. Solenoids controlled by time switches allow delivery of carbon dioxide in any concentration and volume to the rebreathing bag (Fig. 14–7). Although more engineering is needed with this method of preparing the gas mixture for rebreathing, it is recommended because of its speed and ease of operation.
4. Gas mixers of sufficient accuracy are now available commercially; the Wrostoff gas mixer is expensive and more accurate than strictly necessary. Less expensive mixers are part of modern positive-pressure ventilators (e.g., Siemens) and are easily adaptable for the purpose.

BLOOD GAS ANALYSIS

Several electrode systems for the measurement of blood gases and pH are capable of accurate analysis of small samples of blood (Severinghaus, 1962; Adams et al., 1967). I do not attempt to review these systems, all of which use the same analytical principles. In general, it is best to obtain a simple system that is easy to maintain. The accuracy of analysis should be established by tonometry; Pco_2 and Po_2 in the physiological range should be analyzed with an accuracy of $\pm$ 1.5 mm Hg. Some oxygen electrodes read Po_2 in blood a few mm Hg lower than in gas, and a correction is applied for this gas-blood difference once it has been established by tonometry. If very accurate analyses are required, temperature correction is needed in situations in which body temperature rises.

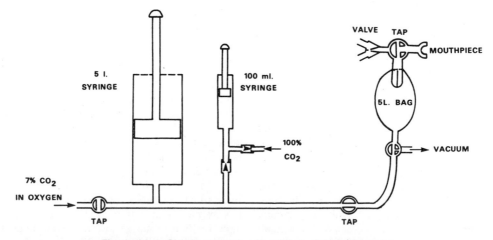

Figure 14–6. Simple apparatus for mixture of rebreathing gas.

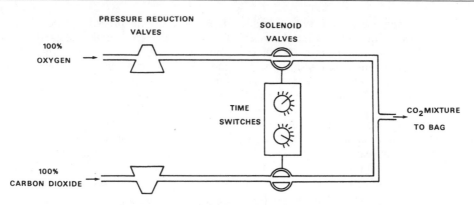

Figure 14–7. Diagram of automatic gas-mixing system.

Several methods exist for measurement of blood oxygen saturation. In general, if P_{O_2} and pH are measured, oxygen saturation may be calculated with reasonable accuracy ($\pm$ 2 per cent). More accurate measurement is seldom required except for specific research reasons. Carbon dioxide content is accurately calculated from measurements of P_{CO_2}, pH, hemoglobin, and oxygen saturation.

Noninvasive Blood Gas Measurement

Although transcutaneous oxygen and carbon dioxide sensors (Parker and Delpy, 1983) have been available for several years, their response times and accuracy are not adequate for use in exercise testing. However, noninvasive measurement of oxygen saturation by ear oximetry is now a well-established method.

Noninvasive Oximetry

A reliable bloodless method for the measurement of arterial oxygen saturation is clearly very helpful in assessing exercise responses (Hansen and Casaburi, 1987), and in one form or another, oximeters have been available for more than 30 years. During the intervening time, it appears that the more precise instruments have fallen by the wayside, probably because they were either too difficult to operate (Lal et al., 1966) or too expensive to be profitable (Saunders et al., 1976). Modern instruments (pulse oximeters) are easy to use and affordable, but the published evidence questions their reliability, accuracy, and precision (Severinghaus et al., 1989; Escourrou et al., 1990). They are most reliable in documenting changes in Sa_{O_2}; comparison with directly sampled arterial blood shows a precision of $\pm$ 4 per cent, but changes in Sa_{O_2} are measured to within $\pm$ 2 per cent (saturation) (Ries et al., 1985; Carlin et al., 1994). Variability is higher in black subjects than in white (Zeballos and Weisman,

1991), and readings are affected by the presence of methemoglobin and carboxyhemoglobin. The latter leads to a problem in smokers, who may have up to 10 per cent carboxyhemoglobin, because the oximeter "sees" carboxyhemoglobin as oxygenated hemoglobin (Tobin, 1988). The reliability of an oximeter in tracking changes in arterial P_{O_2} is easily established by a rebreathing method that compares end-tidal P_{O_2} with the reading of Sa_{O_2} (Lal et al., 1966). Pulse oximeters cost $3000 to $8000 U.S.

BLOOD PRESSURE MEASUREMENT

Although the measurement of systemic arterial pressure by auscultation or palpation is subject to error, for most purposes, changes in systolic pressure with exercise can be measured with sufficient accuracy by trained observers (Perloff et al., 1993). Measurement of diastolic pressure by this method is often unreliable. Automatic cuff inflating and measuring systems are expensive ($3000 U.S.) but may be justified by the laboratory load.

If arterial blood is being sampled with an indwelling catheter, arterial pressure may be measured by use of a pressure transducer and recorder.

Measurement of pulmonary arterial pressure through a thin catheter requires a pressure transducer and accurate calibration; this is a well-established technique that should not be difficult to use in any laboratory in which vascular catheterization is regularly performed.

ELECTROCARDIOGRAPHY

The electrocardiograph is preferred for the measurement of cardiac frequency rather than the less accurate measurement obtained by palpation of the radial or carotid pulse. Rate is measured from a recorder output or may be displayed automatically in digital form. Display of the electrocardiogram is essential in monitoring rhythm and in recognizing changes in the ST segment and T wave: high-quality recordings, free from drift and interference, are necessary for diagnostic use (Pina et al., 1995). These are obtained by reducing skin resistance with abrasion, by using correctly placed electrodes that minimize artefact, and by using appropriate signal conditioning.

A variety of electrodes are available. Best results are obtained from electrodes attached to the skin by circular adhesive pads that leave a gap between the electrode and the skin, which is filled by conducting jelly. Alternatives range from disposable stainless steel mesh electrodes to silver–silver chloride electrodes, which, in our experience, are very satisfactory. The quality of electrocardiogram recordings is influenced by several types of "noise," which need to be reduced to a minimum if recordings are to be interpreted reliably. Cyclic noise at a frequency of 60 cycles per second may be reduced by band pass filters chosen for their ability to attenuate noise without distorting the complexes. Random noise and baseline shift are more difficult to deal with, although they are reduced by good skin preparation; in these types of noise, digital computer smoothing has been found to be a powerful tool. The computer also may be programmed to make measurements of ST depression and its duration (Rautaharju et al., 1971).

A laboratory undertaking exercise testing for coronary artery disease requires a system that is capable of recording good-quality 12-lead electrocardiograms. There are many systems available costing from $8000 to $10,000 U.S. Larger systems provide microprocessor-controlled measurements of cardiac frequency, ST segment changes, and arrhythmias. Cost: $20,000 to $40,000 U.S.

RECORDERS

A recorder is used to collect basic data using the electrical output from the electrocardiograph, oxygen and carbon dioxide analyzers, and a gas meter or spirometer.

Desirable characteristics of a recorder are as follows:

1. At least four, and preferably six channels
2. Direct writing so that data are available immediately
3. Rectilinear writing system
4. Flat frequency response to 50 Hz
5. Resolution greater than 1 per cent of the full-scale deflection
6. Zero suppression

If a large volume of studies is contemplated, the cost of recorder paper may be important, as there is a wide variation among brands. Many recorders meet most of the preceding specifications, and a few meet all. The requirements that may not be immediately obvious are those related to the measurement of carbon dioxide. The reading accuracy for this should be at least 1 mm of pen deflection for 1 mm Hg P_{CO_2}: because the highest levels of P_{CO_2} approach 100 mm Hg during rebreathing, a full-scale deflection of at least 10 cm is required. In order to obtain this, more than one channel of the recorder may be required with zero suppression in one channel. The cost of recorders is generally about $3000 U.S. per channel.

MEASUREMENT OF MUSCLE STRENGTH

Measurement of muscle strength involves the recording of the force exerted in a maximal static or dynamic contraction of the muscles acting across a single joint or several joints involved in some task. Dynamic measurements are preferred, but the differing force-velocity characteristics of different muscles brings up the question of standardization—is one velocity chosen or is the measurement made at the optimal velocity for the movement? The choice is very wide and has to be made on the basis of the application (e.g., patients versus athletes), the complexity of recording (single task versus measurement at differing velocities and joint angles), the time required, and the cost of the equipment. We make no apology for having chosen an inexpensive method that is simple to apply in a wide variety of subjects and takes only a few minutes, even though its precision and scope may be less than with more complex and expensive systems. The following types of assessment may be made.

WEIGHTLIFTING. The maximum weight that can be lifted once (one repetition maximum) is a measure of strength that is often used to prescribe a training weight, but it requires many trials carried out on a weightlifting machine and does not provide a dynamic measurement without complex instrumentation.

ISOMETRIC TESTING. This is easily carried out by use of commercially available dynamometers or strain gauges, but again, the measurement is static and has no velocity component.

ISOKINETIC TESTING. This type of testing is carried out with a system that measures torque at a constant velocity of joint movement; the applied force is matched by a variable electrical resistance imposed by the dynamometer to obtain a constant preset velocity (Perrine, 1986). Several commercially available systems have been extensively validated, such as the Cybex (Sale, 1991) and Kin-com (Murray and Harrison, 1986) systems, but they are expensive (> \$25,000 U.S.). Isokinetic cycle ergometers have been described that control the pedal rate and measure the torque exerted on the pedal crank (McCartney et al., 1983); although normal values are available (Makrides et al., 1985), the system is complex and difficult to add to a routine exercise test protocol. A cheaper (\$6000 U.S.) version of isokinetic dynamometer measures torque during maximal effort at different velocities produced by variable hydraulic resistances, similar in principle to automobile shock absorbers with an adjustable leak. The pressure generated in the cylinders is recorded by transducers, and a microprocessor records the peak pressure at any given resistance setting; in this way, a relatively crude approximation of the more expensive isokinetic systems is obtained. Because the internal surface area of the cylinders remains constant, the pressure (in kilograms per square centimeter) is converted into an equivalent force (kilogram). The peak value is usually, but not always, obtained with the highest resistance (and thus the lowest contraction velocity). However, weak subjects may generate such a low velocity at the high resistances that peak force is recorded with the lower resistances. This system (Hydra-Fitness, Hydra-Gym, Belton, TX) (Sale, 1991) has six settings and can store the peak pressure values at any setting to allow the best value to be chosen. The peak force closely approximates the maximum force recorded with an isometric dynamometer, but the movement makes it more acceptable to obtain peak force in disabled subjects and is thus more reproducible in clinical settings. Measurements are made in leg flexion and extension and arm flexion (pulling) and extension (pushing) and are sufficiently precise for clinical purposes in a routine exercise laboratory.

RESUSCITATION EQUIPMENT

The laboratory should be equipped to meet an emergency, and personnel should be capable of maintaining life until the patient can be managed by a cardiac team (Pina et al., 1995).

The following equipment is required:

1. Drugs for intravenous use: epinephrine, atropine, aminophylline, digoxin, isoprenaline, lidocaine, propranolol, hydrocortisone, procainamide, sodium bicarbonate, calcium gluconate, sublingual nitroglycerin, dopamine, dobutamine, and verapamil
2. Syringes, intravenous infusion sets, and glucose saline
3. Hand-held ventilator, such as the Ambu bag
4. Airways, endotracheal tubes, and laryngoscope
5. Direct-current defibrillator
6. Oxygen

REFERENCES

Adams AP, Morgan-Hughes JO, Sykes MK. pH and blood-gas analysis (methods of measurement and sources of error using electrode systems). Anaesthesia 1967;22:575–597.

Åstrand P-O, Rodahl K. Textbook of Work Physiology. New York: McGraw-Hill Book Co.; 1970.

Bailey JJ, Berson AS, Garson AJ, et al. Recommendations for standardization and specifications in automated electrocardiography: Bandwidth and digital signal processing. A report for health professionals by an ad hoc writing group of the Committee on Electrocardiography and Cardiac Electrophysiology of the Council on Clinical Cardiology, American Heart Association. Circulation 1990;91:730–739.

Beaver WL, Wasserman K, Whipp BJ. On-line computer analysis and breath-by-breath graphical display of exercise function tests. J Appl Physiol 1973;34:128–132.

Carlin BW, Clausen JL, Ries AL. The effects of exercise testing on the prescription of oxygen therapy. Chest 1994;106:361–365.

Cotes JE. Lung Function, 5th ed. Oxford: Blackwell Scientific Publications; 1993.

Crandall CG, Taylor SL, Raven PB. Evaluation of the Cosmed K2 Portable Telemetric Oxygen-Uptake Analyzer. Med Sci Sport Exerc 1994;26:108–111.

Cumming GR, Alexander WD. The calibration of bicycle ergometers. Can J Physiol Pharmacol 1968;46:917–919.

Cunningham DJC, Elliott DH, Lloyd BB, et al. A comparison of the effects of oscillating and steady alveolar partial pressures of oxygen and carbon dioxide on the pulmonary ventilation. J Physiol 1965;179:498–508.

Davies EE, Hahn HL, Spiro SG, et al. A new technique for recording respiratory transients at the start of exercise. Respir Physiol 1974;20:69–79.

Donald KW, Christie RV. A new method of clinical spirometry. Clin Sci 1949;8:21.

Ellis DG, Lampman RM. Lightweight remotely actuated switching valve for rebreathing exercise studies. J Appl Physiol 1980;48:386–388.

Escourrou P, Delaperche MF, Visseaux A. Reliability of pulse oximetry during exercise in pulmonary patients. Chest 1990;97:635–638.

Fedde MR, Pieschl RL. Extreme derangements of acid-base balance in exercise: Advantages and limitations of the Stewart analysis. Can J Appl Physiol 1995;20:369–379.

Hansen JE, Casaburi R. Validity of ear oximetry in clinical exercise testing. Chest 1987;91:333–337.

Huszczuk A, Whipp BJ, Wasserman K. A respiratory gas exchange simulator for routine calibration in metabolic studies. Eur Respir J 1990;3:465–468.

Jones NL. Evaluation of a microprocessor-controlled exercise testing system. J Appl Physiol 1984;57:1312–1318.

Jones NL, Robertson DG, Kane JW. Difference between end-tidal and arterial P_{CO_2} in exercise. J Appl Physiol 1979;47:954–960.

Kane JW. Treadmills and cycle ergometers. In: Laszlo G, Sudlow MF, editors. Measurement in Clinical Respiratory Physiology. London: Academic Press; 1983, pp. 167–184.

Lal S, Gebbie T, Campbell EJM. Simple methods for improving the value of oximetry in the study of pulmonary oxygen uptake. Thorax 1966;21:50–56.

Lenox JB, Koegel E. Evaluation of a new low-resistance breathing valve. J Appl Physiol 1974;37:410–413.

Liese W, Warwick WJ, Cumming G. Water vapour pressure in expired air. Respiration 1974;31:252–261.

Lloyd BB, Wright TA. A four channel tap for use in human respiratory studies. J Physiol (London) 1956;133:34.

Makrides L, Heigenhauser GJF, McCartney N, Jones NL. Maximal short term exercise capacity in healthy subjects aged 15–70. Clin Sci 1985;69:197–205.

McCartney N, Heigenhauser GJF, Sargeant AJ, Jones NL. A constant velocity cycle ergometer for the study of dynamic muscle function. J Appl Physiol 1983;55:212–217.

McKerrow CB, Otis AB. Low resistance valve for hyperventilation. J Appl Physiol 1956;9:497.

Murray DA, Harrison E. Constant velocity dynamometer: An appraisal using mechanical loading. Med Sci Sports Exerc 1986;18:612–624.

Parker D, Delpy DT. Blood gas analysis by invasive and noninvasive techniques. In: Laszlo G, Sudlow MF. Measurement in Clinical Respiratory Physiology. London: Academic Press; 1983, pp. 75–112.

Perloff D, Grim C, Flack J, et al. Human blood pressure determination by sphygmomanometry. Circulation 1993;88:2460–2468.

Perrine JJ. The biophysics of maximal muscle power outputs: Methods and problems of measurement. In: Jones NL, McCartney N, McComas AJ, editors. Human Muscle Power. Champaign, IL: Human Kinetics Publishers; 1986, pp. 15–25.

Pina IL, Balady GJ, Hanson P, et al. Guidelines for clinical exercise testing laboratories: A statement for healthcare professionals from the committee on exercise and cardiac rehabilitation, American Heart Association. Circulation 1995;91:912–921.

Porszasz J, Barstow TJ, Wasserman K. Evaluation of a symmetrically disposed Pitot tube flowmeter for measuring gas flow during exercise. J Appl Physiol 1994;77:2659–2665.

Rautaharju PM, Friedrich H, Wolf H. Measurement and interpretation of exercise electrocardiograms. In: Shephard RJ, editor. Frontiers of Fitness. Springfield, IL: Charles C Thomas Publisher; 1971, pp. 295–315.

Reynolds JA. A method of recording pulmonary ventilation. J Sci Instrum 1968;1:433–450.

Ries AL, Farrow JT, Clausen JL. Accuracy of two ear oximeters at rest and during exercise in pulmonary patients. Am Rev Respir Dis 1985;132:685–689.

Sale DG. Testing strength and power. In: MacDougall JD, Wenger HA, Green HJ, editors. Physiological Testing of the High-Performance Athlete. Champaign, IL: Human Kinetics Publishers; 1991, pp. 21–106.

Saunders NA, Powles ACP, Rebuck AS. Ear oximetry: Accuracy and practicability in the assessment of arterial oxygenation. Am Rev Respir Dis 1976;113:745–749.

Scheid P. Respiratory mass spectrometry. In: Laszlo G, Sudlow MF. Measurement in Clinical Respiratory Physiology. London: Academic Press; 1983, pp. 131–166.

Severinghaus JW. Methods of measurement of blood and gas carbon dioxide during anaesthesia. Anaesthesiology 1960; 21:717–726.

Severinghaus JW. Electrodes for blood and gas P_{CO_2}, P_{O_2} and blood pH. Acta Anaesth Scand 1962;11:208–219.

Severinghaus JW, Naifeh KH, Koh SO. Errors in 14 pulse oximeters during profound hypoxia. J Clin Monit 1989;5:72–81.

Sharrock N, Garrett HL, Mann GV. Practical exercise test for physical fitness and cardiac performance. Am J Cardiol 1972;30:727–732.

Tobin MJ. Respiratory monitoring in the intensive care unit. Am Rev Respir Dis 1988;138:1625–1642.

von Dobeln W. A simple bicycle ergometer. J Appl Physiol 1954;7:222–224.

Wasserman K, Van Kessel AI, Burton G. Interaction of physiological mechanisms during exercise. J Appl Physiol 1967; 22:71–85.

Wilmore JH, Davis JA, Norton AC. An automated system for assessing metabolic and respiratory function during exercise. J Appl Physiol 1976;40:619–624.

Wright BM. A respiratory anemometer. J Physiol (London) 1958;127:25.

Yeh MP, Adams TD, Gardner RM, Yanowitz FG. Turbine flowmeter vs. Fleisch pneumotachometer: A comparative study for exercise testing. J Appl Physiol 1987;63:1289–1295.

Zeballos RJ, Weisman IM. Reliability of noninvasive oximetry in black subjects during exercise and hypoxia. Am Rev Respir Dis 1991;144:1240–1244.

Symbols

The convention established by Pappenheimer and associates (1950) has been followed, with primary symbols (what is measured) and suffixes (where it is measured).

Primary Symbols

C = concentration in blood phase
D = diffusion
F = fractional concentration in dry gas phase
f = frequency
G = any gas
P = pressure in general, including partial pressure
$\dot{Q}$ = volume flow or blood per unit time, including cardiac output
S = oxygen saturation of hemoglobin in per cent
T = time
V = gas volume in general
$\dot{V}$ = volume flow of gas per unit of time

Prefixes and Suffixes

1. Gas Phase
   A = alveolar
   B = barometric
   D = dead space
   E = expired
   I = inspired
   ET = end tidal (e.g., P_{ETCO_2})
   T = tidal (e.g., V_T)

2. Blood Phase
   a = arterial
   c = capillary
   v = venous
   $\bar{v}$ = mixed venous
   c' = end capillary
   p = plasma

3. Miscellaneous Functions
   b = breathing (e.g., f_b)
   c = cardiac (e.g., f_c)
   s = stroke (e.g., V_s)
   tot = total
   VA = venous admixture

Abbreviations

ATP = ambient temperature and pressure
BTPS = body temperature, ambient pressure, saturated with water vapor
STPD = standard temperature (0°C) and pressure (760 mm Hg), dry
FEV_1 = forced expired volume in one second
VC = vital capacity
RV = residual volume
TLC = total lung capacity
MVV = maximal voluntary ventilation
$\dot{V}_{O_2}max$ = maximal oxygen intake (expressed in L/min or mL/min/kg)
met = a multiple of resting metabolic rate

Calculation of Results

The principles underlying calculations have been mentioned previously (see Chapter 9). This section enables you to carry out the calculations, given basic measurements, and discusses all the calculations needed in a steady state exercise test. A recording such as the ones shown in Figures B–1 and B–2 is produced during the test (Chapter 9).

Construction of Calibration Lines for Carbon Dioxide and Oxygen

The upper channel of the recorder covers the range of the three lowest calibrating carbon dioxide mixtures (which contain oxygen at a concentration similar to expired gas), and the lower channel records the higher concentrations of carbon dioxide required for measurements during rebreathing (these calibrating gases contain about 40 per cent oxygen). The deflections are identified and a line is drawn (Fig. B–1) from which unknown carbon dioxide concentrations can be read (mixed expired, end tidal, and rebreathing P_{CO_2}). If the recorder is being used to measure mixed expired oxygen concentration, a similar calibration line is drawn (Fig. B–1).

Measurements (Figs. B–2 and B–3)

1. **Time Factor.** The number of centimeters of recorder paper passing in 1 minute. Because the

recorder speed control may not be accurate, the time factor should be measured by use of the time base, which is accurate.

2. **Volume Factor.** Liters entering the Tissot spirometer or passing through the dry gas meter to produce 1 cm of deflection. If the volume corresponding to one complete revolution of the potentiometer—that is, one complete sweep length (x, liters)—is known, division of that volume by the vertical deflection on the paper of a complete sweep (y, cm) produces the required value (x/y, L/cm).

3. **Time Measurement.** Centimeters of paper for the period of ventilation measurement.

4. **Volume Deflection.** Centimeters of paper measured vertically during the period of collection.

5. **Cardiac Frequency Deflection.** Centimeters of paper, measured horizontally, corresponding to 5 electrocardiographic RR intervals.

6. **Breathing Frequency Measurement.** Number of breaths during collection period.

7. **F_{ECO_2}.** Fractional concentration of carbon dioxide in mixed expired gas (top calibration line).

8. **F_{EO_2}.** Fractional concentration of oxygen in mixed expired gas.

9. **F_{ETCO_2}.** Fractional concentration of carbon dioxide at the mouthpiece at the end of expiration (using top calibration line) averaged for the period of collection.

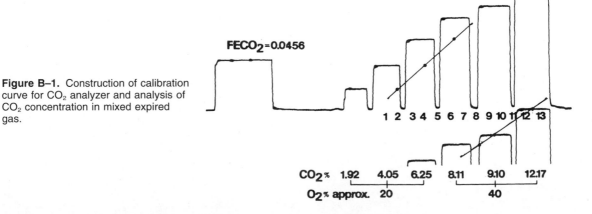

Figure B–1. Construction of calibration curve for CO_2 analyzer and analysis of CO_2 concentration in mixed expired gas.

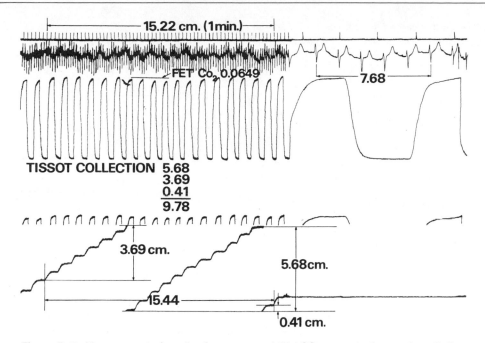

Figure B–2. Measurement of cardiac frequency, end-tidal CO_2 concentration, and ventilation.

10. $F_{ET}CO_2$. Fractional concentration of carbon dioxide at the mouthpiece during a rebreathing equilibrium measurement (see Fig. B–3).
11. P_B. Barometric pressure.
12. T_A. Ambient temperature.
13. $P_{H_2O,T}$. Water vapor pressure of the measured gas, obtained from Table C–2 and corrected for percentage of humidity if not 100 per cent.

Mathematical Description of the Carbon Dioxide Dissociation Curve for Whole Blood

In Chapter 9, a number of shortcuts were presented to enable PCO_2 in mixed venous and arterial blood to be converted into an arteriovenous carbon dioxide content difference. These are based on the relationships derived by McHardy (1967) from the data and equations of Peters and associates in a series of papers published in 1920–1924 and of Visser in 1960. I have reviewed these equations in the light of the more recent study of Loeppky and colleagues (1983) and data generated in our own laboratory from blood sampled in studies of carbon dioxide content at different PCO_2 in vivo (Douglas and co-workers, 1988). On the basis of these studies, I suggest the following approach:

1. Measure PCO_2 and pH in arterial blood and calculate base excess by use of the nomogram or equations of Siggaard-Andersen. Use this value to calculate venous pH (not measured) from mixed venous PCO_2. If a value for arterial pH is not available and one is assumed or estimated from changes in arterial lactate, the same procedure is followed.

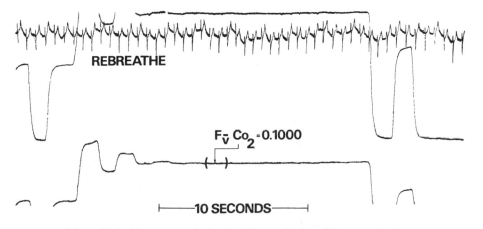

Figure B–3. Measurement of rebreathing equilibrium CO_2 concentration.

2. Calculate plasma carbon dioxide content for arterial and venous blood, from plasma P_{CO_2} and pH:

$$C_{CO_2}(pl) = 2.226 \times 0.0307 \, P_{CO_2} \, (1.0 + 10^{pH-6.1})$$

3. Calculate whole blood carbon dioxide content from $C_{CO_2}(pl)$ by allowing for the effects of oxygen content and pH. Oxygen content is the product of oxygen capacity (Hb $\times$ 1.34 mL/dL) and oxygen saturation. Oxygen saturation is assumed to be 1.0 in mixed venous blood during rebreathing; arterial oxygen saturation is measured or assumed to be 0.95.

Thus three constants require calculation:
a. Effect of hemoglobin (g/dL):

$$K1 = 0.0289 \times Hb$$

b. Effect of oxygen saturation (100 per cent = 1.0):

$$K2 = 1/[3.3582 - (0.456 \times S_{O_2})]$$

c. Effect of pH:

$$K3 = 1/(8.142 - pH)$$

Then

$$C_{CO_2}(bl) = C_{CO_2}(pl) \\ - C_{CO_2}(pl) [K1 \times K2 \times K3].$$

The major advantage of using these equations is that the effects of pH on carbon dioxide content are allowed for; although this is not an important correction for minor degrees of acidosis, it is required for the calculation of cardiac output in heavy exercise. Although they appear complex, the calculations are straightforward when carried out by computer.

Example of Calculations

Workload: 200 kpm/min (see Figs. B–1, B–2, and B–3)

Stage 2 Test Measurements

Barometric pressure	745
Temperature	22°C
BTPS factor	1.0921
Volume factor	1.80
Time factor	15.22
Cardiac frequency deflection	7.68
Volume deflection	9.78
Time deflection	15.44
Number of breaths	18
F_{ECO_2}	0.0456
F_{EO_2}	0.1588
F_{ETCO_2}	0.0649
$F_{\bar{v}CO_2}$	0.1000

Calculations

$$f_c = \frac{50 \times 15.22}{7.68} = 99 \text{ b/min}$$

$$\dot{V}_E \text{ (ATPS)} = \frac{9.78 \times 1.80 \times 15.22}{15.44} = 17.35 \text{ L/min}$$

$$\dot{V}_E \text{ (BTPS)} = 17.35 \times 1.0921 = 18.95 \text{ L/min}$$

$$\dot{V}_E \text{ (STPD)} = 17.35 \times 0.8829 = 15.32 \text{ L/min}$$

$$f_b = \frac{18 \times 15.22}{15.44} = 17.7 \text{ breaths/ min}$$

$$V_T = \frac{18.95}{17.7} \times 1000 = 1070 \text{ mL}$$

$$\dot{V}_{CO_2} = 0.0456 \times 15.32 \times 1000 = 699 \text{ mL/min}$$

$$\dot{V}_{O_2} = 15.32 \left[\frac{0.2093 \times (1 - 0.1588 - 0.0456)}{0.7904} - 0.1588 \right] \\ \times 1000 = 794 \text{ mL/min}$$

$$R = \frac{699}{794} = 0.88$$

$$P_{ECO_2} = 0.0456 \times 698 = 32 \text{ mm Hg}$$

$$P_{ETCO_2} = 0.0649 \times 698 = 45 \text{ mm Hg}$$

$$P_{bag}CO_2 = 0.1000 \times 698 = 69.8 \text{ mm Hg}$$

$$P_{\bar{v}CO_2} = 69.8 - [(0.24 \times 69.8) - 11] = 64.0$$

Derivation of $\dot{Q}_{tot}$ and V_D/V_T from P_{aCO_2} Estimated from P_{ETCO_2} or Measured

Measurements

$$P_{ETCO_2} = 45 \text{ mm Hg}$$

$$V_T = 1070 \text{ mL}$$

$$f_b = 17.7 \text{ breaths/min}$$

$$P_{ECO_2} = 32 \text{ mm Hg}$$

Calculations

$$P_{aCO_2} = 5.5 + (0.9 \times 45) - (0.0021 \times 1070) \\ = 44 \text{ mm Hg}$$

$$V_D = \left(\frac{44 - 32}{44} \times 1070 \right) - 60 \\ = 232 \text{ mL}$$

$$V_D/V_T = \frac{232}{1070} \\ = 0.22$$

$$\log_e CaCO_2 = (\log_e 44 \times 0.396) + 2.38$$
$$= 3.879$$
$$CaCO_2 = 48.4 \text{ mL/100 mL}$$
$$\log_e C\bar{v}CO_2 = (\log_e 64 \times 0.396) + 2.38$$
$$= 4.027$$
$$C\bar{v}CO_2 = 56.1 \text{ mL/100 mL}$$

$$C\bar{v}CO_2 - CaO_2 = 56.1 - 48.4 = 7.7 \text{ mL/100 mL}$$

(No correction required for Hb; SaO_2 assumed 95%)

$$\dot{Q}tot = \frac{699}{7.7} \times 10$$
$$= 9.1 \text{ L/min}$$

$$V_s = \frac{9100}{99}$$
$$= 92 \text{ mL}$$

Additional Calculations Performed When Pao_2 Is Measured

$$PaCO_2 - 44 \text{ mm Hg}$$
$$PaO_2 = 85 \text{ mm Hg}$$

$$pH = 7.40$$
$$SaO_2 = 95.6\%$$
$$Hb = 15.5 \text{ g/100 mL}$$

$$CaO_2 = 0.956 (Hb \times 1.34)$$
$$= 19.8 \text{ mL/100 mL}$$
$$C\bar{v}O_2 = CaCO_2 - \frac{\dot{V}O_2}{\dot{Q}tot}$$
$$= 19.8 - \frac{794}{91}$$
$$= 11.1 \text{ mL/100 mL}$$

$$PAO_2 = [0.2093 \times (745 - 47)] - 44 \left(0.2093 + \frac{0.7904}{0.88}\right)$$
$$= 97 \text{ mm Hg } (Cc'O_2 = 20 \text{ mL/100 mL})$$
$$PA - aO_2 = 12 \text{ mm Hg}$$
$$\dot{Q}VA/\dot{Q}tot = \frac{20.0 - 19.8}{20.0 - 11.1}$$
$$= \frac{0.2}{8.9}$$
$$= 0.02 \ (2\%)$$

Table B–1. EQUATIONS USED IN THE CALCULATION OF RESULTS

Equations	Comments

1. Cardiac frequency (b/min):

$$f_c = \frac{5 \times \text{time factor}}{\text{cm for 5 RR}}$$

Time factor is measurement 1 above in cm for 5 RR intervals.

2. Ventilation (L/min BTPS):

$$\dot{V} \text{ (ATP)} = \frac{\text{vol def} \times \text{vol factor} \times \text{time factor}}{\text{time def}}$$

Conventionally, ventilation is $\dot{V}_E$ expressed at BTPS.

Vol def is measurement 4.
Vol factor is measurement 2.
Time factor is measurement 1.
Time def is measurement 3.

If $\dot{V}_I$ (ATP) is measured,

$$\dot{V}_{E}\text{ATP} = \dot{V}_I \text{ (ATP)} \times \frac{0.7904}{1 - F_{EO_2} - F_{ECO_2}}$$

Corrects $\dot{V}_I$ to $\dot{V}_E$.
Not required if $\dot{V}_E$ is measured.
$0.7094 = 1 - (F_{IO_2} + F_{ICO_2})$.

$$\dot{V}_E \text{ (BTPS)} = \dot{V}_E \text{ (ATP)} \times \frac{273 + 37}{273 + T_A} \times \frac{P_B - P_{H_2O, A}}{P_B - 47}$$

or

$$\dot{V}_E \text{ (BTPS)} = \dot{V}_{E}\text{ATP} \times \text{BTPS factor}$$

Corrects to body temperature, saturated.
T_A is measurement 12.
P_{H_2O} is measurement 13.
Same equation, but BTPS factor taken from Table C–2.

3. Breathing frequency (breaths/min):

$$f_b = \frac{\text{number of breaths} \times \text{time factor}}{\text{time deflection}}$$

Number of breaths is measurement 6.
Time factor is measurement 1.
Time deflection is measurement 3.

4. Tidal volume (mL, BTPS):

$$V_T = \frac{\dot{V}_E \text{ (BTPS)}}{f_b} \times 1000$$

From calculations 2 and 3.

5. Oxygen intake (mL/min, STPD):

Calculate $\dot{V}_I$STPD and $\dot{V}_E$STPD:

$$\dot{V} \text{ (STPD)} = \dot{V} \text{ ATP} \times \frac{P_B - P_{H_2O, A}}{760} \times \frac{273}{273 + T_A}$$

Corrects from ambient conditions, conventionally expressed at ATP (measurements 11, 12, 13), to standard temperature and pressure dry (STPD).

or:

$$\dot{V} \text{ (STPD)} = \dot{V} \text{ (ATP)} \times \text{STPD factor}$$

STPD factor taken from Table C–2.

Then:

$$\dot{V}_{O_2} = 1000\,[\dot{V}_I \text{ (STPD)} \times F_{IO_2}] - (\dot{V}_E\text{STPD} \times F_{EO_2})$$

F_{IO_2} is 0.2093 for air.
F_{EO_2} is measurement 8.

6. Carbon dioxide output (mL/min STPD):

$$\dot{V}_{CO_2} = 1000\,(\dot{V}_I\text{STPD} \times F_{ICO_2}) - (\dot{V}_E\text{STPD} \times F_{ECO_2})$$

Conventionally expressed at STPD.

$\dot{V}_E$STPD is calculation 5.
$\dot{V}_I \times F_{ICO_2}$ is small for room air ($\dot{V}_I \times 0.004$) and usually neglected.
F_{ECO_2} is measurement 7.

7. Respiratory exchange ratio:

$$R = \frac{\dot{V}_{CO_2}}{\dot{V}_{O_2}}$$

Dimensionless.

From calculations 5 and 6.

8. Mixed expired P_{CO_2} (mm Hg):

$$P_{ECO_2} = F_{ECO_2} \times (P_B - 47)$$

Used in calculation 12.

47 is P_{H_2O} at 37°C.
F_{ECO_2} is measurement 7.
Assumes gas analyzed is dry. If not, appropriate corrections are required (i.e., depends on analyzer).

Equations	Comments
9. End-tidal P_{CO_2} (mm Hg): $$P_{ETCO_2} = F_{ETCO_2} (P_B - 47)$$	F_{ETCO_2} is measurement 9. Comments for calculation 8 also apply here.
10. Mixed venous P_{CO_2} (mm Hg): First calculate rebreathing equilibrium P_{CO_2}: $$P_{EqCO_2} = F_{EqCO_2} \times (P_B - 47)$$ Apply alveolar to blood correction factor: $$P_{\bar{V}CO_2} = P_{EqCO_2} - (0.24 \, P_{EqCO_2} - 11)$$	F_{EqCO_2} is measurement 10. Required if rebreathing equilibration method used.
11. Estimation of arterial P_{CO_2} from P_{ETCO_2}: $$P_{aCO_2} = 5.5 + 0.90 \, P_{ETCO_2} - 0.0021 \, V_T$$	May also be derived from P_{ECO_2} by assuming a value for V_D (see calculation 12). This equation should be used only in subjects with normal pulmonary function. *Note:* May be affected by analyzer response time.
12. Dead space (mL BTPS): $$V_D = \frac{P_{aCO_2} - P_{ECO_2}}{P_{aCO_2}} \quad V_T - \text{valve box dead space}$$ The V_D/V_T ratio is obtained by dividing by V_T.	Bohr's equation.
13. Alveolar P_{O_2} (mm Hg): $$P_{AO_2} = F_{IO_2} (P_B - 47) - P_{aCO_2} \left(F_{IO_2} + \frac{1 - (F_{IO_2} + F_{ICO_2})}{R} \right)$$ If air is inspired: $$P_{AO_2} = 0.2093 (P_B - 47) - P_{aCO_2} \left(0.2093 + \frac{0.7904}{R} \right)$$ This value is then used to obtain the alveolar-arterial P_{O_2} difference.	The alveolar air equation.
14. Cardiac output (L/min): $$\dot{Q}tot = \frac{\dot{V}_{CO_2}}{C\bar{v}_{CO_2} - C_{aCO_2}}$$ $$\log_e C\bar{v}_{CO_2} = (\log_e P\bar{v}_{CO_2} \times 0.396) + 2.38$$ $$\log_e C_{aCO_2} = (\log_e P_{aCO_2} \times 0.396) + 2.38$$ If Hb is not 15 g/100 mL, then this value is corrected: $$C\bar{v} - a_{CO_2} \text{ actual} = C_a - \bar{v}_{CO_2} - [(15 - Hb) \times 0.015 \times (P\bar{v}_{CO_2} - P_{aCO_2})]$$ Similarly, if arterial saturation is not 95%, then: $$C\bar{v} - a_{CO_2} \text{ actual} = C\bar{v} - a_{CO_2} - [(95 - S_{aO_2}) \times 0.064]$$	$\dot{V}_{CO_2}$ is calculation 6. Expression of the carbon dioxide dissociation curve for Hb = 15, S_{aO_2} = 100%. Calculates content from $P\bar{v}_{CO_2}$ and P_{aCO_2} (calculations 10 and 11). Assumes $S\bar{v}_{O_2}$ during rebreathing is 100%. Correct for changes in carbon dioxide dissociation curve with change in Hb. Corrects for changes in S_{aO_2}.
15. Arterial oxygen saturation (S_{aO_2}):	Derived from measured P_{aO_2} and pH using Kelman's equation or a standard oxygen dissociation curve.
16. Venous admixture: $$\frac{\dot{Q}_{VA}}{\dot{Q}tot} = \frac{Cc'_{O_2} - C_{aO_2}}{Cc'_{O_2} - C\bar{v}_{O_2}}$$ where: $$C\bar{v}_{O_2} = C_{aO_2} - \frac{\dot{V}_{O_2}}{\dot{Q}tot}$$	Blood P_{aO_2} measurements are converted to oxygen saturation. Mean pulmonary capillary saturation is obtained from P_{AO_2} using Kelman's equation. Oxygen saturation values are converted to oxygen contents by multiplying by Hb $\times$ 1.34 $\times$ 10. Oxygen contents expressed in mL/L.

Note: A program is available to make the calculations above with a small programmable calculator (Powles and Jones, 1982).

Conversion Factors and Constants

Table C–1. CONVERSION OF TRADITIONAL UNITS TO SI (SYSTEME INTERNATIONALE) UNITS

Index	Symbol	Traditional Units	SI Units	Conversion Factor (F)*
Ventilation	$\dot{V}$	1 min^{-1} (L/min)	1 min^{-1}	1
Pressure or tension	P	cm H_2O	kPa	0.098
		mm Hg (or torr)	kPa	0.133
Gas uptake	$\dot{n}$	mL min^{-1} (mL/min)	mmol min^{-1}	22.4^{-1}†
Gas content in blood	C	mL dL^{-1} (mL/100 mL)	mmol L^{-1}	2.24^{-1}†
Gas transfer factor	T	mL min^{-1} torr^{-1} (mL/min/mm Hg)	mmol min^{-1} kPa^{-1}	0.335
Energy expenditure	—	calorie	joule	4.18
Power	W	kgm/min, kpm/min	watt	0.163

*That is, SI = traditional unit × conversion factor.

†For oxygen and most other gases; for carbon dioxide, the factor is 22.26^{-1}, or, in the case of carbon dioxide content in blood, 2.226^{-1}.

Table C–2. FACTORS TO CONVERT VOLUMES MEASURED AT ATPS TO BTPS AND STPD

	Temperature and Water Vapor Pressure at Which Measured					
	20°C 17.5 mm Hg	21°C 18.7 mm Hg	22°C 19.8 mm Hg	23°C 21.1 mm Hg	24°C 22.4 mm Hg	25°C 23.8 mm Hg
	BTPS Factors					
	1.102	*1.096*	*1.091*	*1.085*	*1.080*	*1.075*
P_B	*STPD Factors for Specific P_B*					
730	.87347	.86913	.86476	.860321	.85584	.851305
732	.875922	.871574	.867195	.862748	.858259	.853715
734	.878374	.874017	.869631	.865175	.860678	.856126
736	.880826	.876461	.872066	.867602	.863097	.858537
738	.883278	.878905	.874501	.870029	.865516	.860948
740	.88573	.881348	.876937	.872457	.867935	.863359
742	.888182	.883792	.879372	.874884	.870354	.865769
744	.890634	.886235	.881807	.877311	.872773	.86818
746	.893086	.888679	.884243	.879738	.875192	.870591
748	.895538	.891123	.886678	.882165	.877611	.873002
750	.89799	.893566	.889113	.884592	.88003	.875413
752	.900442	.89601	.891549	.887019	.882448	.877823
754	.902894	.898453	.893984	.889446	.884867	.880234
756	.905346	.900897	.896419	.891873	.887286	.882645
758	.907798	.903341	.898855	.8943	.889705	.885056
760	.91025	.905784	.90129	.896728	.892124	.887467

Table continued on opposite page

Table C–2. FACTORS TO CONVERT VOLUMES MEASURED AT ATPS TO BTPS AND STPD *Continued*

	Temperature and Water Vapor Pressure at Which Measured					
	20°C 17.5 mm Hg	21°C 18.7 mm Hg	22°C 19.8 mm Hg	23°C 21.1 mm Hg	24°C 22.4 mm Hg	25°C 23.8 mm Hg
	BTPS Factors					
	1.102	*1.096*	*1.091*	*1.085*	*1.080*	*1.075*
P_B	STPD Factors for Specific P_B					
762	.912702	.908228	.903725	.899155	.894543	.889877
764	.915154	.910671	.906161	.901582	.896962	.892288
766	.917606	.913115	.908596	.904009	.899381	.894669
768	.920057	.915559	.911031	.906436	.9018	.89711
770	.922509	.918002	.913467	.908863	.904219	.899521
772	.924961	.920446	.915902	.91129	.906638	.901932
774	.927413	.92289	.918337	.913717	.909057	.904342
776	.929865	.925333	.920773	.916144	.911476	.906753
778	.932317	.927777	.923208	.918571	.913895	.909164
780	.934769	.93022	.925643	.920999	.916313	.911575

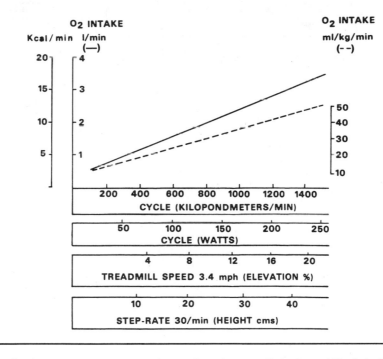

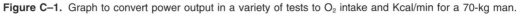

Figure C–1. Graph to convert power output in a variety of tests to O_2 intake and Kcal/min for a 70-kg man.

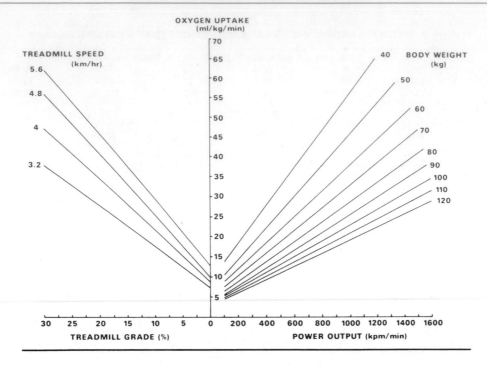

Figure C–2. O_2 uptake in progressive exercise test (stage 1) on cycle ergometer and treadmill in six healthy subjects. (J. Wicks, unpublished data.)

Normal Standards

Table D–1. PREDICTION OF POWER OUTPUT (kpm/min), at MAXIMUM CYCLE EXERCISE

No.	Equation	R	SEE	%
1a.	2526 ht $- 9.08$ A $- 2759$	0.721	245	18
1b.	1266 ht $- 8.27$ A $- 940$	0.648	179	22
1c.	2040 ht $- 8.70$ A $- 288$ S $- 1909$	0.858	216	20
2a.	2169 ht $- 9.63$ A $+ 4.00$ wt $- 2413$	0.727	245	18
2b.	950 ht $- 9.21$ A $+ 6.1$ wt $- 765$	0.668	177	22
2c.	1620 ht $- 9.50$ A $+ 5.60$ wt $- 249$ S $- 1569$	0.863	213	20
3a.	2521 ht$^{1.78}$ $\times$ A$^{-0.46}$			
3b.	1775 ht$^{1.78}$ $\times$ A$^{-0.46}$			

SEE = standard error of the estimate; A = age.

8a.	4.36 ht $- 4.55$ (boys 6–17†)	
8b.	2.25 ht $- 1.84$ (girls 6–17†)	
9a.	0.053 wt $- 0.30$ (boys 6–17‡)	0.94
9b.	0.029 wt $- 0.29$ (girls 6–17‡)	0.86

Equation (a) in a series refers to males, equation (b) to females, and equation (c) to both where a factor is introduced for gender: sex (S) is coded 0 for males, 1 for females. Height (ht) is in meters, weight (wt) is in kilograms. Vital capacity (VC) is in liters BTPS. Thigh volume (TV) (anthropometry) is sum of both thighs in liters. Leisure activity (Lei) is coded 1–4 according to hours of activity per week: 1 = <1; 2 = 1–3, 3 = 3–6; 4 = >6. A = age.

*These equations are for treadmill exercise (Bruce et al., 1973; Drinkwater et al., 1975).

†These are equations of Cooper and Weiler-Ravell (1984), for children.

‡These are equations of Cooper et al. (1984), for children.

Table D–2. PREDICTION EQUATIONS FOR OXYGEN INTAKE (L/min), AT MAXIMUM EXERCISE

No.	Equation	R	SEE	%
1a.	$(60 - 0.55$ A$) \times 0.001$ wt*			
1b.	$(48 - 0.37$ A$) \times 0.001$ wt*			
2a.	5.41 ht $- 0.025$ A $- 5.66$	0.769	0.508	17
2b.	3.01 ht $- 0.017$ A $- 2.56$	0.643	0.389	23
2c.	4.60 ht $- 0.028$ A $- 0.62$ S $- 4.31$	0.869	0.458	20
3a.	3.45 ht $- 0.028$ A $+ 0.022$ wt $- 3.76$	0.799	0.483	16
3b.	2.49 ht $- 0.018$ A $+ 0.010$ wt $- 2.26$	0.654	0.177	10
3c.	3.20 ht $- 0.024$ A $+ 0.019$ wt $- 0.49$ S $- 3.17$	0.881	0.441	19
4.	2.5 ht $- 0.023$ A $+ 0.019$ wt $+ 0.15$ Lei $- 0.54$ S $- 2.32$	0.892	0.415	18
5a.	5.14 ht$^{1.88}$ $\times$ A$^{-0.49}$			
5b.	3.55 ht$^{1.88}$ $\times$ A$^{-0.49}$			
6.	0.74 VC $- 1.04$	0.865	0.473	
7.	0.306 TV $+ 0.08$	0.794	0.588	

Table D–3. PREDICTION OF OTHER VARIABLES AT PEAK EXERCISE

1a. $f_c$max $= 210 - 0.66$ A
1b. $f_c$max $= 350$ ht$^{0.24}$ $\times$ A$^{-0.25}$
2a. Males: $\dot{V}CO_2$max $= 6.23$ ht$^{1.79}$ $\times$ A$^{-0.49}$
2b. Females: $\dot{V}CO_2$max $= 4.22$ ht$^{1.79}$ $\times$ A$^{-0.49}$
3a. Males: $\dot{V}E$max $= 143$ ht$^{0.92}$ $\times$ A$^{-0.29}$
3b. Females: $\dot{V}E$max $= 96$ ht$^{0.92}$ $\times$ A$^{-0.29}$
3c. $\dot{V}E$max $= 10.3 + 26.0$ $\dot{V}CO_2$max
3d. $\dot{V}E$max $= 26.3$ VC $- 34$ L/min
3e. $\dot{V}E$max $= 30.6$ FEV$_1$ $- 29$ L/min (r $= 0.76$)
4a. Males: $V_T$max $= 1.71$ ht$^{1.60}$ $\times$ A$^{-0.12}$
4b. Females: $V_T$max $= 1.18$ ht$^{1.60}$ $\times$ A$^{-0.12}$
4c. $V_T$max $= 0.67$ VC $- 0.64$
5. $f_b$max $= 86$ ht$^{-0.66}$ $\times$ A$^{-0.18}$
6. Females and males: Max dyspnea (Borg rating) $= 14.2$ ht$^{0.70}$ $\times$ A$^{-0.34}$
7a. Males: Max leg effort $= 17.1$ ht$^{0.81}$ $\times$ A$^{-0.35}$
7b. Females: Max leg effort $= 15.6$ ht$^{0.81}$ $\times$ A$^{-0.35}$

Where gender is not indicated, equations apply to both males and females. A = age.

243

Table D–4. PREDICTION OF VARIABLES IN SUBMAXIMAL EXERCISE

Measurements at 300 kpm/min in Age Categories (Females)

Age (yr)	$\dot{V}_{O_2}$ (L/min)	$\dot{V}_{CO_2}$ (L/min)	R	$\dot{V}_E$ (L/min)	V_T (L)	HR (b/min)	BPs (mm Hg)
15–24	0.82	0.67	0.82	20.7	1.10	123	138
SD	0.061	0.062	0.063	2.61	0.104	16.2	*
25–34	0.87	0.72	0.84	21.7	1.23	124	142
SD	0.162	0.114	0.157	2.74	0.305	20.6	*
35–44	0.82	0.71	0.87	23.0	1.26	111	146
SD	0.084	0.053	0.067	2.20	0.231	13.4	*
45–54	0.85	0.70	0.82	22.0	1.31	117	151
SD	0.111	0.093	0.065	4.42	0.213	15.6	*
55–65	0.79	0.69	0.87	22.5	1.08	121	155
SD	0.138	0.132	0.056	5.02	0.269	13.6	*
Total	0.83	0.70	0.85	21.9	1.19	119	133
SD	0.116	0.094	0.089	3.7	0.243	15.9	15.0

Measurements at 300 kpm/min in Age Categories (Males)

Age (yr)	$\dot{V}_{O_2}$ (L/min)	$\dot{V}_{CO_2}$ (L/min)	R	$\dot{V}_E$ (L/min)	V_T (L)	HR (b/min)	BPs (mm Hg)
15–24	1.00	0.82	0.81	22.9	1.60	104	130
SD	0.190	0.166	0.065	4.08	0.859	11.7	13.3
25–34	0.95	0.79	0.83	24.5	1.91	95	127
SD	0.153	0.199	0.128	10.5	0.719	10.1	*
35–44	0.91	0.73	0.81	24.3	1.78	92	125
SD	0.109	0.100	0.077	5.62	0.525	15.5	*
45–54	0.87	0.71	0.82	22.8	1.34	93	125
SD	0.125	0.121	0.074	5.85	0.264	9.7	*
55 +	0.88	0.73	0.83	23.5	1.44	95	167
SD	0.105	0.086	0.073	2.78	0.314	10.9	*
Total	0.92	0.76	0.82	23.6	1.63	96	133
SD	0.146	0.143	0.083	6.37	0.604	12.1	*

Measurements at 300 kpm/min in Height Categories

Height (cm)	$\dot{V}_{O_2}$ (L/min)	$\dot{V}_{CO_2}$ (L/min)	R	$\dot{V}_E$ (L/min)	V_T (L)	HR (b/min) M	HR (b/min) F	BPs (mm Hg)	RPE
<160	0.83	0.74	0.90	22.5	1.14		128	143	3.3
SD	0.152	0.139	0.098	3.89	0.229		11.4	31.8	*
160–165	0.80	0.68	0.85	21.4	1.16		118	143	2.0
SD	0.096	0.090	0.065	4.16	0.232		15.3	28.1	*
165–170	0.82	0.66	0.81	20.9	1.23	97	115	131	1.8
SD	0.112	0.066	0.075	3.47	0.256	15.4	16.3	25.2	*
170–175	0.88	0.72	0.82	22.9	1.48	96	114	130	2.0
SD	0.135	0.121	0.068	4.79	0.330	12.5	21.1	*	*
175–180	0.91	0.71	0.79	22.4	1.60	94		125	2.0
SD	0.066	0.068	0.068	4.46	0.634	17.0		*	*
180–185	0.95	0.80	0.84	25.3	1.51	98		135	1.7
SD	0.081	0.101	0.084	3.71	0.311	11.0		*	*
> 185	1.09	0.93	0.86	28.3	2.27	94		120	1.0
SD	0.178	0.167	0.129	10.1	0.920	11.0		*	*
Total	0.87	0.73	0.83	22.7	1.40	96	119	132	*
SD	0.139	0.124	0.087	5.08	0.502	12.4	15.7	23.2	*

*There were too few observations to calculate SD.

$\dot{V}_{O_2}$ = oxygen intake, $\dot{V}_{CO_2}$ = carbon dioxide output; R = respiratory exchange ratio; $\dot{V}_E$ = minute ventilation; V_T = tidal volume; HR = heart rate; BPs = systolic blood pressure; RPE = rating of perceived exertion (Borg scale).

Table D–4. PREDICTION OF VARIABLES IN SUBMAXIMAL EXERCISE *Continued*

Measurements at 600 kpm/min in Age Categories (Females)

Age (yr)	$\dot{V}_{O_2}$ (L/min)	$\dot{V}_{CO_2}$ (L/min)	R	$\dot{V}_E$ (L/min)	V_T (L)	HR (b/min)	BPs (mm Hg)
15–24	1.30	1.30	0.99	36.1	1.40	156	140
SD	0.129	0.241	0.122	8.65	0.193	15.0	12.4
25–34	1.38	1.27	0.93	36.3	1.70	150	144
SD	0.190	0.149	0.168	7.87	0.280	17.7	16.2
35–44	1.31	1.44	1.10	41.2	1.81	154	152
SD	0.106	0.123	0.123	3.78	0.312	13.8	10.3
45–54	1.35	1.48	1.10	42.3	1.85	151	157
SD	0.120	0.180	0.129	5.38	0.260	12.1	11.3
55–65	1.27	1.53	1.21	46.8	1.76	155	162
SD	0.136	0.199	0.118	8.00	0.271	12.2	20.5
Total	1.32	1.40	1.07	40.4	1.70	153	149
SD	0.137	0.203	0.132	6.95	0.266	14.2	13.8

Measurements at 600 kpm/min in Age Categories (Males)

Age (yr)	$\dot{V}_{O_2}$ (L/min)	$\dot{V}_{CO_2}$ (L/min)	R	$\dot{V}_E$ (L/min)	V_T (L)	HR (b/min)	BPs (mm Hg)
15–24	1.53	1.39	0.92	35.9	2.31	122	152
SD	0.115	0.088	0.073	2.62	1.06	14.6	11.8
25–34	1.48	1.28	0.86	34.0	2.31	112	143
SD	0.093	0.123	0.083	6.00	0.656	12.6	25.9
35–44	1.50	1.32	0.88	37.8	2.35	111	148
SD	0.144	0.075	0.074	5.21	0.656	20.1	10.3
45–54	1.42	1.28	0.90	36.5	1.92	112	157
SD	0.092	0.102	0.065	2.73	0.360	11.6	12.5
54–65	1.35	1.35	1.00	38.7	2.07	123	178
SD	0.140	0.149	0.100	4.32	0.262	13.0	24.9
Total	1.46	1.35	0.91	36.5	2.19	116	154
SD	0.128	0.115	0.089	4.33	0.68	15.0	19.7

Measurements at 600 kpm/min in Height Categories*

Height (cm)	$\dot{V}_{O_2}$ (L/min)	$\dot{V}_{CO_2}$ (L/min)	R	$\dot{V}_E$ (L/min)	V_T (L)	HR (b/min) M	HR (b/min) F	BPs (mm Hg)	RPE
< 160	1.30	1.54	1.19	43.2	1.65		163	159	6.0
SD	0.117	0.199	0.144	6.46	0.196		9.6	13.9	†
160–165	1.30	1.44	1.11	41.7	1.72		153	151	4.7
SD	0.119	0.189	0.138	7.43	0.258		10.8	16.1	†
165–170	1.33	1.29	0.97	36.4	1.78	124	147	144	4.1
SD	0.128	0.178	0.123	6.56	0.391	18.4	12.3	12.3	†
170–175	1.42	1.38	0.98	38.9	1.89	115	144	158	3.9
SD	0.153	0.156	0.148	7.63	0.369	10.8	21.5	31.6	†
175–180	1.51	1.31	0.87	36.8	2.24	114		150	3.0
SD	0.145	0.079	0.077	5.43	0.679	21.7		17.0	†
180–185	1.44	1.32	0.92	37.0	2.01	111		153	3.1
SD	0.086	0.099	0.063	2.41	0.353	11.3		13	
> 185	1.55	1.36	0.88	36.3	2.86	109		149	2.4
SD	0.105	0.113	0.042	4.7	1.109	17.3		18.0	†
Total	1.39	1.36	0.99	38.4	1.96	116	151	151	†
SD	0.148	0.167	0.147	6.49	0.582	15.0	13.0	18.2	†

*There were no significant differences between males and females except for heart rate.

†There were too few observations to calculate SD.

Table D–5. GUIDE TO NORMAL VALUES: STAGE 2 AND STAGE 3 TESTS, MALES AGES 20 to 60 YEARS*

Variable	Symbol		Power Outputs				Variance or SD
			200 (33)	400 (66)	600 (100)	800 (133)	
Power output	W kpm/min	(watts)	200 (33)	400 (66)	600 (100)	800 (133)	
O_2 intake	$\dot{V}O_2$	mL/min	800	1200	1600	2000	10%
CO_2 output	$\dot{V}CO_2$	mL/min	700	1150	1600	2100	10%
Respiratory exchange ratio	R		0.90	0.95	1.00	1.05	10%
Cardiac frequency	f_c	beats/min	95	110	125	140	12%
Ventilation	V_E	L/min	20	32	42	58	15%
Breathing frequency	f_b	breaths/min	18	20	20	24	15%
Tidal volume	V_T	mL	1100	1600	2100	2400	25%
Mixed expired PCO_2	P_ECO_2	mm Hg	30	31	32.5	31	3 mm Hg
End tidal PCO_2	$P_{ET}CO_2$	mm Hg	42	43	44	42	5 mm Hg
Mixed venous PCO_2	$P\bar{V}CO_2$	mm Hg	60	63	66	70	5 mm Hg
Arterial PCO_2	$PaCO_2$	mm Hg	40	40	40	36	2 mm Hg
Dead space/tidal volume	V_D/V_T		.20	.18	.15	.12	.4
Cardiac output	$\dot{Q}tot$	L/min	9.4	11.5	13.5	15.5	2 L/min
Stroke volume	V_s	mL	100	105	110	110	10%
Arterial PO_2	PaO_2	mm Hg	90	92	92	92	4 mm Hg
Alveolar-arterial PO_2 difference	$PA - aO_2$	mm Hg	12	12	14	16	5 mm Hg
Arterial O_2 saturation	SaO_2	%	.963	.965	.965	.960	.005
Venous admixture	$\dot{Q}VA/\dot{Q}tot$	%	4	3	3	3	1
pH	pH		7.40	7.39	7.38	7.35	.02
Bicarbonate	HCO_3^-	mmol/L	24.0	23.5	23.0	21.5	2.0 mmol/L
Lactate	La	mmol/L	1.0	1.5	2.0	3.5	2.0 mmol/L

*Average values representative of healthy nonsmoking males; average weight, 80 kg. Figures are rounded off and variances are also averaged.

Table D-6. GUIDE TO NORMAL VALUES: STAGE 2 AND STAGE 3 TESTS, FEMALES AGES 20 to 50 YEARS*

Variable	Symbol		Power Outputs			Variance or SD
Power output	W kpm/min	(watts)	200 (33)	400 (66)	600 (100)	
O_2 intake	$\dot{V}O_2$	mL/min	800	1200	1550	12%
CO_2 output	$\dot{V}CO_2$	mL/min	720	1180	1630	12%
Respiratory exchange ratio	R		.90	.98	1.05	10%
Cardiac frequency	f_c	beats/min	108	130	155	12%
Ventilation	$\dot{V}E$	L/min	22	33	48	25%
Breathing frequency	f_b	breaths/min	18	19	24	15%
Tidal volume	V_T	mL	1200	1700	2000	25%
Mixed expired P_{CO_2}	$P_{E}CO_2$	mm Hg	28	30	29	3.5 mm Hg
End tidal P_{CO_2}	$P_{ET}CO_2$	mm Hg	40	40	39	5 mm Hg
Mixed venous P_{CO_2}	$P\bar{v}CO_2$	mm Hg	56	61	65	5 mm Hg
Arterial P_{CO_2}	$PaCO_2$	mm Hg	38	36	35	3.5 mm Hg
Dead space/tidal volume	V_D/V_T		.20	.13	.11	.04
Cardiac output	$\dot{Q}tot$	L/min	9	11.5	14	2 L/min
Stroke volume	V_s	mL	85	90	90	15 mL
Arterial P_{O_2}	PaO_2	mm Hg	92	91	92	6 mm Hg
Alveolar-arterial P_{O_2} difference	$PA - aO_2$	mm Hg	14	17	22	4 mm Hg
Arterial O_2 saturation	SaO_2		.965	.965	.961	.010
Venous admixture	$\dot{Q}VA/\dot{Q}tot$	%	3	3	3	1.5
pH	pH		7.40	7.4	7.36	.04
Bicarbonate	HCO_3^-	mmol/L	22.5	22.0	20.0	3 mmol/L
Lactate	La	mmol/L	1.0	2.0	4.0	2 mmol/L

*Average values representative of healthy nonsmoking women; average weight, 60 kg.

Informed Consent

McMaster University Medical Centre Informed Consent for Progressive and for Steady State Exercise Test

Explanation of Progressive Test (Stage 1)

You will perform this test on a cycle ergometer or treadmill. The work will begin at a very easy level and will gradually get more difficult each minute. We would like you to continue exercising until you are limited by fatigue or discomfort.

If the supervising physician sees any reason to stop the test prematurely, he will do so immediately.

Risks and Discomforts

There exists the possibility of certain changes occurring during the test. They include abnormal blood pressure (high or low), fainting, disorders of heartbeat (too rapid, too slow, or ineffective), and, in very rare instances, a heart attack. Every effort will be made to minimize these risks by the preliminary examination and by the observations that are made continuously during the test.

Emergency equipment and trained personnel are available to deal with unusual situations that may arise. If, during the test, you feel some discomfort, continue pedaling but tell the physician, who will advise you; of course, if you feel you must stop, you are at liberty to do so.

Information to Be Obtained from the Test

The results obtained from the exercise test may assist in diagnosis or assessment of your clinical condition.

The results may also be used to evaluate the types of activities you might safely undertake in your daily life.

The physician will be able to give you some indication of how the test went immediately after; however, some of the measurements take time and the full result will be sent, within a few days, to the physician who ordered the test.

Steady State Exercise Test (Stages 2 and 3)

Occasionally more detailed information of your heart and lung function during exercise needs to be obtained. This entails exercising for 6 or 7 minutes at approximately 30 per cent and 60 per cent of the maximum level achieved on your progressive (stage 1) test. The blood sample will be taken from an earlobe on each occasion. The ear will be pricked with a small surgical blade and the blood collected in special tubes. It will also be necessary for you to rebreathe a mixture of oxygen and carbon dioxide for about 15 seconds. There is no danger involved in breathing these gases and it is an easy method to determine heart output.

If you have any doubts or questions about any of these tests, please do not hesitate to ask for more information.

You will be asked to sign a consent form when you come to take the test.

I, _____ _____,

consent to a Stage _____ exercise test (cycle ergometer/treadmill) being carried out on _____, _____.

The nature of this procedure and any risks and discomforts have been explained to me by

Doctor _____

Signature of doctor _____

Signature of patient _____

Signature of witness _____

Dated at _____ this ___ day of _____, 19___.

If patient is unable to consent or is a minor:

Signature _____ Witness _____

Relationship to patient _____

Addresses of Some Manufacturers of Exercise Testing Equipment

Warren E Collins, Inc.
220 Wood Road
Braintree, MA 02184
USA

COSMED S.r.I.
Via dci Piani di Mte. Savello 37
00040 Pavona di Albano
Rome
ITALY

Erich Jaeger
Leibnitzstrasse 7
Hochberg D-97204
GERMANY

Ganshorn ME GmbH
Industriestrasse 6
Niederlauer D-97618
GERMANY

Minato Medical Science Company
3-13-11 Shinkitano
Yodogawa-ku
Osaka 532
JAPAN

P.K. Morgan Ltd.
4 Bloors Lane
Rainham
Kent ME8 7ED
UK

Quinton Instrument Company
3303 Mante Villa Parkway
Bothell, WA 99021-8906
USA

Hans Rudolph, Inc.
7200 Wyandotte
Kansas City, MO 64114
USA

Schiller AG
Altgasse 68
CH-6340 Baar
SWITZERLAND

SensorMedics Corporation
1630 South State College Blvd.
Anaheim, CA 92806
USA

Medical Graphics Corporation
350 Oak Grove Parkway
St. Paul, MN 55127
USA

Vacumed
4488 McGrath Street #102
Ventura, CA 93003
USA

References for Appendices

Åstrand I. Aerobic work capacity in men and women with special reference to age. Acta Physiol Scand Suppl 1960;49:196.

Åstrand P-P. Human physical fitness, with special reference to sex and age. Physiol Rev 1956;36:307–335.

Bruce RA, Kusumi F, Hosmer D. Maximal oxygen intake and nomographic assessment of functional aerobic impairment in cardiovascular disease. Am Heart J 1973;85:546–562.

Cooper DM, Weiler-Ravell D. Gas exchange response to exercise in children. Am Rev Respir Dis 1984; 129:S47–S48.

Cooper DM, Weiler-Ravell D, Whipp BJ, Wasserman K. Aerobic parameters of exercise as a function of body size during growth in children. J Appl Physiol 1984;56:628–634.

Cotes JE. Response to progressive exercise: A three index test. Br J Dis Chest 1972;66:160–184.

Cotes JE, Davies CTM, Edholm OG, et al. Factors relating to the aerobic capacity of 46 healthy British males and females, ages 18 to 28 years. Proc R Soc London B 1969;174:91–114.

Cotes JE, Berry G, Burkinshaw L, et al. Cardiac frequency during submaximal exercise in young adults; relation to lean body mass, total body potassium and amount of leg muscle. Q J Exp Physiol 1973;58:239–250.

Douglas AR, Jones NL, Reed JW. Calculation of whole blood CO_2 content. J Appl Physiol 1988;65:473–477.

Drinkwater BL, Horvath SM, Wells CL: Aerobic power of females, ages 10–68. J Gerontol 1975;30:385–394.

Faulkner JA, Heigenhauser GF, Shork A. The cardiac output-oxygen uptake relationship of men during graded bicycle ergometry. Med Sci Sport 1977;9:143–147.

Gadhoke S, Jones NL. The responses to exercise in boys aged 9 to 15. Clin Sci 1969;37:789–801.

Godfrey S. Manipulation of the indirect Fick Principle by a digital computer program for the calculation of exercise physiology results. Respiration 1970;27:513–532.

Godfrey S, Davies CTM, Wozniak E, et al. Cardiorespiratory response to exercise in normal children. Clin Sci 1971;40:419–431.

Harris EA, Seelye ER, Whitlock RML. Gas exchange during exercise in healthy people. Clin Sci 1976; 51:335–344.

Higgs BE, Clode M, McHardy GJR, et al. Changes in ventilation, gas exchange and circulation during exercise in normal subjects. Clin Sci 1967;32:329–337.

Jones NL, McHardy GJR, Naimark A, et al. Physiological dead space and alveolar-arterial gas pressure differences during exercise. Clin Sci 1966;31:19–29.

Jones NL, Makrides L, Hitchcock C, et al. Normal standards for an incremental progressive cycle ergometer test. Am Rev Respir Dis 1985;131:700–708.

Jones NL, Robertson DG, Kane JW. Difference between end-tidal and arterial P_{CO_2} in exercise. J Appl Physiol 1979;47:954–960.

Kelman GR. Digital computer subroutine for the conversion of oxygen tension into saturation. J Appl Physiol 1966;21:1375–1376.

Lange-Anderson K, Shephard RJ, Denolin H, et al. Fundamentals of Exercise Testing. Geneva: World Health Organization; 1971.

Loeppky JA, Luft UC, Fletcher ER. Quantitative description of the whole blood CO_2 dissociation curve and Haldane effect. Respir Physiol 1983;51:167–181.

McHardy GJR. Relationship between the difference in pressure and content of carbon dioxide in arterial and venous blood. Clin Sci 1967;32:299–309.

Pappenheimer JR, Comroe JH, Cournand A, et al. Standardization of definitions and symbols in respiratory physiology. Fed Proc 1950;9:602.

Powles ACP, Jones NL. A pocket calculator program for noninvasive assessment of cardiorespiratory function. Comput Biol Med 1982;12:163–173.

Radford EP Jr. Ventilation standards for use in artificial respiration. J Appl Physiol 1955;7:451.

Shephard RJ. Endurance Fitness. Toronto: University of Toronto Press; 1969.

Spiro SG. Exercise testing in clinical medicine. Br J Dis Chest 1977;71:145–172.

Spiro SG, Hahn HL, Edwards RHT, et al. Cardiorespiratory adaptations at the start of exercise in normal subjects and in patients with chronic obstructive bronchitis. Clin Sci 1974;47:165–172.

Spiro SG, Juniper E, Bowman P, et al. An increasing work rate test for assessing the physiological strain of submaximal exercise. Clin Sci 1974;46:191–206.

Visser BF. Pulmonary diffusion of CO_2. Phys Med Biol 1960;5:155–166.

Wicks JR, Sutton JR, Oldridge NB, et al. Comparison of the electrocardiographic changes induced by maximum exercise testing with treadmill and cycle ergometer. Circulation 1978;57:1066–1070.

Index

Note: Page numbers in *italics* refer to illustrations;
page numbers followed by t refer to tables.

ISBN 0-7216-6511-X